UNDERSTANDING APHASIA

FOUNDATIONS OF NEUROPSYCHOLOGY

A Series of Textbooks, Monographs, and Treatises

Series Editor

LAIRD S. CERMAK

Memory Disorders Research Center, Boston Veterans Administration, Medical Center, Boston, Massachusetts

UNDERSTANDING APHASIA

Harold Goodglass
Department of Neurology
Aphasia Research Center
Boston University School of Medicine
Boston, Massachusetts

Academic Press
San Diego New York Boston
London Sydney Tokyo Toronto

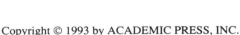
Copyright © 1993 by ACADEMIC PRESS, INC.

All Rights Reserved.
No part of this publication may be reproduced or transmitted in any form or by any
means, electronic or mechanical, including photocopy, recording, or any information
storage and retrieval system, without permission in writing from the publisher.

Academic Press, Inc.
A Division of Harcourt Brace & Company
525 B Street, Suite 1900, San Diego, California 92101-4495

United Kingdom Edition published by
Academic Press Limited
24–28 Oval Road, London NW1 7DX

Library of Congress Cataloging-in-Publication Data

Goodglass, Harold.
    Understanding aphasia / Harold Goodglass
        p. cm. -- (Foundations of neuropsychology series)
    Includes bibliographical references and index.
    ISBN 0-12-290040-5
    1. Aphasia.   I. Title.   II. Series: Foundations of
neuropsychology (San Diego, Calif.)
RC425,G683   1993
616.85' 52--dc20   93-1533
                                                            CIP
PRINTED IN THE UNITED STATES OF AMERICA
          96 97 98   QW   9 8 7 6 5 4 3 2

To Helen

Contents

Chapter 4   *Disorders of Motor Speech Implementation*

Chapter 5   *Disorders of Word Retrieval*

Chapter 6   *Disorders of Syntax and Morphology*

Chapter 7   *Disorders of Auditory Comprehension*

Chapter 8   *Disorders of Repetition*

Chapter 9   *Disorders of Reading*

Chapter 10   *Disorders of Writing*

Chapter 11   *Apraxia and Aphasia*

Chapter 12   *Classification of Aphasia*

Chapter 13   *Relation of Aphasia to Normal Language: Fact and Conjecture*

Preface

The title *Understanding Aphasia* is meant to be taken in its most modest sense, i.e., *toward an understanding of aphasia*. Although I have aimed to bring the reader abreast of current theory and controversy in most aspects of aphasic language impairments, it would be rash to claim that we are anywhere near understanding, at the neural level, the processes by which language is carried out in the normal and damaged adult brain. However, we can claim to be able to describe regularities in the relationship between lesion sites and symptoms produced—regularities that contribute to a plausible but only partial account of the gross neural circuitry of language. Within this generally coarse picture, there are points in which detailed and highly predictable relationships between lesion and deficit can be specified, with corresponding specification of the presumed normal anatomical–functional relationships at these points. I try to show that the aspects of aphasic language impairments that yield to anatomical analysis are essentially those that relate to sensory input channels and motor output channels and the connections between them.

The fascination that the study of aphasia has held for many observers over the past century owes only little to the fact that it may differentially affect auditory comprehension, motor speech production, repetition, reading, or writing. The challenge to understanding comes from the psychological and linguistic factors that may characterize pathological performance within a particular modality or across modalities. The most obvious examples are the impairment of naming and the impairment of syntax, which may affect oral production and written production either selectively or jointly. However, these two instances barely scratch the surface of aphasic phenomena that challenge our ability to find cohesive accounts of them in linguistic or psychological terms.

I have tried to make this book accessible to interested readers who are not in the professions that are most concerned with brain–language relationships. This effort is in the form of a general introduction to aphasia and its history in the first two chapters. This effort continues in the structuring of subsequent chapters, moving from normal language to the phenomenology of aphasic behavior and then to theoretical interpretation in terms of anatomy, psycholinguistic theory, and related research findings.

I have also tried to address the concerns of my colleagues in the field of aphasiology by critically analyzing current theoretical approaches. These criticisms appear mainly in the last two chapters. In these chapters (and elsewhere in the book) I recognize the elegance of the cognitive models that have emerged from studies of occasional patients with highly selective dissociations affecting psycholinguistic elements of language. However, I devote considerable effort to questioning the ultimate fruitfulness of this approach, even when it appears to be justified by dramatic dissociations in some patients. My plea is for further development of interpretations of normal and pathological language as the product of continuously interacting processes. My speculations in this regard go considerably further than I myself am equipped to spell out in any detail. Still, I hope that they are sufficiently cogent to keep alive resistance to the view of language as composed of a series of compartments and processing stages that just happen to have names corresponding to pre-existing psychological and linguistic constructs.

In a sense, this book is more of a personal perspective on aphasia than an exhaustive review of research. Reflecting my career as a clinician, I have dwelled more on the day-in-day-out phenomena of the common variants of aphasic syndromes than the reader is likely to find either in the approaches of cognitive theorists or in the primarily neurologically oriented approaches. I have tried to deal fairly with all the current theoretical trends, but cite specific studies only to the extent that they are needed to give substance to the views that are mentioned. This book is not a substitute for some of the excellent recent treatments of current research in neurolinguistics, such as Caplan's *Language—Structure, Function, and Disorders* and the section on aphasia that I edited in the first and second volumes of Boller and Grafman's *Handbook of Neuropsychology*. However, it does cover much of the same territory in a technically less demanding way.

I am grateful for the supportive counsel that I received from my colleagues Mick Alexander, Martin Albert, David Caplan, Marcel Kinsbourne, and Margaret Naeser, who reviewed parts of this book. The writing of this book was supported in part by Grant DC 00081 from the National Institutes of Health.

Harold Goodglass

Chapter 1

Nature and Scope of the Problem of Aphasia: A Survey

THE CONCEPT OF APHASIA

The term "aphasia" refers to a family of clinically diverse disorders that affect the ability to communicate by oral or written language, or both, following brain damage. A few thumbnail case illustrations may help to bring home the scope of its manifestations.

Case 1. The patient, whose right arm and leg remain paralyzed from a recent stroke, communicates with a small vocabulary of nouns and verbs that he rarely combines into two-word phrases. A typical response to a question, for example, How did you get here today? is "Drivin...wife... yeah...drivin'." These words are produced somewhat effortfully, but are clearly pronounced. He can recite the numbers up to 21 and the days of the week with perfect facility. He understands conversation and commands when they relate to his current situation, but is often left behind by a change in topic. He can read and understand many words and easy sentences, but cannot write more than his name.

Case 2. A patient who suffered an embolic stroke during open-heart surgery produces speech with effortless articulation and grammar, but rarely succeeds in completing a thought because he cannot retrieve the key nouns and verbs of his intended message. He recognizes these words when they are supplied by the examiner, but he cannot repeat them himself. He understands speech almost perfectly, but makes errors in both reading and writing. A sample of his account of his hospital experience goes like this: "I had one of those...they did it on my...my...ort...my art...I can't say it...there are two of them." (Examiner: The aortic valve?) "That right. Then I was in the...where they put three or four people...."

Case 3. This patient proved to have suffered a stroke when he was found confused and unable to make sense in talking. On examination, he is socially appropriate in response to greeting, but answers routine questions with a largely irrelevant and voluble flow of speech. His speech output has no coherent content and is sprinkled with neologisms and incorrectly used words, and although he is attentive and takes turns in conversation, he appears to grasp only fragments of questions and his answers have only tangential allusions to the subject matter. For example, when asked, Who lives at home with you? his response is "My wife, she goes her work to work on it but her heffle is all about it." On testing for comprehension of single words, he can point to only one of six objects that are named for him. He can name none correctly on request. His attempts to write result in a jargon similar to his speech.

These are but a few examples; in some cases, speech production and comprehension are both abolished, whereas in other cases only a single channel is affected. Thus the term "aphasia" is an umbrella concept combining a multiplicity of deficits involving one or more aspects of language use. As we shall see in the next chapter, this concept did not spring up fully formed all at once, but instead evolved over a span of many years.

The principle that accompanied the development of the concept of aphasia is that each of the sensory and motor systems involved in the perception, interpretation, and execution of linguistic acts or symbols is controlled by at least two independently organized brain systems—one controlling the use of these organs in language and one controlling nonlanguage sensory and motor activity. In aphasia, it is possible, for example, for the coordination of tongue, lips, and the phonatory apparatus to be lost in the effort to speak, but not in the act of swallowing, licking the lips, crying, or even singing. Of course, the concept of aphasia does not apply when communication is impeded by paralysis or ataxia of the motor system involved or by primary sensory impairment of audition or vision.

The dissociation between language and nonlanguage functions that became evident in aphasia goes beyond perceptual and motor functions. Memory for the sounds and meanings of words might be lost when memory for all other forms of experience and knowledge appears to be intact. Thus the existence of a specialized cognitive apparatus dedicated exclusively to language appears to be a possibility. Not surprisingly, the distinction between thought and language has not yet yielded to clean, logical analysis and continues to present obstacles to understanding aphasia's relation to normal language that will be touched on in the final chapter.

CEREBRAL DOMINANCE

As though it were not sufficiently remarkable to discover, through aphasia, that the brain has an autonomous subsystem for language, two more related discoveries assured that aphasia would become an entry-way to the understanding of brain function in higher mental processes and to the understanding of normal as well as pathological language. One of these is the phenomenon of cerebral dominance. The study of aphasia led to the discovery that the two grossly symmetrical cerebral hemispheres appeared to have different, genetically preassigned capacities for higher mental functions. There is an almost exclusive relationship between aphasia in any of its forms and injury to the left hemisphere. The recognition of a link between left-handedness and exceptions to the rule of left cerebral dominance for language set in motion another special area of inquiry: the search for and the discovery of functional brain asymmetries for other cognitive operations, some of which are primarily dependent on the left hemisphere, and others on the right. The understanding of cerebral dominance as a psychological and biological phenomenon is now one of the major research topics in neuropsychology.

APHASIC SYMPTOMS AND THEIR LOCALIZATION

The second discovery that emerged is that there is a degree of lawful regularity both in the recurrence of individual deficits and patterns of deficit and in the corresponding lesion sites. Moreover, there is a general consistency between the location of known cortical motor and sensory zones and the lesions producing particular aphasic symptoms. For example, aphasias in which deficits of auditory comprehension are the dominant feature are generally associated with left temporal lobe lesions close to the primary center for audition. Those forms of aphasia that most affect motor articulatory processes have lesions clustering in the lower left frontal lobe, adjacent to the cortical area for the control of oral musculature. Selective deficits involving letter and word recognition involve posterior cerebral lesions bordering on the visual association areas or severing fiber pathways from visual centers of the brain.

A first impression from the foregoing paragraph might be that a complete mapping of the brain's anatomic underpinnings for language is imminent. Correspondingly, one might optimistically anticipate that the psychological structure of language ultimately will be revealed by the lines of cleavage created by injuries to the system. A fuller understanding of the complexities at both the level of anatomo-cinical correlation and that of psycholinguistic analysis now makes it apparent that both of these goals can only be approached through slow, painstaking work in both the behavioral and neuroanatomic areas.

LIMITS TO ANATOMICAL UNDERSTANDING OF NORMAL AND APHASIC LANGUAGE

A transparent relationship between anatomy and behavior is one in which injury to a component of a neuroanatomically modeled system produces a deficit that can be understood and predicted on the basis of the presumed functions of anatomically delineated system components. There are only a small number of disorders in the spectrum of aphasia that are open to this level of understanding. One of these is the (relatively uncommon) phenomenon of pure alexia—loss of the ability to read, with preservation of the ability to write, to spell orally, to speak, and to understand speech. Pure alexia (Dejerine, 1892; Geschwind & Fusillo, 1966) is attributable to a lesion that both damages vision in the right visual field and disconnects visual input from the right cerebral hemisphere to the language processing areas of the left hemisphere. This disconnection is seen as disabling the linguistic processing of visual symbols without affecting other aspects of visual perception.

Most aphasic patients, however, are impaired in many aspects of language. The distinctive syndromes that occur regularly enough to have earned labels (e.g., Broca's aphasia) are identified by *patterns of relative impairment and preservation* among many dimensions of language ability such as word retrieval, articulation, auditory comprehension, and repetition. Some of the individual features that have proven the most stable for purposes of recognizing patterns of aphasia are not derived from preconceived components of language ability, but are empirically observed "positive symptoms" that are typical of people who have suffered injury in particular sites in the language zone. One such feature is *nonfluency* of speech output, characteristic of most aphasics with anterior speech zone lesions. Another is *paragrammatic paraphasia*—the fluently produced, but grammatically and semantically noncoherent output common after temporal lobe lesions.

Thus, the markers that have become indicators of structural lesion sites in the cerebral language system are varied in nature. Some define a channel of sensory input or motor output that is primarily affected. Others refer to psycholinguistically defined operations (e.g., "naming," and "using grammatical forms"). Still others refer to pathological adaptive symptoms (e.g., nonfluency and paragrammatic speech). The first category, that is, the input or output channel that is affected, is the one that has the most understandable relationship to the lesion site. The associations be-tween lesion site and the remaining two categories are based on empiri-cal observation and cannot be deduced from our present understanding of functional anatomy.

As we shall see in detail in the next chapter on the history of aphasia and in Chapter 12 on classification, there has been considerable contro-versy among eminent scholars as to which dimensions of the symptom picture should become criteria for classification. The currently most widely used system of syndrome terminology—the revised "classical" taxonomy promoted by Geschwind, Goodglass, and others from the Boston school of aphasiology—has come under criticism for several rea-sons. One reason is that assignment of a case to a syndrome is not based on rigorous criteria, but rather on a sort of "family resemblance" basis, in which some features are given greater weight than others, but without an explicit basis for this weighting. Another criticism is that the number of instances where the syndrome configuration is at odds with the ob-served lesion is sufficient to undermine confidence in the localizing value of the syndromes.

The refinements in lesion localization currently being made through neuroimaging will almost certainly force an updating of terminology for aphasia. These changes are likely to include greater emphasis on specifi-cation of individual features and less reliance on the syndrome label alone as a means of concisely communicating the essentials of a patient's pattern of language use.

APHASIA AS A CHALLENGE TO COGNITIVE LANGUAGE MODELS

In the earlier examples of aphasic symptoms, we barely touched on the wealth of phenomena that seem to violate and challenge everyday as-sumptions about how language knowledge is organized. These chal-lenges to our understanding may be found at many levels. For example, we are forced to revise our conceptions concerning the information pro-cessing of words in sentences when we see patients who cannot under-stand words in isolation, but who deal with them appropriately in following a command. Our notions as to what makes a word easy or hard are upset when we see patients who can neither read nor repeat such short frequent words as *the* or *with*, but who perform normally with the word *elephant*.

Some of these observations date to the earliest reports about aphasia and are among the first surprises that the aphasia clinician soon comes to regard as commonplace. For example, frequently a patient who cannot voluntarily produce an easy one-word answer may recite a memorized sequence flawlessly in what appears to be a normal speaking style, or he or she may produce an oath easily, or sing both lyrics and melody of familiar songs. Hughlings Jackson (1878) summed up these phenomena by redefining aphasia as not simply a loss of words but a loss of the ability to *propositionize*—that is, to use words for the purpose of conveying information.

Jackson's dictum invoked a new principle: that the *psychological intent* of the utterance is what defines the deficit in aphasia. If this principle were to be applied blindly, it would classify speech acts into two general categories: those that convey a proposition and those that do not. Among the latter would be rote recitation, interjections, filler expressions, and mimicking or repetition of modeled speech. The dichotomy suggested by Jackson's principle does not hold up across all cases or situations, in particular, with regard to repetition. Although it is often nonpropositional in nature, repetition does not have the resistance to aphasia that is often observed in memorized or sung speech. Yet Jackson's rule, however it may be qualified or rephrased, is one of the most stable organizing principles for understanding the conditions for success and failure in performance by aphasic patients.

In the modern taxonomy of aphasia, a major polarity in symptomatology is that between patients who are unable to string words into grammatically organized phrases or sentences and those who cannot supply the information-carrying nouns and verbs for their messages. The former, who are called "agrammatic," typically use one- to three-word noun phrases or verb phrases to express themselves. Their speech is notably lacking in small grammatical words such as prepositions, auxiliary verbs, and articles. The latter, who are called "anomic," typically produce grammatically organized sentences with empty circumlocution taking the place of the words that they cannot retrieve.

A few paragraphs earlier, we learned that brain organization for language is attuned to the propositional versus nonpropositional character of the utterance. Now, a second organizing principle appears to be at work, one which is sensitive to the grammatical or linguistic function of particular words in the message. The lesion that results in the agrammatic syndrome appears to suppress access to grammatical "function words;" the lesion producing the anomic syndrome suppresses access to nouns but leaves the grammatical forms unaffected. It would appear that these phenomena, which are most readily described in linguistic terms, would provide an area of common interest for linguists and neuropsychologists, and one for which linguistic theory may provide insights. Agrammatism, however, has proven particularly recalcitrant to explanation in purely linguistic terms because the particular operations that are impaired vary from patient to patient in a fashion that defies a principled linguistic account (Miceli, Silveri, Romani, & Caramazza, 1989). As we shall elaborate in the chapter on syntax disorders, Chapter 6, this is one of several areas in which there is tension between differing theoretical approaches: the imposition of constructs from theoretical linguistics, the approach of sequential steps of information processing, and the interpretation of surface symptomatology in terms of adaptive strategies on the part of the patient.

A particularly baffling challenge to intuition about language comes from still another type of paradoxical phenomenon—that of category-specific dissociations of word comprehension and word naming. An example that is seen repeatedly in aphasia is a patient's inability to point to parts of her body named by the examiner when she can point to other items named, and when she can point to the same body parts promptly when they are presented in writing. This means that the patient has a word comprehension problem specific to the category of body parts, but only for the auditory and not the graphic input channel. Similar problems affecting other categories (e.g., colors or numbers) have been described. These cases have provoked basic reconsideration of how word naming can be represented in the brain so as to make a particular category inaccessible through one input channel but not another.

We have sampled only a few of the many phenomena observed in aphasia that expose the inadequacy of the categories and assumptions about language knowledge and language use that come not only from naive experience, but also from traditional psychological and linguistic concepts. They have been described here with an emphasis on their paradoxical nature. We shall attempt in the body of this book to use these and other aphasic phenomena to attain an understanding of normal and disordered language that will show some of the symptoms of aphasia to be logical consequences of injury to the system.

CLINICAL ASPECTS

This chapter began with a focus on the nature of aphasia and how it might contribute to an understanding of normal language and brain organization. In a fuller sense, however, any treatment of the problem of aphasia must extend to its applied clinical aspects, where the patient's unique circumstances assume an importance equal to or greater than the brain–language interaction that his or her deficit exemplifies.

Patients with aphasia find themselves abruptly crippled in their ability to interact with or even comprehend those around them. They are often partly or totally immobilized by paralysis. The symptoms of aphasia may be modified or even overshadowed by other behavioral changes induced by the same brain injury; these may include apathy, depression, or euphoria.

Even if it were possible to distinguish sharply the language deficit from other behavioral symptoms in the aphasic patient, the clinical assessment would be grossly inadequate if it did not address nonlinguistic functions and emotional and social factors.

Although aphasia is most commonly seen as a result of stroke in older individuals, strokes of various types leading to aphasia occur in adults of all ages. Other types of brain lesions (e.g., trauma, tumor, or infection) may also produce aphasia in young adults. As a result, the occupational, social, and family circumstances of the patient may vary widely and may play a central role in any therapeutic or rehabilitation plan.

APPROACHES TO EVALUATION AND TREATMENT

In spite of differences in the theoretical orientation of the authors, all aphasia examinations necessarily share a common core of subtests that provide an inventory of such primary language operations as naming, word and sentence comprehension, reading of words and sentences, and writing them to dictation. The theoretical framework of an aphasia examination is intimately related to its author's convictions about the role of taxonomy in aphasia diagnosis, and whether the taxonomy is to be founded on anatomy, on linguistic analysis, or on the expressive and receptive channels that are most affected. With the current advances in the understanding of the anatomy underlying aphasia and the refinement of language information processing models, a new synthesis of these two domains is in the making. The implications of this synthesis for updating both diagnosis and assessment will be developed in the chapter on classification, Chapter 12.

THERAPY AND RECOVERY FROM APHASIA

In our present-day society, it is taken for granted that there is a treatment for every disability. The remediation of aphasia by language therapy is described in writings as early as the sixteenth century (Benton & Joynt, 1960), although the first detailed report on therapeutic approaches is that of Mills in 1904. Since the end of World War II, the availability of language therapy for aphasia has become virtually universal in the urban areas of industrialized countries. Yet, until the 1960s, the effectiveness of such therapy was taken on faith by those who provided it. Even after controlled studies began to be reported that established the utility of language therapy for many aphasic patients, skepticism as to its effectiveness continued among neurologists.

At the root of this skepticism is the fact that some degree of spontaneous recovery is always present and that this recovery can range from a slight improvement in comprehension to nearly complete recovery of all language functions. Recovery can be rapid and complete in the case of a small lesion or of a lesion on the periphery of the language zone. Even though the last 15 years have seen the recognition of other predictors of recovery in addition to lesion size, there remain wide and poorly understood individual differences in both the degree and pattern of spontaneous recovery after a single aphasia-producing episode. Although it has become traditional to say that spontaneous recovery begins to plateau at 2 months and is at an end after 6 months, significant continued improvement over a span of several years is not rare.

The fact of the wide variation in patients' potential for spontaneous improvement has created serious difficulties for the objective evaluation of the results of language therapy. Such studies have had to rely on sheer numbers of subjects to overcome individual variations and have had to assure the unbiased allocation of patients to treated and untreated groups—requirements that have been met only through great organizational effort. Innovations in research methodology have led to the use of "single subject design." There are now abundant case-by-case demonstrations of the effectiveness or lack of effectiveness of particular treatment techniques for particular patients.

THE NATURE OF SPONTANEOUS RECOVERY

Although the anatomical and physiological basis for the spontaneous recovery of language is a matter of speculation, one characteristic of such recovery is clear: the patient experiences a (partial) reconstitution of his or her prior language knowledge and skills. This is true even for recovery that occurs many months after the injury. Thus, we may observe the reemergence of vocabulary that appeared to be long lost and renewed access to grammatical structures that the patient had not been able to produce. Most therapy for aphasia, then, is based on the assumption that it is assisting the patient to retrieve former language knowledge rather than re-teaching the language as though it were new learning.

One account that appears to have face plausibility is that the aphasic patient continues to possess an intact store of language knowledge, and so the disorder is one of access to this knowledge. By this account, recovery is merely the restoration of access to prior linguistic knowledge. In contemporary terminology, aphasia would be considered a disorder of "performance" in which "competence" remains intact (Weigl & Bierwisch, 1970). Indeed, certain aphasic symptoms appear to arise from a failure to activate potential language behavior that becomes available under changed conditions (see Chapter 12 for speech initiation problems in transcortical motor aphasia).

Consideration of clinical facts, however, makes it impossible to accept retention of competence as a general explanation for the reemergence of prior language skills in late recovery. One such fact is that massive destruction of the tissues subserving language commonly results in severe and permanent aphasia. In these cases it appears futile to try to distinguish between a loss of stored representations and a loss of access to them. But the same argument must apply to lesser degrees of destruction, unless one is willing to propose that at some point of increasing damage the representations of language knowledge suddenly disappear, along with access to them. The solution to the problem of recovery awaits a better understanding of how language is implemented neurologically.

Two problem areas, both of great theoretical interest, which are not developed in this book, are dissociations between languages in polyglots with aphasia and aphasia in users of manual sign languages for the deaf. The author has opted not to discuss these problems in detail because of a lack of significant firsthand experience and because they are both extremely well covered in the cited references.

APHASIA IN POLYGLOTS

Most multilingual speakers who become aphasic display a similar level of relative impairment and a similar pattern of impairment in all of their languages. This predominant finding in polyglot aphasics is what one would logically expect. Experience with aphasia in monolingual speakers indicates that it may impact most severely on particular sensory input or motor output modalities (e.g., auditory comprehension, reading, or articulation) and on particular psycholinguistic dimensions (e.g., name retrieval and syntax). Thus, it is natural to anticipate parallel symptoms in all of an affected speaker's languages.

For over a century, however, cases of aphasia in polyglots have been documented in which one of the speaker's languages is much more profoundly affected than the other. In some instances, a relatively disused childhood language remains functional while the currently used adopted adult language is no longer accessible. In other cases, the reverse pattern has been observed. In his excellent review of this problem, Paradis (1989) also describes instances where a patient alternates unpredictably between two languages on different days, only one of them being accessible at a time.

The study of dissocations between the languages of polyglots is still at the stage where its variants are being documented. Although these cases are the exception rather than the rule, they pose a major conundrum that should be addressed in any model of language representation in the brain.

APHASIA IN MANUAL SIGN LANGUAGE

If the preceding phenomenon leaves us with a puzzle to be solved, the present topic is one that has been enlightening for understanding the meaning of a language-competent brain. Until the appearance of some early reports on the effect of brain injury on the sign language of the deaf (Critchley, 1938; Leischner, 1943; Douglass & Richardson, 1959), there was little consideration of the fact that aphasia need not be defined by the auditory–articulatory nature of natural language.

In contrast to oral language, which encodes its messages into auditory segments deployed in time, manual sign languages rely on visually displayed gestural segments, which depend on hand configuration, the character and direction of movement, and the location in space of the gestures. Location of the sign in relation to the body of the signer can define the semantic identity of a particular signed word; it is also used to denote syntactic relationships between the terms of the sentence. Given that the specialized auditory and articulatory capacities of the speaker do not enter into signing, one can ask if the language substrate of sign language is lateralized, like that of hearing persons, and whether the pattern of language breakdown for sign language has any relation either to the subtypes of aphasia or to their intrahemispheric lesion localization in hearing speakers.

The answers to these questions have been provided, in broad outline, by the observations reported by Poizner, Klima, and Bellugi (1987) and Poizner, Bellugi, and Klima (1989). From these authors' case studies of deaf signers with either right- or left-hemisphere strokes, we learn of the amazing degree of analogy between the effects of brain injury on oral language and on signed language. To begin with, loss or impairment of signed language is produced by left-hemisphere, and not by right-hemisphere, damage. Further, as in aphasia of spoken language, injury to the anterior portion of the language zone results in the reduction of signed communication to syntactically unorganized, individual lexical terms. Other forms of sign language aphasia, involving impaired sign comprehension and fluent, but syntactically disordered signing, appear to correspond both in localization and in symptomatology to forms of spoken aphasia.

The phenomena of sign language aphasia suggest that the specialized auditory and articulatory mechanisms of language that have evolved in the left hemisphere are a by-product and not the cause of the lateralization of language. While linguistic analysis (Bellugi, 1980; Padden & Perlmutter, 1987) reveals underlying similarities between the logic structures of oral and signed languages, one must be struck by the disparity in the modes of production and perception, and by the disparity of the modality-specific dimensions that are used to encode information. Whatever is lateralized in language dominance, it must be defined in terms broad enough to encompass at least these two modes of communication.

Chapter 2

Historical Overview

INTRODUCTION

The origins of human language are remote and are assumed to date back many tens of thousands, if not millions, of years. Traumatic brain injuries, as well as lesions produced by infection, tumor, and vascular disease must have been producing aphasia long before any written records were kept. Yet, there is little evidence that anything approaching the present-day concept of aphasia existed before the seventeenth century. To be sure, the loss of speech is recorded in medical writings as early as the Edwin Smith Surgical Papyrus of 3500 BC, but the nature of these cases cannot be discerned from the record.

Benton and Joynt's (1960) review of early descriptions of aphasia brings together virtually all of the known references to the loss of speech and language before the nineteenth century. Prior to the Renaissance, one looks in vain for any clue that observers distinguished between loss of voice or paralysis of the tongue and loss of language. True, the connection between brain injury and speech loss was recognized in the Hippocratic writings of the fifth century BC; however, the Greek terms that were used have been variously translated as "speechless," "voiceless," or "without articulation" (Benton & Joynt, 1960). If any of the ancient Greek clinicians had the concept of language impairment as being distinct from control of phonation or tongue movement, it was not passed on to their successors in the next two millenia. The one exception is a reference to a "learned man of Athens" who had lost his memory for letters after being hit in the head by a stone, but who was otherwise unimpaired.

It is a revealing commentary on communal modes of perceiving and categorizing behavior that a distinction so seemingly obvious now did not have a place in the language or conceptualization of our predecessors. It is not that they were any less capable of perceiving the distinction than we are—principles of language analysis, such as grammar and syntax have a long and venerable history—but the notion of an autonomous system dedicated to language escaped these observers over many centuries. Indeed, as we shall see, it did not emerge as a sudden insight, but evolved in the thinking of clinicians over a period of about 200 years.

CONCEPTIONS OF APHASIA
IN THE POST-RENAISSANCE PERIOD

The period spanning the fifteenth century through most of the eighteenth century was one of accumulating descriptions of aphasic disorders of almost every form that is now recognized. Many of the cases were described as medical curiosities. Still, by the late sixteenth century, there appeared evidence that the language-specific nature of some of these cases was being recognized. These early insights were followed in the next century by case reports that approached modern standards for their analysis of the behavioral deficits exhibited by the patients. Typical clinical descriptions from the late fifteenth century are those of Guainerio (1481, cited in Benton & Joynt, 1960), who made reference to one elderly patient who knew only three words and another who could rarely recall anyone's name. Another physician of the same era, Baverius de Baveriis, attributed his patient's inability to speak to weakness of the nerves that move the tongue.

Benton and Joynt's (1960) citations of sixteenth century authors give evidence of only limited gains in understanding during that century. They include accounts of rapid recovery from aphasia when bone fragments were removed from the brain. More important is a passage quoted from the writing of Johann Schenck von Grafenberg (1585), who points out that in many instances of brain disease, the loss of speech is due to an impairment in the faculty of memory, and not to a paralysis of the tongue. Although Schenck did not yet see the possibility of differentiating memory for language from memory in general, his observation signals a break from the centuries old identification of speech loss with impairment of tongue movement.

It is in the reports of Johann Schmidt (1676) and Peter Rommel (1683) that one encounters the first instances of well-described cases. Schmidt described the case of a patient who recovered from a right-sided paralysis accompanied by speech errors so severe that he could not be understood. As his speech recovered, he continued to suffer from a profound reading impairment, but retained some ability to write. Schmidt contrasted this patient with another, who regained his ability to read after an initial period of alexia. Rommel (1683) gave a vivid description of a woman patient's struggle with a severe nonfluent aphasia, noting with surprise that his patient was unable to utter words spontaneously or by repetition, but was able to recite her prayers by rote, provided that she performed them in the order in which she had learned them. She could not pick up on any one of them out of sequence nor even repeat portions after the examiner. Rommel reported this case as "a rare aphonia," using a term which today would be reserved for a patient who was incapable of phonating. It would appear that by the late seventeenth century, terminology for speech disorders had not been adapted to distinguish between syndromes that were already being distinguished in clinical descriptions.

During the eighteenth century, descriptions of assorted aphasic phenomena multiplied, as did the collections of cases. Many of these descriptions approach the level of behavioral description of Rommel's case; a clear recognition of the autonomy of language-specific deficits from other cognitive and motor control disorders became the rule. Benton and Joynt cite a quotation from the writings of the Duc de Saint Simon in 1718, describing an eminent soldier who was reduced to using a pointer to spell out his messages on an alphabet board because he could neither speak nor write. Linné (1745) gives an account of a patient who could, by himself, neither retrieve nor repeat any name, yet he was able to read them silently with comprehension. A remarkable case of well-preserved singing, of words and music, was described by Dalin (1745) in a patient who was virtually without speech.

A major medical work of the later eighteenth century was Morgagni's *De Sedibus et Causis Morborum per Anatomia Instigatis* (*The Seats and Causes of Disease Investigated by Anatomy*, 1769). The great Italian anatomist included many cases of aphasia arising from brain disease of assorted etiologies. Although Morgagni refers to the right hemiplegia or left cerebral disease that accompanied some of these cases, he seems not to have noticed the constancy of this association.

A landmark contribution to concepts of aphasia appeared in the form of a chapter titled "Die Sprachamnesie" by Gesner (1770). In this chapter, Gesner describes and analyzes the symptoms of several patients who had lost different aspects of language, but retained the use of the motor and articulatory aspects of speech. Two of these patients spoke and wrote only in a neologistic jargon; another suffered a sudden inability to read along with a loss of speech, both of which recovered in a few days. Gesner's final case contains a self-report by a teacher who, to his great frustration, persisted in producing unintended words with each attempt at oral reading, although he could read silently with comprehension.

Gesner's interpretation, more than those of any of his contemporaries or predecessors, anticipates nineteenth century thought. He notes that the disorders of his patients are specific to language—that the memory for words is autonomous from other types of memory and from other cognitive abilities. He proposed the theory that his patients had lost the association between an image or idea and its linguistic sign.

EARLY NINETEENTH CENTURY THOUGHT ON APHASIA

As we have seen, the progression from scattered case reports of aphasia as medical curiosities to the recognition of these disorders as specific to language emerged gradually from the writings of physicians of various European countries. By 1800, considerations about the loss of language moved into a new phase to which the French were major contributors.

With the writings of Franz Gall in the early 1800s, the problem of aphasia became a focus of intellectual speculation, both in relation to its bearing on the psychology of language and its implications for brain organization. This was a period of controversy as to whether the cerebral hemispheres functioned as a whole, as Flourens contended, or whether the brain was subdivided into different functional areas. Gall's phrenology was, of course, the antithesis of Flourens' position. Even though Gall's model of the brain as a mosaic of regions subserving various faculties and personality traits has come to be regarded as charlatanism, Gall was also an accomplished anatomist and a serious theoretician. His belief that the seat of language was behind the eyes in the prefrontal zones of both hemispheres is the best known element in his mosaic of faculties. According to Ombredane's review (1951), Gall conceived of the faculty of language as comprising two components: memory for words and the feeling for language (sens du language). Gall also published a number of clinical cases, among which were two aphasic patients whom he cited in support of his localizationist theory. One was a patient who developed a severe speech output disorder as the aftermath of a stroke. He pointed to his forehead as the source of his troubles. Perhaps Gall took this patient's gesture as vindicating his own theory. The other patient developed a severe word-finding disorder and right-sided weakness as the result of a stab wound with a fencing foil that penetrated the prefrontal zone.

One of Gall's admirers was Jean-Baptiste Bouillaud, an articulate and controversial participant in the debate on the organization of language in the brain—a debate that until the 1860s was largely conducted among members of various French medical societies. Bouillaud's 1825 paper was written to stand as a confirmation of Gall's anatomical theory of language. This and subsequent contributions brought Bouillaud under attack because of his dogmatic style and poor anatomical documentation. Yet Bouillaud had supporters, among them Aubertin and Gratiolet, who published clinical reports endorsing Bouillaud's position. Whatever his shortcomings in other regards, Bouillaud must be credited with presenting ideas on the biology of language that were advanced for his time. He pointed out that the organs of articulation—tongue, lips, and glottis—could have perfectly preserved function in their nonspeech activity, while their motor control for speech was abolished. Bouillaud proposed dual neural control systems for these organs, one for the learned activity of speech and one for the instinctive behavior of eating and swallowing. He was one of the earliest writers to distinguish between aphasic syndromes involving a breakdown of motor speech mechanisms and those that appeared as an amnesia for words. In this regard, he anticipated the dichotomous forms of aphasia later described by Broca, Wernicke, Baillarger, and Bastian.

The contribution of Jacques Lordat (1843) is sometimes referred to as merely an early self-description of aphasia. Lordat, professor on the faculty at Montpellier, had indeed suffered a transient episode of severe aphasia, and his introspections figured prominently in the account of aphasia that he published and lectured on extensively to medical students. Lordat's analysis of the speech process was remarkably advanced for its time. It anticipated the ideas expressed 70 years later by Arnold Pick, but it was peripheral to the main controversies of the time concerning the localization of language and received only minor notice. Lordat analyzed the generation of a spoken message into 10 stages. The first stage involved the mobilization of the intent to speak and the delimitation of the thought to be expressed; the second was the differentiation of the general idea into more elementary thoughts, whose sequential arrangement and interrelationships could then be processed rapidly. A later stage was termed by Lordat as the "corporealization" (*corporification*) of the ideas, followed by the stringing together of the sounds, and finally, their motor realization.

When Lordat wrote and gave his lectures, the term "aphasia" had not yet been coined. He used the term "alalia" to refer to his own and other clinical cases. His attribution of specific aphasic symptoms to failures at particular stages of his model is strikingly similar to contemporary analysis. For example, the failure to mobilize the sound sequence corresponding to a corporealized idea was "verbal amnesia." In his personal experience with aphasia, this disorder also took the form of producing unintended or transposed sound sequences. Lordat termed failure at the stage of motor implementation as "verbal asynergy."

FROM BROCA (1861) TO WORLD WAR II

Broca's (1861) report that a lesion of the foot of the third frontal convolution is responsible for the loss of articulate speech has come to be perceived as a turning point in the history of aphasia. That report, and the succession of confirming cases, was the first of three major discoveries in a span of less than 15 years. The second was the report, also by Broca, that language impairment followed lesions of the left, but not the right hemisphere. The third event was Carl Wernicke's (1874) monograph describing aphasia of the posterior first temporal gyrus, known as "sensory" aphasia or Wernicke's aphasia.

During this period, the intellectual climate assumed a state that was to change little, in principle, for the next 85 years. Language was distinguished (by most authors) from other human cognitive functions; the left cerebral hemisphere was readily accepted as providing its major biological substrate. There was a consensus that the dissociations of language skills produced by aphasia could somehow help in understanding the psychology of normal language. Correlations between aphasic symptoms and sites of brain injury were seen as the route to understanding the anatomical organization of language in the normal brain. Whereas new clinical observations brought greater sophistication to bear on these problems, the trend in thinking that was current in 1935 was already discernible in 1875.

In his original report in 1861, Broca was quite specific in saying that he was dealing with the loss of articulate speech—that is, a defect in the motor realization of language. This disorder, which he called "aphemia," he attributed to a lesion of the foot of the third frontal convolution. The term "aphemia" soon gave way, under the philological arguments of Trousseau, to the term "aphasia," which was quickly and universally adopted. Broca also recognized another form of language disorder that he referred to as "verbal amnesia"—a disorder in which motor speech production was intact, but words could not be recalled or were inappropriately used. He did not propose a lesion site for verbal amnesia.

As a result of Broca's report, in 1865, of the constant association of aphasia with left-hemisphere injury, there came to light an earlier unpublished manuscript by Marc Dax, dating to 1836, in which the identical insight had been gained through the collection of a series of about 40 cases. Both Dax's and Broca's treatment of these data were cautious and circumspect, but it was Broca who also noted that there were exceptions to this rule of left cerebral dominance for language, and that these cases tended to be left-handed.

As we have seen, Broca was not the first to distinguish between the loss of motor speech production and the loss of the association between concept and word. Baillarger (cited by Lecours, Lhermitte, & Bryans, 1983) appears to have been the first to apply the word "aphasia" to these two very disparate manifestations. "Simple aphasia" referred to the loss of speech and writing. The other category involved "a perversion of the language faculty in which patients produce unintended words but cannot access the words that they need." Hughlings Jackson (1915, pp. 8–9) also recognized two main forms of language impairment—one in which speech is severely damaged or absent and the other in which there is copious but erroneous output. The English neurologist, Bastian (1869), also distinguished between "aphasia" in the sense of Broca's "aphemia" and what he called "amnesia" in the same sense as Broca's "verbal amnesia."

The description by Wernicke of sensory aphasia in his 1874 monograph arrived at a point when the groundwork for this contribution had already been laid. The clinical features noted by Baillarger, Broca, Bastian, and Jackson were the very ones that characterized the speech output of sensory aphasia. Wernicke, however, emphasized the impairment of auditory language comprehension and showed that this complex of deficits results from a lesion of the posterior portion of the first left temporal gyrus. In his view, the destruction of auditory language processing was responsible for erroneous speech output and patients' unawareness of their errors.

Wernicke's work was extremely influential in a number of respects. His mapping of psychological processes onto anatomical data was rigorously reasoned. Building on Meynert's postulation of a fiber bundle connecting the first temporal gyrus to the motor speech zone, Wernicke proposed a model in which this connection played a vital role. In Wernicke's view, Broca's anterior speech zone was the seat of learned motor articulatory patterns, whereas the posterior first temporal gyrus was the center for auditory word images. The connection between these two centers was vital for conveying word images to the motor speech area for production. Wernicke predicted that a lesion confined to this fiber bundle would produce an aphasia in which motor speech skills and auditory comprehension are preserved, but word retrieval would fail and speech errors would appear.

Wernicke's schema was elaborated by Lichtheim (1884) by means of a simple model (Fig. 2.1) that is the basis for the classical anatomical–connectionist model of aphasic syndromes. In Lichtheim's formulation, subsequently endorsed by Wernicke, the lesion of the pathway connecting the auditory and the motor speech centers produces an aphasia for

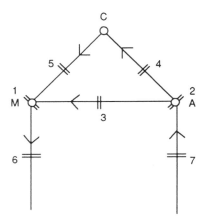

Figure 2.1. The Wernicke–Lichtheim schema. M, motor articulatory center; A, center for auditory word images; C, conceptual center. Possible lesions sites are numbered 1 through 7.

repetition, termed *conduction* aphasia *(Leitungsaphasie)*. The Wernicke–Lichtheim schema includes a node representing the store of conceptual knowledge that gives meaning to the word images of the auditory center, provided that the pathways from this center are functional. The output from the conceptual center provides the messages that are to be implemented through the motor speech area. Damage to the pathways leading into or out of the conceptual store results in two different forms of aphasia, transcortical sensory and transcortical motor aphasia, but both are characterized by preserved repetition ability. (A more detailed review of the syndromes arising from this schema is provided in Chapter 12.)

The classical typology of the aphasias was passed along to the clinicians of the twentieth century with minor modifications of the original Wernicke–Lichtheim model. The eminent French neurologist Dejerine (1901), for example, accepted the roles of Broca's and Wernicke's areas, but rejected the idea of a "conceptual center" to which no anatomical structure could be assigned. Dejerine's thinking was influenced by the progress in anatomy that was made in the intervening years. Taking into account the long and short cortico-cortical connections between the various sectors of the language zone, he held that any lesion in the perisylvian region had some impact on multiple language modalities, although a particular language channel might be predominantly affected. Thus, he did not accept the purity of the syndromes predicted by the Wernicke–Lichtheim model, nor did he accept the notion of transcortical aphasia, as predicted by that model.

Dejerine was sensitive to the role of the corpus callosum as the communication channel between the two hemispheres, and to the necessity of taking into account the bilateral innervation of the oral motor apparatus. His contribution on the clinicopathology of pure word-blindness directly implicates the corpus callosum. His description of alexia with agraphia and its anatomical basis was the occasion for his postulating a visual–verbal zone in the angular gyrus of the left hemisphere. Dejerine accepted the clinical reality of pure single modality forms of aphasia such as word-deafness, subcortical ("pure") motor aphasia, and word-blindness when lesions were located at the periphery of the language zone in such a way that they could produce a disconnection affecting only a single input or output channel.

Kussmaul (1881) identified two forms of deficit; "agrammatism" and "amnesia for words," as autonomous forms that were included under the heading of "aphasia." Both of these were subjected to further scrutiny in the ensuing years at the clinical descriptive level and by psychological interpretation. Pitres (1898) elaborated on the syndrome of amnesic aphasia, or pure word-finding difficulty. Although he conceived of it as a dissociation between a concept center and a store of word images, he did not propose a lesion site for it.

Agrammatism was a particularly intriguing disorder, restricted to a small proportion of patients who adopted a pattern of speech in which they communicated chiefly with nouns or very brief phrases and who appeared to be unable to use the purely grammatical elements of speech, such as auxiliary verbs, noun and verb inflections, or prepositions. Although agrammatism had been described before Kussmaul, it remained for the scholars of the early twentieth century (Pick, 1913; Salomon, 1914; Kleist, 1916; Isserlin, 1922) to carry out detailed clinical and psychological analyses.

THE REJECTION OF ASSOCIATIONISM

The names most prominently associated with the reaction against models based on anatomic centers and interconnections are those of Marie (1906) and Head (1926). This alternative viewpoint, often referred to as "noetic," links the impairment of language to the impairment of an underlying intellectual capacity. Special terms that have been assigned to this impairment are "asymbolia" (Finkelnburg, 1870) and impaired "abstract attitude" (Goldstein, 1948). In fact, credit for originating this approach ought to be given to Hughlings Jackson. Jackson wrote about aphasia over a 30-year period, starting in 1863. Beyond recognizing the dominance of the left hemisphere and the perisylvian location of the language zone, he was little concerned with issues of localization of function. On this topic, the farthest he commited himself was to write, "the nearer the disease is to the corpus striatum, the more likely is the defect of articulation to be the most striking thing, and the farther off, the more likely is it to be mistakes of words" (Jackson, 1866).

Jackson attempted to apply general psychological principles to the manifestations of aphasia, whatever their particular form. He was strongly influenced in his thinking by the philosopher Herbert Spencer, and he attempted to show that certain general principles of neural activity could be seen as expressed across many systems, including language and perception. The distinction between automatic and volitional behavior was a salient principle in Jackson's view, and he considered these two forms of activity to have different underlying neural organizations. In aphasia, the automatic mode was represented by the production of interjections or the recitation of memorized sequences or passages. Aphasia, Jackson emphasized, was not the loss of words, but the loss of the ability to use words to convey information or to "propositionize." An aphasic might be unable to produce a word in answer to a simple question, but is able to say the word flawlessly as part of a memorized passage. These observations of Jackson's fit so well to everyday clinical observation that they are virtually axiomatic for contemporary clinicians who deal with aphasic patients and their origin may be forgotten.

Jackson saw a relationship between cerebral dominance and the concept of automatic, nonpropositional speech. Given the observation that many totally aphasic patients with extensive left hemisphere destruction continue to produce memorized speech and swearwords, Jackson suggested that the right hemisphere alone might mediate those productions. It was Jackson, too, who pointed out the fallacy of attributing a damaged language skill to the site of the lesion that produced the impairment. Goldstein's later distinction between abstract and concrete behavior borrows heavily from the Jacksonian principle.

In addition to Jackson, two other names deserve to be mentioned as early contributors to the noetic viewpoint. Trousseau (1864), who is remembered for having coined the term "aphasia," adopted the view that most aphasic patients had severe intellectual impairment. Finkelnburg (1870) considered aphasia to be only one manifestation of an "asymbolia," or inability to manipulate symbols for communication. The identical underlying deficit made it difficult for individuals who were aphasic to express their ideas by gesture or pantomime.

The most dramatic challenge to the associationist view by a proponent of the noetic viewpoint came with Marie's (1906) publication of a series of articles in which he argued that there was only one basic aphasic disorder, namely that of Wernicke. Moreover, Marie argued that aphasia was a disorder of the intellect that had a special manifestation in language. The difficulty in speech output seen in Broca's patients was simply the combination of aphasia with dysarthria (a specific disorder of articulatory control). Marie's view was quickly challenged by other contemporaries, notably Dejerine. Nevertheless, the noetic viewpoint was to attract adherents well into the twentieth century.

Pick and von Monakow, among the early twentieth century neurologists, developed views on aphasia that had no link to the anatomic—associationist tradition. Pick's early work was, in fact, totally along the lines of that tradition, but he abandoned that approach in favor of a psychological and linguistic analysis of normal and aphasic language, applying it as well to the study of the development of language in children. One of his major works was a monograph on agrammatism, which took the form of a step-by-step analysis of the process of formulating and producing a sentence. Pick was well versed in the linguistics of his era and well acquainted with the clinical varieties of aphasia, including agrammatism. Yet his approach differed, in principle, little from Lordat's intuitive self-analysis. Like Lordat's, Pick's work is a pre-experimental precursor of the information processing approach to be found in contemporary cognitive psychology.

Von Monakow (1914) regarded most linguistic acts as requiring the interaction of many neural networks, so that the functional localization of individual language skills was of little concern to him. He introduced the concept of "diaschisis," which recognized the depressing effect of a cerebral lesion on functions that depend on structures remote from the lesion site.

Henry Head's two-volume *Aphasia and Kindred Disorders of Speech* (1926) combined a sarcastic attack on the "diagram makers" of the associationistic tradition with an effort at a totally psychological taxonomy of the aphasias. Head was, in a sense, the successor to Hughlings Jackson. In fact, it was Head who collected Jackson's long neglected work, republished them in the journal *Brain,* and restored Jackson's views to an audience that was now primed to appreciate them. Head viewed aphasia as a disorder of symbolic formulation and expression that extended beyond language to any behavior in which some symbol plays a part between its initiation and its realization. As an example of loss of symbolic representation in a nonlanguage task, he gave the example of a patient who could toss an object into a basket when the basket was in view, but could not retain a mental representation of the basket when the view of it was obstructed.

Head's view of aphasia as an impairment of symbolic function was certainly congruent with Jackson's dictum that the aphasic had not lost words so much as the ability to propositionize with them. It was even close to the view presented by Finkelnburg in his influential paper of 1870, setting forth the concept of "asymbolia" as the disorder underlying all impairments of symbol use, whether linguistic or nonlinguistic.

Head offered a classification of the aphasias under four categories representing disruptions of different aspects of language. Head's "verbal aphasia" is closest to the traditional motor or Broca's aphasia, with the major impact of the disorder falling on motor realization of the utterance. His definition of "syntactic aphasia" resembles most closely the traditional Wernicke's aphasia, whereas his "nominal aphasia" is virtually identical to amnesic aphasia, as described by Pitres. It is striking that in spite of his borrowing a terminology from the vocabulary of linguistics, Head was impressed by the same configurations of concurring symptoms that had impressed his predecessors of the anatomic–associationistic school. Yet Head's syndrome descriptions were often vague and included features whose meaning was unclear or could not be generalized across patients. Ten years later, his admirers, Weisenburg and Mcbride, (1935) acknowledged that his classification had failed to arouse support "because it does not outline types which can be generally observed."

It is worth commenting on the fourth of Head's aphasia types, which he called "semantic aphasia." This was an entirely novel perception of a variety of language processing difficulties—this aphasia spares the basic skills of phonology, syntax, and word retrieval, as well as word comprehension, but impairs the capacity to draw inferences beyond the literal meaning of the word. It is notable that the same term was independently resurrected by Luria (1970) with a symptomatology closely resembling that proposed by Head.

In the United States, neurologist Theodore Weisenburg, working with psychologist Katherine McBride, carried out an extensive study of aphasia that culminated in an influential book reviewing the history and clinical features of the disorder from the perspective of their investigation (Weisenburg & McBride, 1935). They administered a battery of standardized intelligence and language achievement tests to see whether the results of such a study would lead to an objective classification. Their selection of a study population set a standard never before (and rarely since) met in the collection of clinical data of this type. They screened 234 aphasic patients to select 60 individuals presenting a variety of aphasic disturbances of both tumor and vascular etiologies that were uncomplicated by other cognitive problems, and were under 60 years of age. These were compared to several different nonaphasic control groups, both brain-injured and normal. After a thoughtful consideration of all the alternative classification systems that had been offered up to then, they concluded that their data could support only three major types of aphasia: predominantly expressive, predominantly receptive, and amnesic. The overlap in the impairments observed in their patients precluded their acceptance of the more fine-grained varieties of the classical authors.

Although Weisenburg and McBride's philosophical approach was clearly in the noetic tradition, they were dissatisfied with the explanatory principles that had grown out of that tradition—such principles as automatic versus volitional, or the impairment of symbolic formulation—to account for aphasic disorders. Even though they saw the relevance of both of these ideas, they concluded that one must take into account the impairment of specific skills and specific sensory or motor channels. They viewed their approach as empirical and pragmatic, and made no commitment to any theory, model, or anatomical account.

Kurt Goldstein occupies a dual role in the recent history of aphasia. Schooled in the classical German anatomic tradition, even his latest major work on aphasia (1948) presents a classification and view of anatomic localization that accepts that general framework, although differing in the interpretation of particular syndromes. At the same time, Goldstein is regarded as one of the strongest voices of the noetic movement. Goldstein emphasized the pervasive effect of changes in the aphasic patient's intellectual and adaptive capacities which he felt interacted with and even determined the form of their language behavior. Goldstein introduced the concept of "abstract behavior," sometimes referred to as "categorical" behavior. The loss of the capacity for abstract behavior abolishes the ability to deal with symbols, to pretend, or to deal with a hypothetical situation, and to shift from one task to another.

The loss of abstract behavior became, in Goldstein's view, an explanation for a number of specific linguistic symptoms. For example, agrammatism was due to the abstract nature of grammatical morphemes; amnesic aphasia was the result of the patient's inability to conceive of the object's name as an arbitrary label that stands for the object. Because the patient suffering a loss of abstract behavior cannot conceive of categories, they would be unable to cope with the several sorting tests that he developed with his collaborators, Egon Weigl and Martin Scheerer.

Goldstein did not regard the loss of abstract behavior to be an explanation for all aspects of aphasia. He referred to the specific components, such as articulation, syntax, reading, writing, and auditory comprehension as the "instrumentalities" of language that could be affected independently of the capacity for abstract behavior. Even naming could be impaired, as an instrumentality of language, in patients who did not suffer from the loss of abstract behavior. Such a patient, however, did not have true "amnesic aphasia," as Goldstein defined the term.

Although Goldstein's taxonomy of aphasia accounted for the same major syndromes as the Wernicke–Lichtheim model, there were some differences in his approach. He related symptoms to lesion sites, but he did not indulge in efforts to localize functions nor engage in any form of associationistic model building. Although he recognized the symptomatology of the syndromes of conduction aphasia and transcortical motor aphasia, he rejected the associationistic account of these phenomena. Goldstein preferred the term "central aphasia" instead of conduction aphasia and he considered the symptomatology of the classical transcortical motor aphasia to be the result of a nonlinguistic impairment affecting the initiation of speech.

Théophile Alajouanine (1890–1980) was the leading French aphasiologist in the period leading up to World War II and until his retirement from the Salpêtriere Hospital in Paris, where he held the prestigious position formerly occupied by Charcot. Alajouanine initiated the trend of cross-disciplinary neurolinguistic research by bringing the collaboration of André Ombredane, a psychologist, and Marguerite Durand, a linguist, to bear on the analysis of a clearly defined problem in aphasia, that of the breakdown of articulation (Alajouanine *et al.*, 1939). Alajouanine's influence was expressed both through his emphasis on the psycholinguistic features of aphasia and their anatomical foundations, and through his training and collaboration with other neurologists who have achieved prominence in contemporary aphasiology, such as François Lhermitte and André-Roch Lecours.

APHASIA AFTER WORLD WAR II

The Second World War produced several converging influences that accelerated both basic research on aphasia and the efforts to rehabilitate aphasic patients. The sudden flow of brain-injured soldiers with aphasia into military and veterans' hospitals was met with an expansion of funding for the training of clinicians—both psychologists and speech pathologists—and for research on language and brain function. When the flow of war-injured veterans subsided, there was already in place a knowledgeable and experienced professional cadre ready to deal with the "normal" intake of patients with stroke-induced aphasia.

The birth of the field of psycholinguistics in the 1950s and its mergence with the approaches of information processing and cognitive psychology in the next two decades brought about the first significant shift in 90

years in the type of questions that began to be asked in the study of aphasia. The influence of psycholinguistics and the experimental method was
pervasive, and it became part of the training of speech pathologists, as
well as of psychologists.

The change in the approach to aphasia cannot be reduced to a single
factor, nor did it totally replace earlier approaches. A major element of it
was the introduction of the experimental method. Semianecdotal accounts of single cases and small series of cases began to be replaced by
formal, controlled experiments involving groups of comparable patients.
Individual case studies were likely to consist of formal experiments carried out with the patient, or a series of test procedures administered under controlled conditions and providing enough of a sample to permit a
statistical analysis. High standards for statistical significance and rigor of
experimental methodology became, within a few years, requirements for
a report to be accepted for publication.

A second aspect of the new approach was that formal models of language processes or of language impairment became the basis for making
predictions that could be experimentally tested. The study of aphasia began to attract theorists from the fields of linguistics and normal psycholinguistics who viewed it as a testing ground for theories derived
from studies of normal language. It would have been impossible for an
intuitive analysis like that of Pick to obtain a serious hearing in the zeit-
geist of the second half of this century.

The changes in the approach to aphasia research did not just spring
into existence; therefore it is helpful to trace them through the work of
the leaders in the field from the 1950s through the 1980s.

POST-WORLD WAR II TAXONOMIES OF APHASIA

The early twentieth century heard a number of influential voices
against anatomic associationism—those of Marie in France, Head in Eng-
land, and Weisenburg and McBride in the United States. In the mid-
century period, a number of alternative approaches to a taxonomy of
aphasia blossomed and faded. This was a period when, in response to
the exuberant growth of aphasia rehabilitation, various standardized
tests for aphasia were published by authors whose differing rationales
were reflected in the makeup of their tests. Some leading figures in the
postwar period are discussed here.

Eberhard Bay, a German neurologist, rejected both the anatomic association theories and the newer classifications based on psychological
and linguistic factors. He held that neither approach could provide an

unambiguous basis for classification (Bay, 1964). Instead, he argued that aphasia is an indivisible entity, which always entails a breakdown in conceptual thinking. Different cases of aphasia can be distinguished by differences in the level of severity and by the presence or absence of particular accompanying features, such as dysarthria, reading impairment, euphoria, and so forth. Bay's approach thus echoed that of Marie in almost all essentials.

Hildred Schuell was an American speech pathologist and director of the aphasia rehabilitation program in the Minneapolis Veterans Administration Hospital. She carried out formal studies on varieties of speech errors of aphasics and was widely regarded and highly influential in advancing the teaching of aphasia therapy techniques and in promoting treatment for aphasic patients. In 1953, she published her *Minnesota Test for the Differential Diagnosis of Aphasia* (MTDDA), a comprehensive survey of language skills in all modalities. Her test included highly analytic procedures, such as speech–sound discrimination, and extremely complex performances of functional competence (e.g., "Name three things that a good citizen should do").

Schuell collaborated with psychologist J. J. Jenkins in carrying out a factor analysis of patients' performance on the MTDDA. They interpreted their results as showing that a single general language factor accounts for virtually all of the deficits of aphasics. On this basis, they espoused a view that was not too divergent from that of Marie and the other noeticists.

Schuell did offer a typology of aphasia with five subcategories, but these were neither psycholinguistically nor anatomically based. Rather, Schuell's typology was based in part on severity and in part on how the language problem interacted with sensorimotor impairments. This typology had limited acceptance and did not survive.

Roman Jakobson, a Russian-born linguist, devoted himself to a wide range of issues related to the properties of language and their interaction with various human activities, from poetry to the acquisition and loss of language. He developed the concept that any phoneme can be uniquely defined as a configuration of distinctive features, of which there are a finite number. This notion became one of the foundations of modern phonology.

Jakobson's interest in aphasia as a field that could be illuminated by linguistic principles, became manifest early in his career. He believed that both language acquisition and language breakdown were governed by certain universal principles. One of these is that the very properties of a phoneme that leads to its early appearance in children's speech, also make it likely that it would appear almost universally in the phoneme repertory of all the world's languages. At the other extreme, phonemes perfected late in children's speech were likely to be in the phoneme repertory of the fewest languages. In 1941, he published a widely known monograph in which he claimed that the same principle extended to the loss of phonemes by aphasic patients—namely that the latest to be acquired would be most vulnerable to loss after brain damage, whereas the earliest learned would survive the best. This monograph, appropriately titled *Kindersprache, Aphasie und allgemeine Lautgesetze* (*Child Language, Aphasia, and General Sound Laws*), has not stood up to subsequent clinical observation, but with it Jakobson established the interest of linguistics in the biology of language and set the stage for other linguists who followed in his steps several decades later.

In 1956, Jakobson and Halle published a monograph in which a concept appeared that has remained influential in the classification of aphasia. Drawing on the polarity, well known in linguistics, between paradigmatic and syntagmatic aspects of language, they showed that this could be applied to the major dichotomy among types of aphasia. "Paradigmatic" relations are those between a symbol and its referent. Jakobson called the breakdown of this function "similarity disorder" and its prototypical manifestation in aphasia was in anomic aphasia, the inability to access the names of concepts while the syntax of sentences is preserved. "Syntagmatic" relations are those between the elements in a string of linguistic segments, such as between a word and those that precede and follow it in a sentence. Jakobson called the breakdown of this function "contiguity disorder" and its prototypical manifestation took the form of agrammatism.

Jakobson used the principle of contiguity disorder to account for and even to make predictions concerning the order of difficulty of particular syntactic structures. For example, utterances that were free of syntactic links, such as free-standing nouns, would be most robust. He deduced that in languages that use noun inflections, the nominative case should replace oblique cases. Inflections that signaled a syntactic relation (e.g., the possessive *s*) would be more fragile than those that modified word meaning without reference to other words (e.g., the plural *s*). Jakobson's views on agrammatism strongly influenced Luria and are reflected as well in the research of Wepman and Goodglass.

Joseph Wepman was an American psychologist whose career in aphasiology began with his service during World War II. He exerted considerable influence on American speech pathology through his views on the treatment of aphasia, the classification of aphasia, and the assessment of aphasic deficits. Nowhere in Wepman's work is there any concern with the neuroanatomical correlates of aphasia, except for a passage in his book *Recovery from Aphasia*, suggesting that disorders following right-hemisphere lesions do not affect language, so much as they affect articulation.

Wepman's views on the types of aphasia are couched entirely in terms of psycholinguistic functions. His typology is based on the work of American philosopher Charles Morris (1938), in which three types of relationships are proposed in the use of signs: "semantic" relations are those between a sign and its referent; "syntactic" relations are those of signs to each other; and "pragmatic" relations are those between sign and interpreter.

Wepman adapted these concepts to his taxonomy of the aphasias. Thus, Wepman's semantic aphasia entailed a breakdown in the association between the referent and its name, corresponding to the classical anomic or amnesic aphasia; his syntactic aphasia involved a loss of the word-to-word relationships of the traditional agrammatism (Jakobson's "contiguity disorder"). Wepman's pragmatic aphasia is less easily related to traditional categories and less easily defined. It refers to a category of aphasic patients who speak with a fluent output that has a normal balance of nouns to verbs and grammatical words, but who produce speech that has no relationship to any discernible subject matter; it may include neologisms, and no meaning can be extracted from it. Wepman also proposed varieties that he called "jargon aphasia" and "global aphasia."

Wepman's classification was adopted by a limited following and soon was abandoned. In part, this lack of acceptance is due to his renaming the symptoms of agrammatism and anomia with terms that were not as descriptive as the more traditional ones, and because the subtypes "pragmatic" and "jargon" were not easily distinguished in clinical observation, and both were within the range of variation of the classical Wernicke's aphasia.

Wepman and Jones (1961) published an examination for aphasia that had quite a different rationale from that put forth in Wepman's classification system. For purposes of measurement, they defined a series of language operations in terms of the combinations of sensory input and motor output channels that were involved in any task. Wepman and Jones submitted the results of their examination, carried out on a population of aphasic patients, to a factor analysis and drew a conclusion directly contradictory to that of Schuell and Jenkins. Rather than only one factor, they proposed that there were five autonomous components of language that could be damaged: visual-to-oral transmission, aural-to-oral and aural-to-graphic transmission, and matching to either oral or visual stimulation.

ANATOMICAL ASSOCIATIONISM IN THE LATE TWENTIETH CENTURY

Although the twentieth century scholars whose views have been cited here did not explicitly acknowledge the historical roots of their work, it appears that, with the exception of Jakobson, they were, for the most part, echoing nineteenth and early twentieth century authorities. Bay and Schuell seemed to be restating Marie's position; Wepman is quite reminiscent of Henry Head, who also eschewed anatomy in favor of a purely psycholinguistic basis for classification.

Two major figures, Luria and Geschwind, played a major role in reasserting the importance of anatomy for understanding the phenomena of aphasia in finer detail. Both were sophisticated in their appreciation of psycholinguistic factors that could not be fully accounted for in anatomical terms. Their influence led to the assignment of equal importance to these two aspects of the investigation of aphasia, which is the hallmark of the current era.

Luria published his *Traumatic Aphasia* in the original Russian in 1947. His viewpoint became well known outside of the Soviet Union with the English edition of *Higher Cortical Functions in Man* in 1966, and with the English language translation of *Traumatic Aphasia* in 1970. Luria preserves the gross anatomo-functional distinction between the impairment of motor–articulatory aspects of speech, associated with anterior speech zone injury and impairments of auditory language processing, and sound-to-meaning associations, arising from temporal lobe injury. Luria introduced distinctions within the motor and sensory categories that arose from his view of the relationship between primary motor and sensory centers, the secondary zones adjacent to them, and tertiary areas that combined input from multiple secondary zones. At various points, psychological constructs, such as "inner speech" that he borrowed from his mentor, Vigotsky, are assigned a mediating role.

Luria proposed a subdivision of motor aphasia into two subtypes: afferent and efferent motor aphasia. Afferent, or kinesthetic motor aphasia is attributed to a loss of the sensory feedback controlling articulatory movements caused by injury immediately posterior to the lower rolandic fissure. This disorder is manifested by difficulty in assuming individual articulatory positions. Efferent motor aphasia, resulting from a lesion in the traditional Broca's area, is manifested by the inability to produce the transition from one articulatory movement to the next. In the receptive sphere, Luria makes another dichotomy: that between sensory acoustic aphasia of the superior temporal gyrus (the traditional Wernicke's area) and sensory amnestic aphastia, associated with injury of the middle and inferior temporal gyri, near the temporo-parietal junction.

In the sensory acoustic form, the basic problem is one of "phonemic hearing"—the ability to discriminate between the sounds of the speaker's language. In the amnestic form, sound discrimination is intact, but its link to word meaning is disturbed, at times totally "alienated"— the patient may repeat a word that he has just heard without appearing to derive any meaning from it. Both word comprehension and word retrieval are disturbed in both forms of sensory aphasia but, according to Luria, for different underlying reasons.

Luria's "dynamic aphasia" is the transcortical motor aphasia of the classical typology. It is characterized by a poverty of spontaneous speech and the inability to formulate ideas, attributed by Luria to the effect of prefrontal injury on self-initiated behavior. As in the transcortical syndrome, the patient's ability to repeat is preserved and he or she is often able to give brief factual responses.

The sixth syndrome in Luria's typology is "semantic aphasia," a form in which the elementary language processes of auditory processing and motor articulation are preserved, but the patient is deficient in grasping and manipulating relationships between concepts, particularly "logico-grammatical" relationships. It is associated with problems in calculation and in visuo-spatial processing and is attributed to injury of the parieto-occipital region, a tertiary association area. As noted in describing Henry Head's typology, the designation "semantic aphasia," the locus of lesion, and the symptomatology are virtually identical in the taxonomies of these two authors, although it is not identified as a syndrome by any other writers. Wepman used the same term in an entirely different sense.

Luria departs from the approach of the classical associationists in his avoidance of the concept of disconnection between centers and the theoretical consequences of the disconnection concept. For example, he makes no note concerning the preservation or loss of the ability to repeat, and he rejects the notion of conduction aphasia. Although repetition failure is a feature of both forms of his motor aphasia and both forms of his sensory aphasia, it is attributed to the basic deficit underlying each of those four subtypes of aphasia.

Luria leaned heavily on neural physiology in his account of the varieties of aphasia and disturbances of related higher functions. Yet he was also cognizant of the psychological and psycholinguistic factors that could not be reduced to anatomical terms. His linguistic outlook is strongly influenced by that of Jakobson. For example, the breakdown of syntactic expression in efferent motor aphasia (i.e., agrammatism) is assigned to the loss of the predicative function of speech and the preservation of the more robust nominative function. He cautioned against any effort to account for aphasia in either totally anatomical terms or linguistic terms, but he incorporated the thinking of both of these disciplines in his primarily anatomo-physiological approach.

Norman Geschwind was equally sensitive to the features of aphasic symptomatology that demanded description in psycholinguistic or psychological terms. However, unlike Luria, his major explanatory efforts concentrated on those symptoms that could be accounted for in terms of the transmission of information between the major motor and sensory processing centers. His 1965 paper "Disconnexion syndromes in animals and man" was a statement of principles that appeared over and over in his subsequent work. It was preceded by another important paper "A human cerebral disconnection syndrome" (Geschwind & Kaplan, 1962) in which he revived the awareness of the syndrome of the interrupted corpus callosum, calling attention to Liepmann's earlier demonstration of the effects of hemispheric disconnection produced by a natural lesion. Geschwind and Kaplan showed, for the first time, that the interruption of pathways through the corpus callosum could prevent tactile information that was available in the right hemisphere from reaching the language zone in the left hemisphere. The result was that objects palpated and recognized by the left hand could not be named; that is, there was a unilateral tactile anomia. Geschwind and Kaplan's patient could demonstrate that he had, in fact, recognized the objects placed in his left hand; although he could not name them, he could draw them with his left hand.

In his 1965 article, Geschwind argued that the principle of disconnection between right and left hemispheres could be applied to some lesions that were confined to the left hemisphere. If properly situated, such lesions could produce a disconnection, within the language zone of the left hemisphere, between two centers in different parts of the language zone. He argued that conduction aphasia was the result of such a disconnection. In 1968, he published another influential paper with Quadfasel and Segarra, describing a syndrome termed "isolation of the speech area" that provided a basis for reconciling the classical interpretation of transcortical aphasia with the anatomy and physiology of the brain. Specifically, they argued that the physiology of brain circulation permitted the development of lesions that essentially isolated Wernicke's and Broca's areas from the rest of the brain, allowing certain elementary language skills such as repetition and meaningless recitation to be preserved without any input to or output from the thinking and experiencing part of the brain.

Geschwind deserves credit for introducing the terms "fluent" and "nonfluent" to designate the two major subtypes of aphasic syndromes.

Earlier in this chapter, the conceptual roots for this distinction were traced back to the writings of Bouillaud and many authors who followed him. But none before Geschwind thought to apply these two simple and clearly descriptive terms to label forms of aphasia. They quickly came into general use, displacing the ambiguous terms "expressive" and "receptive."

It is fair to say that Geschwind's explanatory accounts are largely confined to mechanisms of information transmission to the neglect of the operations of processing mechanisms. It would be a mistake to see Geschwind as opposing the psycholinguistic analysis of language, because he endorsed this enthusiastically and made many clinical observations of the psycholinguistic character of particular syndromes. Unlike Luria, however, he produced little speculation on the relation between these factors and anatomical structures. Geschwind was particularly influential in advancing the detailed correlation of specific components of aphasic syndromes with careful analysis of lesions. He was a dynamic teacher and spokesman for the neurology of behavior as a subspecialty. The Aphasia Research Center that he organized in 1965 at the Boston Veterans Administration Hospital trained most of the senior behavioral neurologists in the United States and many practicing in Europe.

THE CONTEMPORARY SCENE: 1970–1990

We have already noted that objective measurement and statistical standards as bases for judging the validity of tests and experimental observation became part of aphasiology in the early post-World War II era. American psychologist Arthur Benton, with his students and collaborators, pioneered in the development of testing instruments in many areas of neuropsychology, memory and face recognition as well as aphasia, with his *Neurosensory Center Comprehensive Examination for Aphasia* (Spreen & Benton, 1977) and his *Multilingual Examination for Aphasia* (Benton & Hamsher, 1989). Benton's collaboration with a number of leading European neuropsychologists played a role in the introduction of objective measurement methods in their work. De Renzi and Vignolo, who founded a productive school of aphasia research in Milan, for example, published the popular Token Test for the measurement of auditory language comprehension in aphasia.

Other European leaders whose work reflected the new demand for objective data that could be replicated by others were Henry Hécaen in Paris and Klaus Poeck in Aachen, Germany. Hécaen, working at the Saint Anne Hospital, was the hub of an interdisciplinary group that included linguists, psychologists, and neurologists. His work on cerebral dominance and many aspects of aphasia and related disorders earned him the status of the dean of European neuropsychology, until his death in 1983. He founded the journal *Neuropsychologia* in 1963. Within a few years, two new journals, *Cortex*, founded by DeRenzi in 1964 and *Brain and Language*, founded by Whitaker in 1974, became the major exchange media for articles on brain–language relationships for the rapidly burgeoning international community of aphasiologists.

Just as far-reaching as the introduction of objective methods in measurement and experimental analysis of symptoms was the approach of the newly developing field of cognitive psychology that brought about the creation of "cognitive neurolinguistics." Cognitive psychology is devoted to the analysis of human mental processes, such as perception, memory, and language in terms of the step-by-step unfolding of the work of specifiable subsystems whose operating characteristics are the subject of experimental study. Although Lordat and Pick can be regarded as precursors of this approach, they did not conceive of the essential feature of contemporary cognitive psychology: that any model that is offered have specific performance implications that can be tested in the laboratory. Competing theories must stand the test of experimental verification. It is no longer sufficient to offer an intuitively plausible account as a retrospective explanation of clinical observations.

Experimental verification, in the case of an aphasic symptom such as agrammatism, may take the form of a sentence production test that incorporates particular grammatical operations about which the theory makes a prediction. For example, to test Jakobson's prediction that constructions signaling a syntactic link between words (e.g., the English possessive 's) would be more vulnerable than constructions that were purely semantic in nature (e.g., the plural *s* or *es*), Goodglass and Hunt (1958) and Goodglass and Gleason (1960) created a series of sentence completion frames in which aphasic subjects were required to supply a word that carried either a plural or a possessive marker.

Another type of experimental foundation for a model of language processing is represented by the collection of speech error data from normal speakers in everyday discourse. The theoretical questions at issue in these investigations are what are the elementary segments that are assembled in the planning of an utterance and in what order are they retrieved for insertion in the speech stream? Shattuck-Hufnagel (1983), for example, shows that in a large body of speech error data, inadvertent exchanges between parts of words (often called "spoonerisms") overwhelmingly involve a single phoneme (vowel or consonant) rather than a syllable or a consonant cluster. This would argue for the individual phoneme, rather than the syllable, as the building block in the assembly of sounds to form words. It was also observed that inflectional forms (such as *ing* or *ed*) may become detached from their intended roots and appear on another word in the sentence. This was taken as evidence that the retrieval of lexical terms and the insertion of grammatical morphology follow separate tracks in sentence planning. It must be stressed that the use of this type of evidence is based on the accumulation of a large body of speech error data, not on casual anecdotal observation.

The area of reading is one in which the approach of cognitive psychology has been particularly successful in combining aphasic symptomatology with evidence from normal reading to develop a model that links the abnormal to the presumed normal process. Normal reading is presumed, in folk psychology, to entail associating a sound to each letter in sequence, assembling these sounds mentally (or in oral reading), and then interpreting the meaning of the word so perceived. A somewhat more sophisticated view makes provision for the reading of abbreviations and irregular words that cannot be assembled sound by sound. In 1973, Marshall and Newcombe described and analyzed the characteristics of a form of reading disorder seen in certain aphasic patients that shed a new light on the mechanisms of reading—both in aphasic and normal readers. "Deep dyslexia" is a disorder in which patients have no capacity to associate sounds to letters (termed grapheme-phoneme conversion), are unable to read aloud any grammatical words (articles, prepositions, or auxiliary verbs), and often misread nouns, verbs, or adjectives by substituting a semantically related, but visually completely unrelated word. Such a patient, for example, might read aloud the sentence "the early bird catches the worm" by saying "soon robin capture bug." The analysis of this disorder led to experiments in which patients of this type were given lists of words controlled for frequency, part of speech, length, regularity of spelling, abstractness, and picturability. From an analysis of the types and frequency of errors made in each category of words, a picture emerged that led to a more sophisticated model of the normal reading process and its aberrations in aphasia. (This will be developed in detail in the chapter on disorders of reading, Chapter 9.)

A characteristic of the models produced by many cognitive psychologists is their representation of operations in the processing of a linguistic task in the form of a flow chart made up of boxes that represent separate processing operations and arrows connecting them that represent the path of information flow. In some cases, such as oral reading, there may be several concurrent, alternative pathways reaching an output product through different possible processes. Aphasic symptoms of particular types are expected if a particular pathway is disabled. It is characteristic of contemporary cognitive psychology that predictions of the model are tested and retested on additional patients, and that the models are modified for further verification when discrepant performances are documented by such case studies.

The mapping of linguistic processes onto flow chart diagrams is characteristic of a group of English cognitive psychologists. Other investigators have been concerned with the internal operating characteristics of the processes that are represented by the variously labeled boxes. The investigation of ongoing language processes has become feasible with the advent of electronic apparatus and computers that can probe events as they actually take place "in real time." These techniques have served to investigate long standing questions, but they have also led to the emergence of new theoretical issues. An example of a modern technique that is widely used in research on aphasia is "primed lexical decision." A lexical decision task requires a subject to react to a presented letter string or utterance by pressing a "yes" button if the stimulus is a real word, and pressing a "no" button if it is a nonword. It is a well-established finding that "yes" reactions are faster for words that have been primed by the previous presentation of a related word than for test words that follow an unrelated prime. Milberg and Blumstein (1981) reasoned that the demonstration of a priming effect of this type in aphasics would be evidence that the patient had carried out semantic processing of the priming and target words. By demonstrating priming in patients who were clinically severely deficient in auditory comprehension, they established that some form of semantic processing of auditory input was nevertheless being carried out.

Much of the theorizing about language in aphasia is colored by the analogy of the computer. Such terms as information input, storage, retrieval, and storage buffers are evidence of this influence. Current approaches to the modeling of language processes are influenced by two conflicting views of brain mechanisms for language. One is based on the notion that cognitive processes, with particular reference to language, are implemented by self-contained "modules" (Fodor, 1983). A module is unaffected by any conscious effort or contextual influences.

A competing approach, termed "parallel distributed processing," PDP (McClelland & Rumelhart, 1986), is based on computer-modeled demonstrations that complex, seemingly "rule-governed" behavior may be generated by the interaction of a large number of elementary associative connections that change in their associative strength and reinforcing or inhibitory effects during the learning process. In this view, a "representation" is not stored as an abstract unit of latent knowledge or rules, but is a probabilistic pattern of neural activity that is regenerated on each occasion of use. The PDP approach has particular appeal to neuroscientists working in the borderland between neural representation and the output of complex behavior. This approach is represented, for example, in Damasio's (1990) proposal to dispense with the notion that an integration of multimodal information in a parietal lobe convergence zone underlies the concepts and memories of language. Instead, Damasio suggests that association areas such as the parietal lobe serve to coordinate the activation of elementary sensory and motor units that remain widely distributed in their respective primary motor and sensory areas.

The current scene, then, is marked by three parallel lines of research. At the level of clinical behavioral observation, new phenomena are still to be described and subjected to systematic study with methods that did not exist at the beginning of this century. At the level of information processing analysis of cognitive psychology, theoretical models of language processing impairments are subjected to experimental testing. At the level of anatomy and physiology, finer analyses of structural and metabolic changes are being carried out with such brain imaging techniques as the CT scan, magnetic resonance scanning, and positron emission tomography (PET).

Chapter 3

Anatomy of Language

The anatomy of the language system is inferred entirely from the relationship between lesions of particular regions and the corresponding deficits that appear in patients who have suffered these lesions. Strictly speaking, as Hughlings Jackson (1874) pointed out, such correlations give the localization for a symptom, but not necessarily for the injured function. That is, a complex function such as naming may depend on interconnections between multiple regions and may thus be totally disrupted by lesions at various points in the system; none of the regions, either individually or jointly, can be considered a "naming center." Nevertheless, a plausible anatomic framework for language has developed. This model is based in part on the tracing of connections involving sensory or motor zones the functions of which are relatively "hard wired." It is also based in part on the analysis of symptoms that have an exclusive and fairly consistent relation to the integrity versus injury of particular structures.

For practical purposes, it is valid to describe the anatomy of language as lying entirely in the left cerebral hemisphere because injuries to the right hemisphere rarely produce clinically noticeable defects in basic language skills. In the small proportion (estimates range from 3% to 9%) of adults whose language is mediated by the right hemisphere, the same anatomical organization appears to hold for the majority of individuals (see Alexander *et al.*, 1989, discussed in last section of this chapter).

The language zone, as seen on the lateral surface of the brain (Fig. 3.1), extends forward to the third frontal convolution and posteriorly to include the angular gyrus of the parietal lobe. Its vertical extent is from the inferior temporal gyrus to the supramarginal gyrus. Anteriorly, a restricted cortical zone in the posterior portion of the second frontal convolution (Exner's writing center) has been repeatedly implicated in selective disorders of writing. It is the upper limit of the anterior portion of the language area. A separate structure, the supplementary motor area, appears to be vital for the initiation of language output. This region

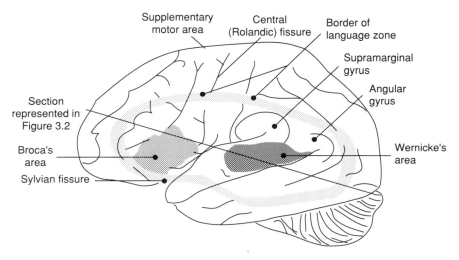

Figure 3.1. Lateral view of left cerebral hemisphere.

lies on the lip of the mesial surface of the frontal lobe, anterior to the Rolandic fissure.

The language zone cannot be described simply with reference to the preceding surface topology. Normal language function requires the integrity of a subcortical region extending inward to the lateral ventricles, along virtually the entire front to back extent of the cortical language zone. Within this zone are gray matter structures, for example putamen, insula, and thalamus, as well as fiber pathways, whose specific contributions to language functions are understood to varying degrees (Fig. 3.2). Language functions are distributed discontinuously through the broad perisylvian region just delineated. Some areas, such as the anterior temporal lobe, appear to have little influence on language; others produce purely motor effects on the mechanics of articulation without affecting higher level "linguistic" aspects of speech output.

THE CLASSICAL VIEW

The anatomic model for language (Fig. 2.1) first proposed by Wernicke (1874) and Lichtheim (1885) was elaborated by Geschwind (1970) in a formulation that is disarmingly logical and compelling. According to this model, the auditory patterns that are endowed with meaning are stored in Wernicke's area in the left temporal lobe (Fig. 3.2). They are activated

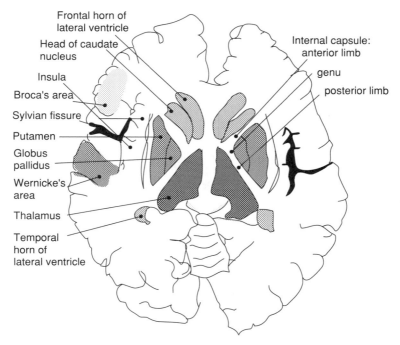

Figure 3.2 Horizontal section of brain at level intersecting the language zone. Level of cut shown in Fig. 3.1.

when a spoken word is recognized or when an intended word is to be spoken. For the intended word to be uttered, its auditory form is conveyed from Wernicke's area to Broca's area, which is in the lower posterior frontal lobe. The pathway for this information transfer is a fiber bundle—the arcuate fasciculus—that includes connections between Wernicke's and Broca's areas. Broca's area, according to Geschwind's summary, would be the storehouse for the codes that convert the auditorily patterned input to the motor articulatory code that mediates speech production. Hence, a lesion of Broca's area would produce reduction of speech output with severely impaired articulatory control. A lesion of the arcuate fasciculus would disable the repetition of auditorily perceived words without affecting either the articulation of spontaneous speech or the auditory comprehension of speech because both Broca's and Wernicke's areas are spared.

By this model, the processing of written language begins with the perception of written words in the primary visual cortex and the visual association areas of the occipital lobe. This information is conveyed to the angular gyrus of the parietal lobe where the letters are recognized as forming words. The angular gyrus, situated between the visual and auditory association areas, is in an ideal location to bring about the auditory–visual associations that are basic to reading and writing. In fact, lesions of this area commonly result in the loss of ability in both reading and writing (alexia with agraphia). According to the traditional model, for a written word to be read aloud, it remains only for the sound of the name to be activated in Wernicke's area and for the impulse to be transferred over the arcuate fasciculus to Broca's area, and then to the motor cortex for implementation.

The straightforward serial processing model proposed by Geschwind has considerable support in a number of clinically observed disorders as they relate to the functional anatomy of the language system. But it also comes into conflict with other clinical observations and with more sophisticated views of possible information processing mechanisms used by the brain. Progress toward understanding the relationship between anatomy and language functions requires a more fine-grained analysis of anatomical detail on the one hand, and language processes on the other. In this chapter we show that current knowledge of anatomic–behavioral correlations paints a more complex and less complete picture of the brain as a language processor than that proposed by the classical model.

THE AUDITORY RECEPTIVE COMPONENT

All processing of auditory signals, whether linguistic or nonlinguistic depends on a bilaterally organized chain of connections from the cochlea of the inner ear through a series of brain-stem nuclei, to the medial geniculate bodies of the thalamus, to the two Heschl's gyri, small cortical structures lying in the depths of the Sylvian fissures, on the upper surface of each temporal lobe. The work of recognizing and retaining the auditorily encoded features of heard language depends on the region close to and predominantly posterior to Heschl's gyrus of the left cerebral hemisphere. The portion of the left superior temporal gyrus, extending back from Heschl's gyrus to the end of the Sylvian fissure is "Wernicke's area"—the region which, when damaged in adults, produces the most severe impairments of auditory language processing, without significant effect on primary auditory functions.

There are, however, subcortical connections that affect the input to Wernicke's area and hence affect auditory comprehension. One of these, the tract from the medial geniculate body to Heschl's gyrus, passes through the anterior temporal isthmus, a small white-matter zone between the temporal horn of the lateral ventricle and the posterior end of the Sylvian fissure (Nielsen, 1946). The temporal isthmus is commonly injured as a result of left subcortical lesions, rendering the patient dependent on the right temporal lobe for auditory processing. Wernicke's area then becomes dependent on auditory signals conveyed from its homologous zone in the right hemisphere, via the corpus callosum. The pathway taken by these signals runs deep in the parietal lobe, near the posterior border of the lateral ventricle. A sufficiently extensive subcortical lesion can severely compromise the auditory language system, without impinging on Wernicke's cortical area (Naeser *et al.*, 1982).

It is important to realize that association areas, such as Wernicke's area, do not have anatomically sharply defined borders. The concentration of auditory processing in this zone appears to be a function of maturation over the first 15–20 years of life because severe selective comprehension deficits from focal temporal lobe lesions do not occur in children. In this respect, the auditory language association areas differ from the primary auditory processing system, which is "hard-wired" with fixed structures and connections from early life.

Of the basic language operations, auditory language processing is the one which is least an exclusively left-hemisphere prerogative. There is usually at least minimal residual comprehension, mediated by the right hemisphere, when the entire language zone on the left is destroyed and no expressive language is possible. Such residual comprehension may be limited to the recognition of the semantic category of a word that has been heard or only to an appreciation that it is a word of one's language. The degree to which the right temporal lobe can carry residual auditory functions or recover them after a period is a matter of individual differences, possibly genetic in origin. Naeser *et al.* (1987) reported that lesions that destroy Wernicke's area completely or nearly so result in lasting, severe deficits of auditory comprehension, whereas those that spare half of that region produce an initial deficit that recovers to functional levels.

PURE WORD-DEAFNESS

This uncommon disorder is manifested by a severe loss of comprehension of speech, even though speech production, reading, and writing are minimally affected or normal. In functional terms, it appears to spare the higher language processes that depend on Wernicke's area, while depriving Wernicke's area of all auditory input. Anatomically, it requires a left temporal lesion that isolates Wernicke's area both from the adjacent

Heschl's gyrus and from the transcallosal pathway from the right hemisphere. Alternatively, a bilateral lesion may produce the same effect.

Pure word-deafness has, in fact, been found as a sequel of both unilateral and bilateral temporal lobe lesions. To date, the precise anatomy of these lesions has not been sufficiently delineated to confirm the proposed anatomical basis of the disorder.

THE MOTOR ARTICULATORY COMPONENT

Anatomical Extent

The cortical zone that primarily subserves the execution of speech movements occupies the lower posterior portion of the left frontal lobe (Fig. 3.2). At its anterior border is the foot of the third frontal convolution, defined by Broca as the seat of articulate speech and referred to now as "Broca's area." It is subdivided into the *pars triangularis* and, immediately posteriorly, the *pars opercularis*, the portion of frontal lobe that overhangs the insula. The motor speech zone extends posteriorly along the lower frontal lobe to the Rolandic fissure. Subcortically, it involves both fiber pathways and gray matter structures at various levels of depth from immediately subcortical, down to the left lateral ventricle.

The initiation and maintenance of speech flow may be affected independently of the articulation of speech, per se. Speech initiation depends on the integrity of frontal lobe cortical structures that are at a distance from Broca's area: that is, the left supplementary motor area and the cingulate gyrus and their connections to the caudate nucleus. Injury to the supplementary motor area or to the fibers descending from it results initially in complete muteness, which recovers after some weeks to halting, effortfully initiated speech.

Permanently impaired speech initiation, however, involves more than a single cerebral structure. Naeser *et al*, (1989) found that permanent loss of voluntary speech resulted from combined lesions of two deep whitematter structures. One is the medial subcallosal fasciculus, a narrow fiber bundle that serves as a funnel for communication with the cingulate gyrus and the supplementary motor area. The second is the middle portion of the periventricular white matter (PVWM). The PVWM is a region adjacent to the lateral ventricle in which at least five partially traced fiber tracts are comingled; among these are descending motor and ascending sensory tracts for the mouth area, posterior–anterior cortico-cortical long tracts, callosal pathways, thalamo-cortical pathways, and the body of the caudate nucleus. Lesions in this area, therefore, produce disconnections in a number of systems, whose individual contributions to articulatory disorders are not yet parceled out.

The major channel for motor tracts descending from the cortex to the brain stem is the internal capsule, L-shaped in cross section at the level of Broca's area. The corner or "genu" (knee) of the internal capsule is the point at which an impinging lesion damages articulatory outflow, perhaps originating in the motor cortex for mouth and tongue.

The specific role of Broca's area in the speech output system has yet to be fully clarified. Until 1978, many writers unquestioningly followed Broca's dictum that the foot of the third frontal convolution was the seat of articulate speech; that a lesion of that zone would produce a lasting aphasia of the type that Broca had described. Mohr *et al.* (1978) reported that lesions limited to this area and its immediately subjacent white matter produced at most a very transient disturbance of speech production. Broca's aphasia required a much deeper lesion, and usually one also extending posteriorly to the foot of the motor strip.

There is some evidence that lesions that involve both the cortical Broca's area and subcortex down to the lateral border of the left frontal horn result in a distinctly different production pattern from the purely subcortical lesions. When the cortex is involved, the disorder impacts on the sentence structure as well as on the availability of grammatical words in the intended message. Production tends to be limited to the major nouns and occasional verbs, uttered in brief word groups. This is the output pattern of "agrammatic Broca's aphasia." The cortex of Broca's area appears, then, to be a necessary but not sufficient part of the anatomy of this disorder. Agrammatic aphasia is not simply a disorder of motor implementation, for in most instances patients show a similar difficulty in writing. The significance of linguistic and cognitive factors in agrammatism will be further developed in Chapter 6.

Role of the Basal Ganglia

The deep gray-matter structures of the frontal lobe—the putamen and globus pallidus, lying lateral to the internal capsule, and the caudate nucleus, situated between the capsule and the frontal horn of the ventricle—are generally implicated in any deep lesions of the anterior speech zone. Sometimes a lesion is confined to one of these structures without impinging on adjacent white matter. Because of the intimate anatomical associations in this zone, it has been difficult to determine what, if any, role these nuclei (i.e., the basal ganglia) play in language. Careful comparison of the effects of lesions that did or did not include basal ganglia led Alexander, Naeser, and Palumbo (1987) and Alexander and Naeser (1988) to conclude that they play little or no role in the symptomatology of aphasia. The production deficits observed in the presence of basal ganglion lesions are probably due to the injury of adjacent white matter, internal capsule and periventricular white matter.

ANATOMICAL INTERDEPENDENCE VERSUS AUTONOMY OF MOTOR IMPLEMENTATION FROM "INNER SPEECH" PROCESSES

Throughout virtually all of the frontal motor speech system, as described, aphasic impairments of motor implementation are closely associated with impairments of word retrieval and speech formulation. Such a close association could signify that motor implementation and inner language are two aspects of a single process, and this is the conclusion that would result if one examined correlations across large numbers of subjects.

Alternatively, multiple independent subsystems for motor control and for language formulation could have such interwoven neuronal networks in this region that it would be impossible to injure one system alone or to exempt a single function from damage by any lesion. For example, it has been noted that considerable differentiation in degree and quality of motor output disturbances may result from very small differences in extent of lesion site within white matter: a small, deep white-matter lesion adjacent to the lateral border of the frontal horn may implicate the medial subcallosal fasciculus and profoundly reduce speech output. Restriction of the depth of a lesion involving Broca's area may allow recovery of useful telegraphic speech, rather than severely limit output. Second, there are individual cases that show considerable dissociation of particular language components: sparing of functional writing at the word or even the sentence level in some patients with Broca's aphasia and remarkable sparing of naming ability in other patients of this type.

Inspection of the lesions of such cases provides no encouragement that each of these variations is explainable by a lesion difference specific to the case—much less to a localization principle generalizable across patients. Rather, it appears likely that these cases illustrate differences in possible organizations of language functions that may be established by different brains. A position like this, which allows for individual variations in the organization of subsystems, implies some autonomy in their neural representation. It also places limits on our expectancy of discovering a distinct lesion difference for every variation in patterns of dissociation among language functions.

PURE ARTICULATORY IMPAIRMENT

Although we have emphasized the intimate association between the anatomy of motor speech implementation and that of inner speech, there is a point at which the motor component diverges from the language system and where a lesion affects only articulatory movements. A lesion in the outflow path of speech, such as the genu of the internal capsule or further downstream at the level of the brain stem, has no linguistic component and affects purely the motor realization. Within the cerebral speech zone, this divergence becomes apparent with restricted white-matter lesions that undercut the foot of the motor strip, presumably damaging the input to the motor cortex for the articulatory apparatus. The resulting articulatory impairment is almost devoid of linguistic features; that is, the patient can write normally. As speech production improves to slow and awkward articulatory output, it is clear that access to vocabulary and syntax is unaffected. This pattern of almost pure articulatory impairment is called *aphemia* (adopting Broca's original term for aphasia). It has also been referred to as "subcortical motor aphasia" and as "cortical dysarthria."

THE ANATOMY OF REPETITION AND PHONETIC SEQUENCING

The notion that there is a specific anatomical circuit for repetition developed originally from Lichtheim's (1884) deduction that repetition should be specifically affected if a lesion were to disconnect the auditory from the motor speech center. However, when the clinical phenomenon of conduction aphasia was observed, one of its salient features was the disordered selection and sequencing of syllables and phonemes, which might result in multiple self-corrective efforts at a single target (e.g., "paker . . . no . . . saker . . . taper" for "paper"). Because these phonological intrusions and substitutions occur equally in tests of object naming, in free conversation, and repetition, it is not clear that conduction aphasia can be defined in terms of the core deficit of repetition. In any case, the anatomical basis for a selective disorder of repetition is identical with that which produces impairment of phonemic selection and sequencing—the twin features that mark conduction aphasia.

Geschwind's (1965) review of the anatomy of this disorder is predicated on the hypothesis that it is, in fact, due to a disconnection of auditory association cortex from Broca's area. The anatomical structure involved is the arcuate fasciculus, a bundle of fibers originating in the upper temporal lobe and following an arching path subcortically around the posterior end of the Sylvian fissure, passing deep to the supramarginal gyrus and then forward to the anterior speech zone. A large proportion of cases of conduction aphasia have lesions in the supramarginal gyrus, but many implicate the temporal lobe and the insula.

Not all investigators subscribe to the idea that the symptoms of conduction aphasia are caused by a disconnection between Wernicke's and Broca's areas. Goldstein (1948), for example, accepted the existence of the syndrome, which he preferred to call "central aphasia"; however, he attributed it to an insular lesion. Damasio and Damasio (1989) rejected the classical view that conduction aphasia represents a disconnection within a simple repetition circuit. Instead, they see the disorder as disrupting the perception and short-term storage of phoneme strings and their assembly for production. They maintain that the cortex of the perisylvian language zone is always involved and that white matter involvement is not the primary factor.

THE ANATOMY OF NAMING

Pure anomia, the inability to evoke the phonological form of a concept to be named, may appear in patients who have virtually normal facility in articulation, sentence construction, and auditory comprehension. The lesion site most often cited in association with this disorder is the temporo-parietal junction; that is, the zone just posterior to the end of the Sylvian fissure that bridges the temporal and parietal lobes, including the angular gyrus. Geschwind (1965) suggests that the angular gyrus is a phylogenetically new association area, unique to man, and that it makes it possible for us to have names for concepts by serving as a polysensory convergence area. However, pure anomia is not restricted to lesions of the temporo-parietal junction. It is seen in conjunction with injury to the posterior portion of the middle and inferior temporal gyrus and, less frequently, with subcortical lesions of the frontal lobe.

However, the idea that any one or all three of these areas constitutes a naming center is overruled by an unavoidable fact about naming disorders—namely, that impaired word retrieval is virtually universal in most forms of aphasia. The forms of pure anomia that have been cited are unique, not because of the severity of the name retrieval problem observed in these cases, but because they are uncontaminated by difficulties in motor speech production, sentence construction, auditory comprehension, or by intrusion of unintended speech errors.

There are, however, two subgroups of patients that provide clues to the anatomical link between the preverbal representation of concepts and the activation of corresponding phonological patterns. One of these are individuals whose failure to retrieve names goes along with a corresponding inability to derive any meaning from the spoken name (in spite of perfectly preserved repetition—without comprehension). This disorder characteristically appears in those *transcortical sensory aphasics* who have a lesion in the region between the postero-lateral thalamus and the inferior temporo-occipital zone. This area appears to serve as the channel for the input of visually and, perhaps, tactually based semantic representations to the language system (Alexander, Hiltbronner, & Fischer, 1989). Alexander *et al.* also suggest that various sensory components of the semantic representation may suffer dissociations from each other with lesions in this area. Luria (1966) also implicates the temporo-occipital region in the loss of word meaning.

The second subgroup of patients are those with "optic aphasia," the inability to name objects presented visually despite preserved visual acuity and with preservation of the ability to name using definitions or by touch. Although optic aphasia is a rare disorder, it is always associated with a parieto-occipital or occipital lesion, a lesion which presumably interrupts input from visual association areas at a point sufficiently "upstream" toward the source of visual information that it does not affect any other sense modalities. It appears, then, that the anatomic channels through which the various sensory components of conceptual representations communicate with the language system occupy a region low in the parieto-occipito-temporal region where lesions are likely to produce either a severe two-way dissociation of name from concept, a naming difficulty selective to a single sensory modality (particularly visual), or dissociations of a single sensory modality from the rest of the conceptual representation (e.g., visual agnosia). Once the language system is engaged in a word retrieval effort, however, the entire perisylvian zone participates in a broadly distributed network. As we interpret the evidence, the broad zone that is active during naming includes areas that overlap with other language components, as well as areas in which there is little or no overlap. The latter areas are the sites that may produce pure anomia. Finer differentiation of aspects of naming within this anatomical zone must remain tentative for the present. The data bearing on this issue are developed in Chapter 5.

THE ANATOMY OF READING

Reading depends on the activation of linguistic and conceptual associations through visually perceived graphic symbols. The anatomy of the visual system and of visual perceptual disorders have been particularly well studied. The distance separating the primary visual and visual association areas from the perisylvian language area has made it easier to discern the anatomy of some types of reading disorders than is the case for analogous disorders in the auditory sphere.

Segregation of Visual Half-Fields to Opposite Cerebral Hemispheres

A fundamental difference between the visual and auditory systems is that visual input from each side of the visual field is segregated along the entire path: hemiretina, optic nerve, thalamus, and optic radiation that is transmitted exclusively to the visual cortex of the opposite hemisphere. The boundary between the half-fields on the retina is sharply defined at the midline. The visual association areas of the two hemispheres are linked, however, through the posterior portion (the splenium) of the corpus callosum. Although the sharing of visual information across the corpus callosum is virtually instantaneous, it is nevertheless the case that visual stimuli from the left side of the visual field can be *efficiently* processed linguistically only by virtue of this callosal pathway. This aspect of visual functional anatomy is fundamental for the understanding of certain forms of reading disorders. The word *efficiently* is emphasized because a limited level of processing of written language is often possible in the right hemisphere (see Chapters 9 and 13).

Pure Word-Blindness

Injury to the splenium of the corpus callosum is rarely encountered without damage to adjacent visual association cortex, except as a result of surgery. The effect of such injury, however, is to deprive the language zone in the left hemisphere of access to words that fall in the left visual field. The patient sees, but cannot read this material, unless she turns her gaze to bring it into the right visual field. In this case, she is said to have a left hemialexia. More commonly, the splenium is damaged along with the left visual association cortex, which renders the patient blind in the right visual field (right hemianopia). Now she can see print only via the right visual cortex, but cannot interpret its meaning. No other aspects of language need be involved—not even writing. Pure word-blindness may also be produced by a lesion within the left parieto-occipital white matter, so placed as to block the pathway between the visual association cortex and the region of the angular gyrus, which appears to serve as the gateway to the language system for graphic material.

Alexia with Agraphia

The angular gyrus and the white matter below it appear to be uniquely important for all aspects of graphic language that involve its linkage to writing, to spoken language, and to word meaning. Injury to this area disrupts not only the ability to understand the written word, but also disrupts related knowledge such as oral spelling and letter–sound correspondence, and therefore disrupts the ability to write.

Aphasic Alexia

Lesions that totally spare the region of the angular gyrus rarely produce a profound alexia to the level of recognizing letters and primer words. On the other hand, reading comprehension is rarely completely spared in aphasia. Patients who have a marked reduction of auditory comprehension associated with extensive subcortical white matter involvement usually have commensurate reduction of reading comprehension. The neural circuitry involved in reading comprehension is obscure at present, and has not been extensively investigated. It is plausible to argue that reading comprehension is so functionally related to auditory comprehension that injury to the latter also damages the former. It is not uncommon to find Wernicke's aphasics with severe impairment of speech comprehension and a functional, if not normal, level of reading. Hécaen (1969) observed that Wernicke's aphasics whose lesions did not extend posteriorly beyond the Sylvian fissure retained considerable reading ability, whereas those with posterior extension were more likely to be severely alexic. It is reasonable to presume that Wernicke's aphasia need not entail severe reduction of reading, unless the lesion involves the pathways to the angular gyrus. Similarly, reading comprehension to the sentence and paragraph level is often spared in Broca's aphasics who do not also have a large and deep subcortical extension of their lesion.

WRITING

Although writing is the most vulnerable of all the language modalities to impairment in aphasia, isolated loss of writing ability (pure agraphia) from focal brain injury is rarely described. Exner's (1881) assertion that the foot of the second convolution is a lesion site for pure agraphia has had some support from subsequent observations. Other sites have been reported as associated with pure agraphia in scattered cases. For example, Roeltgen, Sevush, and Heilman (1983) described a patient with an insular lesion, possibly extending into the supramarginal gyrus, whose only linguistic deficit was in spelling nonwords. Impaired writing, including failure to recall the movements for forming individual letters, is seen with both severe Broca's aphasia and with angular gyrus lesions. Roeltgen and Heilman (1984) found that posterior angular gyrus lesions were characteristic of individuals who had particular difficulty with whole-word retrieval, causing them to misspell irregular words by direct applications of letter-to-sound rules.

OTHER ANATOMIC CONSIDERATIONS

Vascular Supply of the Language Zone and its Pathology

By far the most frequent etiology for aphasia is stroke—usually in the form of a thrombotic or embolic occlusion of a blood vessel that supplies a critical portion of the language zone. Such an occlusion results in an infarction, an area of tissue that has died because of the loss of its blood supply. The anatomy of the vascular system, although subject to structural variations among individuals, is sufficiently uniform so that the pattern of infarction following occlusion of many vessels is fairly uniform. A third form of stroke, cerebral hemorrhage, is also less predictable than occlusive stroke as to the pattern of the resulting long-term functional loss.

The zone of destruction produced by an occlusion corresponds to the area perfused by the damaged artery and need not correspond to a particular functional area. Hence, the pattern of deficit observed in cases of vascular aphasia are, in a sense, artifacts of the region irrigated by the occluded vessel. Certain sites in the cerebral vasculature are particularly prone to occlusion, others are rarely or never affected. Consequently, some forms of aphasia are much more common than others. Nevertheless, the damage produced by a limited occlusive stroke is the best source of information on the effect of a lesion because it leaves a well-defined zone of infarction, without damage to other structures, as in the case of penetrating or closed head injuries.

Each cerebral hemisphere is supplied by three major arteries: the anterior, middle, and posterior cerebral arteries (ACA, MCA, and PCA). It is the middle cerebral artery and its branches that supply almost the entire language zone and that are particularly vulnerable to occlusive stroke. The blood supply reaches the brain through the internal carotid artery on each side and the basilar artery posteriorly. Each internal carotid gives rise to the anterior and middle cerebral arteries, whereas the basilar artery bifurcates to form the two posterior cerebral arteries. The entire system is linked into a ring (the Circle of Willis) by the anterior communicating artery in front and the posterior communicating arteries laterally (see Fig. 3.3). The Circle of Willis makes it possible for a deficiency in blood supply in a major artery on one side to be compensated for by the circulation from the opposite side. Such deficiencies typically occur because of plaques that form in the carotid artery, reducing the flow into the internal carotid on that side. However, the degree to which such compensation is effective varies from individual to individual, and is quite sensitive to small differences in the diameter of the arteries and in their branching patterns. It is for this reason that the actual

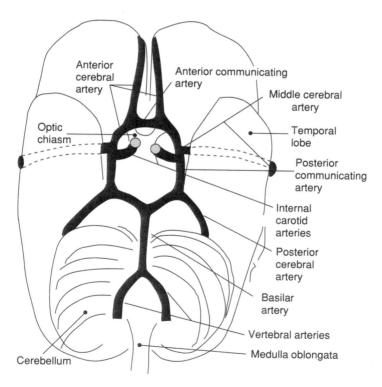

Figure 3.3 Schematic diagram of Circle of Willis and major cerebral arteries, seen from below.

damage resulting from an occlusion or partial blockage (stenosis) of the carotid artery is hard to predict.

The MCA has two major branches, referred to as the *upper* and *lower* divisions. The upper division chiefly supplies the anterior speech zone, including Broca's area. The inferior branch of the upper division of the MCA irrigates the supramarginal gyrus; occlusions of this branch may result in conduction aphasia. The lower division follows a more horizontal course along the Sylvian fissure and is responsible for the blood supply to the temporal and parietal lobes. Occlusions involving branches of the lower division result in forms of fluent aphasia, such as Wernicke's aphasia, conduction aphasia, or anomic aphasia. An important group of small vessels are the lenticulo-striate arteries which arise from the MCA, close to its origin, and provide the blood supply for the basal ganglia and the white matter tracts surrounding them.

The ACA is less vulnerable to stroke than is the MCA. Its territory includes the supplementary motor area, along with the bulk of the frontal lobe which is anterior and superior to Broca's area. Lesions of the ACA territory may affect the initiation of speech, but have little impact on the elementary skills of language.

The territory of the PCA, in addition to all of the occipital lobe, extends forward along the inferior temporal lobe to include the hippocampus, a mesial temporal lobe structure that plays a vital role in memory. Occlusions of the PCA are often associated with disease of the basilar artery. The sudden onset of pure word-blindness is an almost certain indicator of an occlusion in PCA territory. Severe impairment of memory is a frequently associated symptom.

Border Zone Infarcts

Each of the three major cerebral arteries enters its territory with large branches, which divide into finer and finer arterioles toward the periphery of the territory. The border zones between the territories of the MCA and the two other arteries derive their blood supply from intermingled small peripheral branches of the two neighboring arterial systems. When there is a marked insufficiency of blood because of stenosis of a major artery, it is the border zone that suffers the impact. Infarcts may develop at one or more points along the roughly arc-shaped region that encompasses the anterior and posterior border zones of the MCA. Because these strokes do not impinge on the immediate perisylvian portion of the speech zone, they may produce forms of aphasia in which repetition is unaffected (transcortical motor or transcortical sensory aphasia, and anomic aphasia).

The Role of the Thalamus

Several of the thalamic nuclei, particularly the posterolateral and pulvinar, have been shown to have extensive projections to the language association areas (Peters, 1979). Thus, it is not surprising that lesions involving the thalamus have repeatedly been reported to produce aphasic symptoms. Yet it is extremely difficult to isolate the contribution of the thalamus to language processing; the symptoms that do appear are not unique to thalamic injury. Often, they are confounded by other byproducts of thalamic damage, such as confusion and memory loss. One recurring pattern has been described in association with hemorrhage; it consists of fluent, paraphasic speech output, with impaired naming and impaired auditory comprehension, but preserved repetition (Cappa & Vignolo, 1979; Alexander & LoVerme, 1980). Alexander (1989) reports that language symptoms have cleared up, essentially completely, within months in the cases of thalamic infarction and hemorrhage that he has followed. In particular, one case that had recovered normal language was found, on postmortem, to have suffered complete destruction of the pulvinar and posterior thalamus.

CEREBRAL DOMINANCE

In the century and a half since the discovery that language processing is dominated by the left cerebral hemisphere, little or no progress has been made toward understanding what property of the left hemisphere gives it an advantage (in most individuals) over the right hemisphere in acquiring these functions. The hypotheses that this property is simply a larger volume of tissue in the language zone of the left hemisphere, or a greater density of dendrites in portions of the left hemisphere have gained little support from correlations with language performance.

Three forms of evidence must be taken into account in developing a theory for the mechanism for language dominance:

1. *Developmental.* There is considerable plasticity in the early years that permits the child born with a defective left hemisphere to develop essentially normal language competence with only the right hemisphere functional (although subtle deficits in syntactic processing may be detected with special tests; Dennis and Kohn, 1975). Children who become aphasic as a result of left-brain injury before puberty regain functional language to a level of proficiency rarely seen in adults with similar damage. In cases with major injury, this recovery is almost certainly mediated by the right hemisphere. The age of puberty is offered only as an arbitrary boundary,

because the capacity for rapid reconstitution of language appears to decrease in later childhood and declines to adult levels by late adolescence. (see discussion by Lenneberg, 1967.)

2. *Differential hemispheric control of particular language components.* It has been noted that some patients retain limited one-word auditory comprehension after massive destruction of the left hemisphere language zone, indicating that word comprehension is at least partially subserved by the right hemisphere when word production in a propositional sense is no longer possible. Limited one-word reading comprehension has been demonstrated in the isolated right hemisphere of patients who have undergone section of the corpus callosum (Gazzaniga *et al.*, 1965). However, Zaidel and Peters (1981) showed that such individuals were unable to make judgments about the sounds of written words that are "seen" only by the right hemisphere; that is, they appear to grasp word semantics, but not word phonology. When tested with the left hemisphere only, they demonstrated awareness of both sound and meaning. (Note that these observations were made in individuals who had acquired normal reading with a fully functional left hemisphere. Dissociation of phonology from meaning during word reading is not characteristic of children who acquire language with the right hemisphere because of early left hemisphere injury.)

In the foregoing examples, we referred to a small subset of language components for which many individuals have some limited functional control in the right hemisphere, although not at the level of competence of the left hemisphere. There is, however, one component—sentence prosody—for which most people appear to have right hemisphere superiority. Blumstein and Cooper (1974) used a series of sentences spoken with the intonation of a question or a command, or neutral declarative, and passed them through a low-pass filter so that only the intonation could be perceived, but the words were unintelligible. Subjects heard competing pairs of intonation patterns dichotically and were required to match them with symbols corresponding to the sentence type. Significantly higher accuracy scores for the left ear indicated a right hemisphere advantage for this task. The production of speech intonation is abolished by deep right-frontal lesions, resulting in speech output that is on a monotone (Ross, 1981).

Several investigators (Heilman, Scholes, & Watson, 1975; Tucker, Watson, & Heilman, 1977) have also found that the interpretation of emotional prosody is significantly more impaired in right-brain injured than left-brain injured patients. Ross (1981) reports that posterior right hemisphere lesions interfere with the interpretation of the emotional tone of sentences, as it is extracted from the speaker's intonation, whereas lesions deep in the anterior portion of the right hemisphere may abolish the ability to control the production of speech intonation.

3. *Opposite lateralization types in humans and their relationship to handedness.* By 1865, Broca realized that there were exceptions to the general rule that aphasia appeared as a consequence of damage in the left cerebral hemisphere, but not the right. He noted that the small minority of individuals who became aphasic following right cerebral damage were likely to be left-handed. These observations quickly blossomed into the "classical doctrine of cerebral dominance," which held that the control of language lay in the cerebral hemisphere opposite the preferred hand. Exceptions to this rule were considered to be cases of "crossed aphasia." The classical doctrine was abandoned after studies by Goodglass and Quadfasel (1954), Penfield and Roberts (1959), and Hécaen and Ajuriaguerra (1963), among others, showed that at least half of left-handers with aphasia had left hemisphere lesions. Subsequent series in which both positive and negative cases were included indicated that the great majority of left-handers who become aphasic have had left hemisphere lesions. On the basis of the incidence of transient aphasia induced by the Wada Test (injection of sodium amytal into the left and right internal carotid arteries), Milner (1975) reported the following figures for left handers: 69% became aphasic following injection of the left brain only; 13% following injection on each side; and 18% following injection of the right side only. Naeser and Borod (1986) found a total of 31 left-handed aphasics in a restrospective survey of admissions to the Palo Alto and Boston VA Hospitals from 1975 to 1983. Only four (13%) of these had had right cerebral strokes; the remainder had left-sided strokes. As these figures indicate, there is only a ballpark consensus among various recent estimates of the percentage of left-handed individuals who may be subject to aphasia as a result of right-brain injury. An important reason for this lack of precision is that the criteria for classifying people as right-handed, left-handed, or ambidextrous are not standard across studies. As Annett (1985) and others have pointed out, a strict criterion, such as "exclusive use of the left hand," results in a very small percentage of people being identified as left-handed. Handedness questionnaires provide data that permit the investigator to set differing cutoff points for classifying individuals as left-handed. Many of the clinical studies cited simply rely on the patient's self-report as to his or her preferred hand.

Although the proportion of left-handers who are susceptible to aphasia following right-sided brain injury is much smaller than the 50% estimate of Goodglass and Quadfasel (1954), it is still many times the frequency of this form of brain organization in right-handers. The term "crossed aphasia" is now reserved for right-handers who suffer aphasia following right cerebral injury. The incidence of crossed aphasia is generally estimated at about 1%. Thus, while the "classical doctrine" of cerebral dominance is defunct, there is a clear association between the probability of being left-handed and the probability of having right cerebral language dominance. The implication of the existence of bilateral language representation in some left-handers is that they may be more susceptible to aphasia from a lesion on either side. Also, they may recover more quickly from such aphasias. There are some reports consistent with each of these interferences, but the literature is far from agreement. An excellent review of this topic is to be found in the chapter by Joanette (1990).

The literature on aphasia following right hemisphere lesions includes repeated references to striking dissociations involving the impairment of particular language components (e.g., articulation and syntax), whereas others (e.g., auditory comprehension) are often exempt from damage. Alexander, Fischette, and Fischer (1989) undertook a survey of the literature on crossed aphasia to resolve conflicting opinions as to whether the patterns of language impairment observed in these cases were generally congruent with the patterns to be expected in similar left cerebral lesions or whether they were atypical. Of 34 cases that were described in sufficient detail to make a judgment, Alexander *et al.* considered 22 cases to display a pattern of language that was congruent with the lesion location, had it been in the left hemisphere. Twelve (35%) showed anomalies. In each anomalous case, there was a fluent aphasia, often with paraphasia, in spite of a predominantly anterior lesion which would have been expected to produce a nonfluent disorder. Further, 11 of these patients had severe jargon agraphia—in some instances disproportionately severe in comparison to the patients' speech impairment. Limb praxis was rarely affected. Alexander *et al.* suggest that crossed aphasia often produces dissociations among typically left hemisphere components such that some are affected by the right hemisphere lesion, whereas others apparently continue to function in the intact left hemisphere. They consider semantic and phonological functions to be particularly subject to dissociation. Control of purposeful movement (praxis) seems to remain under the control of the left hemisphere in right-handers with crossed aphasia.

ANNETT'S "RIGHT SHIFT" THEORY OF THE GENETICS OF LATERALITY

Since the lateralization of language cannot be determined in an individual with certainty without invasive interference with brain function (e.g., Wada Test or a naturally occurring stroke), there is no way of directly investigating the genetics of language dominance. Such studies can, however, be carried out with respect to hand preference, both by studying family histories and by the administration of tests of manual skill. Studies of sizable samples by Chamberlain (1928) and by Rife (1940) have shown that matings between two left-handed parents produced no more than about 50% left-handed offspring.

Annett (1985) offers a theory that accounts for these data and that is applicable to interpreting the dissociations seen in crossed aphasia. The "right shift" theory owes its name to the fact that there is a bias toward right-hand advantage in population samples of manual skills tested in the right and left hands. Annett proposes that a single "right shift" gene (*rs+*), transmitted in Mendelian fashion results in a bias toward left hemisphere lateralization of each of the human capacities that have been observed to exhibit left cerebral dominance. This bias is operative both in persons whose genotype is *rs++* and *rs+ −*. The right shift gene is absent (*rs − −*) when neither parent contributed an *rs+* gene. Right shift bias interacts with random intrauterine, experiential and environmental influences to increase the likelihood of left cerebral lateralization of the cerebral substrate for a number of developing capacities, among them hand preference. The absence of a right shift gene (i.e., the *rs −* genotype) allows lateralization to be determined totally by random, nongenetic influences. These random influences may act independently on hand preference and on language. There is no gene for left-handedness; left-handedness has a 50-50 probability of developing in a population of *rs − −* individuals. By the same token, having a *rs++* genotype does not dictate left hemisphere dominance, but merely a greatly increased probability that such dominance will be expressed in the face of competing random influences. The population of manifest left-handers includes 50% of individuals with the *rs −* genotype, plus those individuals with the *rs+* gene for whom nongenetic influences overcame the right shift bias. Calculations based on the incidence of aphasia following right-brain injury led Annett to propose the following distribution of genotypes in the population: 32% *rs++*; 49% *rs+ −*; and 19% *rs − −*.

According to Right Shift theory, the occurrence of aphasia following right cerebral injury is a strong indicator of an *rs − −* genotype, which signifies that there is no genetic bias for the lateralization of language on either side. If one grants, as Alexander, Fischette, and Fisher (1989) proposes, that certain subcomponents of language are free to lateralize independently of others, the analysis of patterns of dissociation in crossed aphasia may yield new understanding concerning which components obligatorily cluster in the same hemisphere.

ANATOMICAL EXPRESSION OF LATERALITY IN THE BRAIN

Acting on suggestions by prior observers (e.g., Von Bonin, 1962), Geschwind and Levitsky (1968) carried out a statistical analysis of left–right asymmetries in the temporal speech zone of 100 brain specimens. The area investigated was the planum temporale, the portion of the upper surface of the temporal lobe that lies posterior to Heschl's transverse gyrus. Sixty-five percent of brains had a larger area of planum on the left, and only 11% had a larger planum on the right. Twenty-four percent showed no difference between sides. Numerous subsequent studies, summarized by Witelson and Kigar (1988), have shown a range from 60% to 83% of larger areas on the left. Associated with the left–right asymmetry of the planum temporale is a difference in the shape of the Sylvian fissure, which has a shorter horizontal extent in the right hemisphere and angles upwards and back on that side, more than on the left.

Comparisons of left- and right-handers with respect to anatomical asymmetry have generally shown greater disparities among the right-handed than among the left-handed. However, efforts to correlate anatomical asymmetry with speech lateralization have yielded mixed results—virtually every positive result being offset by a negative one. It may prove parsimonious to treat anatomic brain asymmetry as one additional autonomous factor that is subject to the influence of the Right Shift gene, keeping in mind, however, that the distribution of left–right brain asymmetries does not quite correspond to the theoretical distribution of *rs*++, *rs*+ −, and *rs* − − genotypes.

Chapter 4

Disorders of Motor
Speech Implementation

In reviewing disorders of the motor realization of speech output in aphasia, we are confronted with some impairments that are independent of the linguistic structure of the utterance, as well as those that are intimately bound to the nature of the intended communicative act. Several levels of impairment may coexist in any aphasic patient, particularly in patients with injury in the pre-rolandic speech zone. It is necessary to identify the impairments and the way they interact in their clinical presentation. Also, within the scope of language-related disorders, there are some that affect the articulatory realization of phonemes and syllables and others that bear on the implementation of larger message units. Among the latter, are disorders affecting sentence prosody and fluency.

In outline, then, this chapter deals with the following aspects of motor speech implementation.

Sublinguistic features:

A survey of speech motor control
Hypophonia
Dysarthria
Oral apraxia and its interaction with language

Aphasic articulatory impairments:

The syndrome of phonetic disintegration
Phonemic versus phonetic disorders

Motor implementation beyond the segmental level:

Impaired initiation
Prosody and its disorders
Nonfluency versus fluency in aphasia

SUBLINGUISTIC DISORDERS

Speech motor control

The motor realization of speech involves the smooth coordination of a number of separate neuromuscular systems—some of which operate totally outside of conscious control. Every voluntary speech act sets into motion an interlocking pattern of neuromuscular activity.

Closest to our awareness are the rapid and finely adjusted movements of the tongue and lips as they modify the shape of the vocal tract, to block or constrict it at various points. These are the adjustments that give vowels and consonants their unique pattern of acoustic characteristics that makes them understandable as speech. Outside of our awareness are the coordinated movements of the uvula that open or block the nasal passage to create the distinction between nasal and oral consonants and vowels. In close coordination with the articulators at the upper end of the vocal tract is the action of the larynx, the movement of the muscles controlling the approximation and separation of the vocal cords, and thus the voicing or devoicing of the speech sound currently being produced.

Two other coordinated systems are at work in speech production. One controls the respiratory patterns that activate the vocal cords, modifying volume and phrasal patterns of speech, and the other controls the tension of the vocal cords so as to vary the fundamental frequency, giving melodic shape to words and sentences.

Sensory feedback and monitoring enter this process at many points. The precision and timing of articulatory movements rely on the position and touch receptors of lips, tongue, and palate. The rhythm and timing of speech is affected by rhythmic cues in auditorily perceived speech output. Voice volume is also modulated by external auditory feedback. Interference with or injury to any one of these feedback or receptor systems produces disorders that are characteristic for that system.

Daunting as it is to contemplate the many levels of neural command that come into synchronized play with every speech act, there are two more aspects of coordination that even the notion of synchrony does not do justice to. One is the fact that the lead time required between the initiation of neural activity in each system and the moment of a synchronously executed speech event is different from system to system. The second aspect is that linguistic planning units extend across phoneme, syllable, and even word boundaries. For instance, in motor speech production, there is the phenomenon of "coarticulation." For example, in pronouncing the word "tune," we round our lips for the vowel *u* even before producing the preceding consonant, *t*. Coarticulation can be detected in almost every phoneme sequence in normal speech.

What is surprising, in a survey of disorders of these systems, is how robust the coordinating mechanisms are even when affected by brain lesions. We shall examine some of the more common forms of breakdown, both in individual subsystems and in coordination, touching mainly on those that are often observed in conjunction with aphasia.

Hypophonia

A common accompaniment to aphasia is pathologically reduced voice volume, or "hypophonia." Hypophonia is often observed in aphasia resulting from deep subcortical lesions, but it may also appear as an isolated symptom without any aphasic features. The severely hypophonic patient may be unable to speak above a whisper. More commonly, the patient phonates appropriately, but cannot obtain normal volume, even when trying to shout.

When hypophonia occurs, it is almost invariably in association with deep anterior lesions involving the basal ganglia. It is most predictably present when these lesions are bilateral, but it is also observed after unilateral anterior lesions. There are other reasons for hypophonia besides focal destructive lesions. It is a common feature in parkinsonism. It may also be a feature of depression that varies with the patient's mood.

Dysarthria

The mark of articulatory impairment as a manifestation of aphasia is that the impairment varies in severity under specifiable conditions. For example, normally we observe facilitation during the production of familiar or memorized utterances, or by providing a model for imitation; we also observe improvement in successive attempts after a distorted production on first try. This variability in speech production provides evidence that the strength and coordination of the muscle groups involved are adequate for the intended articulatory gesture.

The term "dysarthria," on the other hand, is applied to defects of articulation that are caused by impaired motor strength, impaired coordination, or structural defects of the articulatory apparatus. Dysarthria is unaffected by the automaticity or familiarity of the utterance or by having a model to imitate. It persists unchanged when the patient recites memorized passages or reads aloud.

An exception to the rule that dysarthria is constant under all speech conditions is the case of slurred articulation. Slurring, as a manifestation of dysarthria, may be improved by concentration and an effort to slow down, especially when it appears in conjunction with cluttered, over-rapid speech.

Among the causes of dysarthria that may accompany aphasia are injuries of the brain stem or of the cerebellum, which are more likely in patients who have had a head injury than in stroke patients. However, dysarthria without aphasia may also result from injuries in the left anterior speech zone at a few points that do not impinge on the linguistic form of the message, including sites that interrupt sensory feedback from the articulators. Damage to a portion of the internal capsule or to subcortical connections close to the foot of the motor strip may produce such an effect. The latter lesion may result in what has been variously called "subcortical motor aphasia," "cortical dysarthria," or "aphemia." Aphemia is similar to dysarthria in that it is consistent across various speech conditions. However, patients with aphemia characteristically speak with equal syllabic length and stress on each syllable of a word. That is, they have lost word prosody. Prosody and other interesting and distinctive interactions with linguistic structure are discussed later in this chapter.

Dysarthria and aphasia-based disorders of articulation can exist side by side. In some patients, the specific sound distortions caused by dysarthria may persist unchanged at the same time that other aspects of articulation improve dramatically during the recitation of memorized passages. Often the distinction between aphasic and dysarthric features is murky.

Aphasic Articulatory Breakdown and Oral (Bucco-Facial) Apraxia

"Apraxia," the loss or impairment of volitional control of purposeful movements, usually impairs limb movements in gesture and pantomime, or in object manipulation. Apraxia can also affect the execution of deliberate oral movements. This form of the disorder is referred to as "bucco-facial apraxia." Although bucco-facial and limb apraxia are often commensurate in severity, they may vary independently, bucco-facial apraxia being more severe with lesions of the anterior speech zone. These relationships were well documented by De Renzi, Pieczuro, and Vignolo (1966). Chapter 11 of this book is devoted entirely to apraxia.

Bucco-facial apraxia not only interferes with the performance of lip and tongue gestures (e.g., protruding tongue, licking lips, and so on), but it also renders the patient incapable of executing on command a number of gestures involving respiratory control, such as sniffing, blowing, or coughing. (Although these movements cannot be performed on command, they occur normally in spontaneous real-life contexts.)

The interaction between bucco-facial apraxia, as a nonlinguistic disorder, and aphasic articulatory breakdown is still to be sorted out. The two disorders may dissociate in either direction. That is, some patients who cannot cough, sniff, or blow on request, may articulate speech with normal or near normal facility. On the other hand, patients with profound articulatory impairments have been observed to produce all nonspeech oral movements with alacrity. It must be acknowledged, however, that these dissociations are the exception. In most instances, patients who cannot assume the articulatory positions for speech sounds are equally at a loss in their efforts to execute nonlanguage movements on request or by imitation. On observing individuals with global impairments of oral praxis, it is difficult to escape the interpretation that a single disorder is at the root of both linguistic and nonlinguistic motor failures. Yet the knowledge that either of these failures may exist in isolation leaves open the possibility that there are two coexisting impairments in these individuals.

Apraxia of Speech

More than one author has drawn parallels between aphasic disorders in the sphere of language, apraxia in the sphere of purposeful movement, and agnosia as a disorder in the recognition of once-familiar sensory percepts. All of these have in common the fact that they affect high-order processes in the presence of adequate primary sensory or primary motor functions. Furthermore, all of these disorders show variability as a function of context, familiarity, or type of material. Aphasia, which entails both receptive processing and motor execution, differs from the other two disorders only in that by definition it involves disorders specific to language use, whereas the terms "apraxia" and "agnosia" are customarily restricted to nonlanguage activities.

It is a simple exercise to relabel each symptom of aphasia as a special form of apraxia or agnosia by appending the qualifier "verbal" or "speech." For example, we could refer to impaired auditory comprehension as "auditory verbal agnosia," to impaired reading as "visual verbal agnosia," and to impaired articulation as "oral verbal apraxia." These terms appear in the glossary of J. M. Nielsen's (1946) text on aphasia. They represent no more than an alternative basis for terminology that dispenses with the concept of language as the defining criterion of aphasia. The major categories of higher functional disorders are reduced to two—one of input (agnosia) and one of output (apraxia).

The distinction between a linguistically based and a motor praxic impairment of the articulatory apparatus continues to be a point of controversy. One problem in making such a distinction is that the surface appearance of the disorder always suggests impaired motor control. For

example, Liepmann, known for the earliest in-depth clinical and anatomical analysis of apraxia is reported by Buckingham (1991) to have
considered motor aphasia as an apraxia of the glossolabiopharyngeal
apparatus. Buckingham also cites Kleist's characterization of the articulatory errors in conduction aphasia as an "ideokinetic apraxia for the for-
mation of speech sounds." Another influential voice on this issue has
been that of Kimura, who has argued in a number of publications (1976,
1979) that spoken language has its origin in the specialization of the left
hemisphere for the control of sequential movements. She equates apraxia
with a disorder of movement sequencing. With Mateer (Mateer and
Kimura, 1977), she reported that aphasics were impaired in nonverbal
oral movements in comparison with other brain damaged subjects.

In the United States, Frederick Darley of the Mayo Clinic and his collaborators (e.g., Johns and Darley, 1970; Johns and LaPointe, 1976) popu-
larized "apraxia of speech" as an umbrella term for the articulatory
disorders of aphasia, excluding only those that were of dysarthric origin.

The author argues for reserving the term "apraxia" for disorders of
purposeful movement that are not specific to language and for avoiding
the term "apraxia of speech." One reason relates to the logical consistency of terminology. The usefulness of the term "aphasia," as distinct
from "agnosia" and "apraxia" is well established in most sensory and
motor domains. The criterion for defining a deficit as aphasic requires
that it be limited to the production or interpretation of linguistic symbols,
varying as a function of the communicative context in which the symbols occur. The criterion is readily applied in every linguistic use, although, granted, it is difficult to meet in the realm of speech production
because identical errors of articulatory realization may result from
dysarthric, apraxic, or language specific causes. The diagnosis can be
made only by observing whether the disorder is sensitive to parameters
of linguistic automaticity, familiarity, and communicative load. These
and related sources of variation related to aphasia will be discussed in
the section on aphasia of phonetic realization.

APHASIA OF PHONETIC REALIZATION

In 1939, Alajouanine, Ombredane, and Durand used the term, "phonetic disintegration" to characterize the breakdown of articulation in
aphasia. Their analysis, although guided by linguistic categories, was primarily descriptive. They noted that motor weakness, dystonic innervation of articulatory muscles, and apraxic elements combined to produce

an array of characteristic distortions of articulatory implementation. The approach of Alajouanine *et al.* reflects the ambiguity of attempting to distinguish between the language dependent, the praxis related, and the purely motor-based contributions to impaired articulation.

In the present treatment, we share the use of the term "phonetic." Here, it refers to the fact that the disorder affects the manipulations of the articulators by which individual sounds are generated, resulting in aberrations in the acoustic product. We shall distinguish it from a phonemic breakdown, in which there is a disorder in the selection and ordering of phonemic targets while facility in the realization of speech sounds, correct or incorrect, is maintained.

Although the disorder of phonetic realization is usually cited as the major feature of Broca's aphasia, it is usually equally present in global aphasia and in subcortical aphasias involving the capsular-putaminal region. It may range in severity from a complete inability to direct the articulators in the formation of individual speechlike sounds to residual forms, in which there is only a trace of awkwardness. It is most useful to describe the appearance of the disorder in patients who have regained some articulatory control.

The detailed symptomatology in cases with phonetic breakdown varies considerably among patients in the diagnostic groups affected. Some features are almost universal; others appear only in a subset of patients. The overall speech pattern is nonfluent. That is, to the extent that speech is produced, it comes forth in short utterances of one to four words. Articulatory placement is variably slowed and awkward, sometimes to the point of unintelligibility, but the ease of production may vary from one utterance to another, or between the words in a single utterance, depending on their familiarity or predictability.

Communicative Context, Familiarity, and Automaticity

Even at early and severe levels of aphasic phonetic breakdown, it is often possible to have a patient count aloud with normal or only mildly affected articulation. The beginning of the number series is the best preserved. As the patient attempts to go beyond the most overlearned opening portion of the series, articulation again degenerates. Providing the patient with lipreading and auditory cues for the first sounds of succeeding numbers permits the maintenance of articulatory facility for a longer string. Similarly, expletives, profanity, and stereotyped verbal formulas (e.g., "I know it") seem to find an outflow channel that either overcomes or circumvents the incapacity to produce speech movements of a communicative type. This is the phenomenon first noted by Jackson that led him to distinguish between the propositional and nonpropositional use of words.

But communicative intent is not necessarily inhibiting, as compared to parrot like repetition. In working with one severe, globally impaired aphasic patient, the author was totally unable to elicit from him the repetition of the words "yes" or "no." Yet this patient would reliably and appropriately say "yes" or "no" when asked simple factual questions (e.g., Is this [ashtray] made of wood? [No]; Is this a pen? [Yes]). Having used the word as a response, he was unable to say it again immediately afterward. It might be suggested that simple affirmation or negation has the force of an expletive. In fact, these were the only communicative utterances he ever produced. Yet the example shows that the categorial definitions that we devise to account for aphasic behavior are only approximations to nature's categories.

Familiarity with and personal relevance of the verbal content are other factors that become apparent early in recovery from speech output disorders. Whether asked to repeat or to provide one-word answers, the patient with Broca's aphasia typically first regains articulatory mastery of a small vocabulary of words, while continuing to display extreme difficulty with other words that may be only slightly less familiar. The author's colleague, N. Helm-Estabrooks, has repeatedly demonstrated that severe Broca's aphasics may break through their articulatory barrier to say "pizza" or "beer," when they cannot yet intelligibly repeat the more neutral word "table."

Improvement with Imitation and Repeated Attempts

The articulatory failures of Broca's aphasics behave like failures of motor memory that can be refreshed or reconstituted by either an external reminder or by the patient's own kinesthetic experience during initial attempts. A severely distorted production may approach closer and closer to normal when the patient is encouraged to make several additional attempts, or does so on his or her own.

Recurrent Stereotyped Utterances

Although still incapable of retrieving the motor plans for purposeful speech movements, many patients have a recurring utterance that appears immune to their speech output problems and often seems to block their efforts to achieve an intended articulatory target. A number of quite different types of recurring utterances have been noted, beginning with

Broca's famous patient whose only vocalization was "Tan." A nonexhaustive list of such behavior includes:

1. Single syllable or short multisyllable, meaningless forms that are produced in the same way on each effort to speak (e.g., "walla-walla").
2. Continuous output of a chain of repeated syllables, sometimes produced with sentencelike prosody.
3. A real word or short phrase that intrudes with each effort to speak, without any relevance to the subject matter at hand. Some recent examples from the author's clinic are "television" and "gotta go." Rare instances have been described (Head, 1926) of patients whose unique production was a word or phrase that seemed to be linked to an event at the moment of their stroke.

Recurring utterances, even sentencelike reiterations of the same syllables, are a familiar symptom in global aphasics. Poeck, DeBleser, and von Keyserlingk (1984) found no distinctions, anatomically or behaviorally, between those global aphasics who used recurring utterances and those who did not.

Recurring utterances may also persist in patients who are not global, but who are recovering some speech output. This behavior has been observed in patients originally treated with melodic intonation therapy (Albert *et al.*, 1973). The first of these patients was a woman who produced the same polysyllabic nonsense utterance with each effort to repeat or to respond to a question, even though she had good auditory comprehension. Her first controlled voluntary utterance appeared with the facilitation of a simple intoned melody. However, the patient's subsequent recovery left persisting difficulties in phonetic realization and nonfluent, telegraphic speech. In this and other cases, the pseudofluency of the recurrent syllables is not a harbinger of later fluency in speech recovery, nor is the ease of production of the stereotyped utterance any sign of potential for recovery of articulatory facility.

Characteristic Articulatory Behavior Caused by Disorders of Phonetic Realization

Beyond the overall characterization of speech movements as slow and awkward, there are a number of quasi-rulelike features that describe this behavior.

Greater vulnerability of consonants than vowels

When a word is even minimally intelligible, it is rare to hear gross departures from the target in the value of the vowel, even though consonants may be badly malformed. In occasional patients, however, vowels may be shortened and dipthongs reduced. Such vowel changes may contribute to the impression of a foreign accent—the "foreign accent syndrome." For example, Blumstein *et al.* (1987) reported a patient whose only residual impairment from a transient aphasia was a subtle change in articulation and speech prosody that gave her what struck listeners as a French or Scandinavian accent. Phonological analysis revealed characteristic shortening and loss of diphthongization of vowels. Changes in speech prosody were the dominant feature in the famous case of Monrad-Krohn (1947) of a native Norwegian speaker who was mistaken for a German after her recovery from aphasia.

The relative vulnerability of consonants in comparison to vowels may be related to the speed of the required movements, particularly in shifts from one consonant to another in comparison to the nearly steady state of vowels.

Reduction of phonetic complexity

It is characteristic for Broca's aphasics to reduce the complexity of consonant sequences in one of several ways. Consonant blends (e.g., *pl* and *tr*) or combinations (e.g., *st* and *sp*) may be reduced by omitting the continuant and retaining only the stop consonant—a maneuver that least affects intelligibility. Thus, "play" may become "p'ay," "train" becomes "t'ain," and "spoon" becomes "poon." Affricates, such as *ch*, may be similarly reduced (e.g., "church" becomes "t'urch"). Another device is the insertion of an epenthetic neutral vowel between combinations of two stop consonants, for example, "captain" becomes /kæp ət ən/. The same device may be used between words when a final stop consonant is followed by an initial consonant in the next word.

Perseveration

Perseveration of initial stop consonants may intrude in the same position in a following word (e.g., "cold potato" becomes "cold cotato") or replace a subsequent stop consonant in the same word.

Disturbance in the force and timing of movements

Among the most readily recognized impairments that contribute to articulatory "awkwardness" are the excessive force in the closure of voiceless stop consonants and the excessive force and duration of the plosive release of the stop. This common feature of Broca's aphasics' speech results in increased voice onset time (VOT).

PHONETIC BREAKDOWN AND VOT

Voice onset time refers to the interval between the release of articulatory closure at the lips, alveolar ridge, or velum (corresponding, respectively, to the consonants p/b, t/d, and k/g) and the onset of vocal cord vibration for the following vowel. A normal English speaker perceives consonants with short VOTs (< 20 msec) as voiced (i.e., b, d, or g) and those with VOTs longer than 40 msecs as voiceless. The English speaker/listener is extremely sensitive to minor variations in VOT near the border zone of 20–40 msecs, where a small change will cause the perceived consonant to switch between voiced and voiceless. Large variations in VOT go unrecognized if they are on the same side of the border value. That is, the speaker/listener appears to have divided the physical acoustic parameters into categories that correspond to different sounds. These divisions develop early in the acquisition of one's own language ("categorical perception"; Liberman *et al.* 1967) and differ somewhat from language to language.

Voice onset time is an easily measurable and sensitive indicator of phonetic articulatory impairment. Other movements of the articulators (e.g., velar closing) are more difficult to measure.

Acoustic measurement of VOTs for voiced and voiceless target sounds produced by Broca's aphasics have shown a poorly defined border, with many voiced targets extending into the range of unvoiced consonants. Such a breakdown of the VOT categorical boundary was not observed in Wernicke's aphasics (Blumstein *et al.*, 1977; Hoit-Dalgaard *et al.*, 1983; Shewan *et al.*, 1984). Using fiber optic techniques, Itoh *et al.* (1979, 1983) found a similar dissociation between Broca's and Wernicke's aphasics in the coordination of velar opening with other articulatory movements. Their subject had phonetic production difficulties and lowered his velum out of synchrony with other articulatory components of the target letter, *n*. Velar movement errors of Wernicke's aphasics, however, were not errors of synchronization, but corresponded to complete phoneme substitution. That is, they were phonemic, rather than phonetic errors.

Alajouanine *et al.* (1939) also noted how frequently voiced target consonants were produced as unvoiced (i.e., with delayed VOTs). In the framework of linguistic markedness theory (Jakobson and Halle, 1956), the absence of voicing corresponds to the "unmarked" or basic form of a contrasting pair of sounds. Thus, a *p* is unmarked for voicing, whereas a *b* is marked. The unmarked form usually corresponds to the earliest sound acquired in development and the phonetically least complex. The fact that Broca's aphasics tend to shift voiced to unvoiced consonants is one of numerous instances in which error tendencies in aphasia move toward the simpler form.

Summarizing the work on phonetic breakdown in aphasia, Blumstein (1988) points out that the failures in articulatory timing by Broca's aphasics always involve the coordination between two different articulators. More importantly, however, they are not a simple motor breakdown, but are determined by the speech context. For example, English voiced fricatives (e.g., *v*) are shorter than unvoiced ones (*f*). Vowels followed by an unvoiced consonant (e.g., pl*a*te) are shorter than those followed by a voiced consonant (e.g., pl*a*yed). These subtle timing differences are maintained by Broca's aphasics in spite of other failures of coordination.

PHONEMIC BREAKDOWN

The preceding section reviewed articulatory failures linked to physical implementation of target sounds. The contrasting mechanism for articulatory errors results in the facile production of mistargeted sounds—that is, of phonemes or syllables that are substituted or omitted, or else transposed from their intended position in a word. These errors are likely to occur in a context of normal articulatory facility. They are referred to as "phonemic" in the sense that they correspond to the linguistic level of phonology. Phonology deals with the sound-units (or phonemes) of a language as they are conceived by a competent speaker/hearer. It is not concerned with the physical structures and acoustic waveforms that create these sounds. Phonemic errors (referred to as "phonemic" or "literal" paraphasias) are made characteristically by patients with lesions of the posterior speech zone who have Wernicke's or conduction aphasia. They also occur frequently in patients who have phonetic articulatory problems, as observed in Broca's aphasia and aphasia from lesions of the anterior subcortical speech area.

PHONEMIC PARAPHASIA VERSUS PHONETIC MISARTICULATION

For definitional purposes, a literal (or phonemic) paraphasia is any well-formed sound or syllable that is out of place (substituted or transposed) in an otherwise recognizable target word. Within this general definition, we observe patterns that are distinctive for various types of aphasia. Without taking into account these distinctive clinical presentations, one would have to say that phonemic paraphasias are common in aphasic patients of almost any type. For example, phonemic paraphasias occur frequently in the context of the phonetically disordered awkward speech of Broca's aphasics. In some instances, the listener cannot tell whether such errors represent phonetically based coordination failures that happen to sound like an incorrectly chosen phoneme.

For conduction aphasics, literal paraphasias are the dominant or exclusive form of word production error, and they are heard in a context of otherwise facile articulation. Conduction aphasics typically monitor these errors and attempt to self-correct the same word repeatedly. They may not lose the basic phonological framework of the word form during their repeated corrections, but may correct one part of a word while spoiling another part that was previously correct. For example, "I came into the hospital for some tecs . . . some secs . . . tesk T E S . . . tests."

A different clinical context for phonemic paraphasia is heard in the speech of Wernicke's aphasics. These patients often recover some of the phonological fragments of a word, filling the rest of the production with paraphasic elements that may have no relation to the target. However, the model that guides these utterances is fleeting and unstable. An initial stab at a word may come close, but drift into completely unrelated neologisms on subsequent attempts. Documented illustrations of such behavior may be found in Joanette *et al.* (1980) and Miller and Ellis (1987).

PROSODY

The term prosody refers to a group of features, including stress-pattern (or meter), word grouping, melodic contour, and changes in voice volume, that may be imposed on units of word, phrase, or sentence length. They are also called "suprasegmental features" because the units they modify are more than a phonemic segment in length.

Although loosely grouped under the single term "prosody," these various features play different roles at the word, phrase, and sentence levels. Every one of them may be affected in various forms of speech-output disturbance.

Word Prosody

This is word rhythm, determined by the number of syllable beats and the position of primary and, in longer words, secondary stress. Word stress is usually marked by both an increase in volume, vowel duration, and a rise in pitch on the stressed syllable. The pitch marking, however, is variable. In some pragmatic speech contexts (e.g., a questioning tone), a drop in pitch may take the place of a rise. There are many instances in which different stress patterns signal totally different meanings for words with similar phonemic structures (e.g., verb versus cognate noun, as in (*pro*test/pro*test*). In English, many nouns are reduced to the neutral "schwa" (/ə/) in an unstressed position.

For many patients with Broca's aphasia, word prosody may be maintained in spite of severe phonetic distortions at the segment level. There are, however, forms of phonetic breakdown in which the stress pattern gives way to a syllable by syllable delivery, with each syllable receiving almost equal stress and each vowel receiving its full value instead of being reduced to a "schwa." In this output, the restoration of full vowel value shows that the problem is not merely one of motor control or apraxia, but is instead an adaptation that interacts with the aphasic speaker's access to the "citation form" of a normally unstressed syllable.

Syllable by syllable delivery is associated with extreme difficulty in making transitions between a stop consonant and any other consonant. The epenthetic /ə/ is often used at these transitions. This form of prosodic breakdown is a constant feature of patients with "aphemia" (see Chapters 3 and 12). It also appears sporadically during the speech of some Broca's aphasics.

Syntax-Marking Prosody

The relationships between the words and phrases of a sentence and the pragmatic function of the entire sentence are marked by differences in stress and duration of words, by pauses at particular phrasal junctures, and by the melodic contour superimposed on the entire sentence. For example, in English, grammatical functors are typically short and unstressed in contrast to the lexical terms that they connect. Compound and complex spoken sentences would often be unintelligible to the listener if phrasal groupings were not set off by rising or falling pitch just before the break. We would often not distinguish a statement from a command or a question without the overall sentence melody, typically falling toward the end of a statement or rising at the end of a yes–no question.

Obviously, the pauses created by word-finding difficulty, articulatory struggle, and midsentence word-initiation efforts play havoc with syntax-marking prosody, even with the simplified and fragmented sentences produced by Broca's aphasics. Yet, in spite of these problems, the overall pitch contour of their utterances is surprisingly robust. In a study by Danley, DeVilliers, and Cooper 1979), Broca's aphasics were found to preserve the falling pitch that marks the end of a declarative utterance. They also moved to a higher pitch level at the beginning of a new utterance.

However, this evidence of sentence planning was absent in longer sentences (over seven words).

Danley and Shapiro (1982) examined five types of sentential prosodic signals in oral sentence reading of five Broca's aphasics, each of whom had agrammatic, phonetically disordered speech output. These five features were

Fo declination. The progressive decline in fundamental frequency (Fo) from the beginning to the end of a sentence.

Continuation rise. The brief elevation in Fo on the last word preceding a syntactic juncture that signals both the end of a semantic word grouping and that there is more to follow.

Fo resetting. The establishment of a new Fo level at the beginning of a sentence or immediately after a continuation rise.

Sentence terminal contour. The relatively sharp fall in Fo in the last word of a declarative sentence.

Utterance final lengthening. Prolongation of the final word in a sentence.

All of the intonational signals were found to be present in the speech of the Broca's aphasics, except for the lengthening of the last word of the sentence. However, unlike the control subjects, Broca's aphasics did not adapt their initial Fo resetting to the length of the planned utterance. These results indicate that the intonational aspect of utterance planning is typically largely preserved in spite of the presence of agrammatism and phonetic output disorders. It is available to signal the grouping of thought units within the sentence, even when the individual words are widely spaced. The dysprosody of these patients lies in the interruption of the speech rhythm caused by articulatory, word-finding, and speech formulation blocks. This dysprosody is naturally much more apparent in free conversation than in oral reading—the task used by Danley and Shapiro. In free speech, there are many more sentence fragments, false starts, and backtracking, all of which contribute to interruptions of speech rhythm.

NONFLUENCY AND FLUENCY IN APHASIA

In Chapter 2, we examined the historical origin of the dichotomy between nonfluent and fluent forms of aphasia and the reasons for the adoption of these terms in place of the formerly popular terms expressive versus receptive (or motor versus sensory). The fluency–nonfluency distinction has its greatest value in communicating the global characteristics of the speech output pattern, which often serves as an effective "first cut" in diagnostic classification, and in predicting whether the patient's lesion is anterior or posterior to the Rolandic fissure.

Like many words that are borrowed from everyday vocabulary for a specialized technical meaning, the terms "fluent" and "nonfluent" have been widely misapplied under the misapprehension that they correspond to the user's nontechnical criterion for fluency. For example, patients who produce a continuous mumble or a continuous iteration of a stereotyped utterance have been mislabeled as "fluent aphasics." The application of the fluency–nonfluency concept to the classification of aphasia will be developed further in Chapter 12.

In their 1964 article, Goodglass, Quadfasel, and Timberlake showed that aphasics could be dichotomized on the basis of the number of words that they could typically utter as an uninterrupted string. Short-phrase dominant (nonfluent) aphasics rarely exceeded three to four words per utterance group. Long-phrase dominant (fluent) aphasics could frequently run on without interruption in strings of five or more words. The dichotomy was truly bimodal, with the great bulk of patients falling in the two modal groups and very few in between. Thus, in its technical meaning in aphasia, fluency is not a continuous variable, but falls into one of two states.

It must be recognized that in present usage, fluency and nonfluency are purely empirically based, and not theoretical constructs. Nonfluency is often defined in terms of a combination of articulatory problems, such as agrammatism and short word groupings, which tend to occur together in Broca's aphasics. However, in all likelihood, this concurrence is due to the fact that articulatory difficulty and agrammatism may each be a cause of short and choppy speech output groupings. These components, while tending to be correlated, also vary autonomously. There is still a need for a careful analysis of the basis for nonfluency in terms of individual factors and their anatomic bases.

Chapter 5

Disorders of Word Retrieval

Clinical observations of aphasic patients have revealed a treasure trove of phenomena that in different ways reflect disorders in the retrieval of the names of objects and other concepts. Some of these point to a deceptively simple picture—for example, that "naming" is a discrete language function that can be selectively damaged by certain focal lesions. Other observations are not only challenges to such views, but defy any current theories about the organization of cognitive functions. Among such challenges is the observation that some patients may be more successful in naming words of a particular category (e.g., parts of the body) than any other word category, yet inferior in identifying those objects on auditory presentation.

Anomia, or impaired access to one's vocabulary, is virtually universal in aphasia, with the exception of those "pure" forms that affect only a single input or output channel. In fact, the degree of word-finding impairment tells more about the general severity of the aphasia than about its type. Such a statement may seem to be at odds with the fact that "anomic aphasia" is defined as a pure disorder of word retrieval, whereas Broca's aphasia is described in terms of the impairment of articulation and syntax. This chapter presents the argument that the main differences among subtypes of aphasia, including the two just mentioned, do not depend on the level of the patient's word retrieval ability, but on the prominence of other impairments—for example, those of syntax, fluency, auditory comprehension, and so on—in relation to the word retrieval difficulty. Although the degree of word-finding ability may not, by itself, provide interesting differences related to the lesion site, the different ways in which patients fail does give clues concerning both the normal cognitive apparatus for naming and the dissociations within this apparatus that are brought about by brain damage.

CLINICAL FORMS OF ANOMIA

In describing the symptomatology of anomia it is indispensible to define the various error types that commonly appear in aphasic speech.

Paraphasia

Collectively, the term "paraphasia" is applied to any unintended error of word or sound choice (except those at the phonetic level of articulation as discussed in Chapter 4).

Verbal Paraphasia

Verbal paraphasia is the unintended use of another word in lieu of the target. Most verbal paraphasias have a clear meaning relationship to the desired word and represent the same part of speech. Hence they are commonly referred to as "semantic paraphasias" (e.g., I went to the store . . . no, the movies). They may be recognized and self-corrected, as in the foregoing example, or uttered without awareness of the error. Verbal paraphasias may also be unrelated to the meaning of the target, or occur as perseverations of a previously used word (paraphasic perseveration.) Examples of verbal paraphasias obtained in a picture-naming test from two aphasic patients follow:

	TARGET WORD	RESPONSE
Mr. W. (Broca)	stethoscope	"telescope—not right"
	asparagus	"carrot—no"
	pinwheel	"kite"
	nozzle	"hose—no"
Father L. (Wernicke)	seahorse	"mandarin"
	globe	"atlas"
	stethoscope	"octopus—no"
	hourglass	"it's a weather"

Semantic paraphasias may be generated through a number of different mechanisms. One that is common in normal speech is simple lack of knowledge. For example, many people do not know exactly how a beaver, a woodchuck, or a badger differ in appearance. Saying "woodchuck" in response to a picture of a beaver may be a normal error, even when produced by an aphasic patient. Yet, aphasia also may produce a pathological breakdown in the semantic boundaries between meaning-related words that were premorbidly clearly distinguished. For example, the response "It's a weather" to the picture of an hourglass suggests a blurring of distinctions between measuring devices related to time, weather, and so on.

Yet in many instances semantic misnaming occurs in spite of demonstrable preservation of the concept structure of the target word. When Mr. W., the Broca's aphasic, immediately rejects his response with "no" or "not right," it is clear that he has recognized the disparity between the uttered word and the meaning of the target. In one instance this was also true for the Wernicke aphasic. However, it is interesting to note that the response "octopus" to the stethoscope was a perseveration from the presentation of a picture of an octopus earlier in the series. The semantic disparity between the two words was great enough for him to have detected it after hearing his paraphasic production. It is rare to find a patient whose naming goes awry in exactly the same way on each occasion. In general, however, we have found that Broca's aphasics are more likely than any other group to signal their perception of a semantic mismatch by appending "no" to their responses (Kohn and Goodglass, 1985).

Semantic paraphasia is distinguishable from the use of one-word circumlocutory comments that patients sometimes use to tell something about the meaning of a word that they cannot retrieve. For example, it is not unusual for a patient, unable to name the picture of a cigarette, to say, "Well ... smoking," as though to convey the message "I can't get the name of it, but it's for smoking." As a rule of thumb, it may be assumed that a response to an object picture with a word that is not a noun is not intended as a name for the object, but is a one-word circumlocution.

Phonemic Paraphasia

Phonemic paraphasia, also called "literal paraphasia," is the production of unintended sounds or syllables in the utterance of a partially recognizable word (e.g., "paker" for "paper" "sisperos" for "rhinoceros").

Phonosemantic Blends

It is often the case that a phonemic sound substitution results in another real word, related in sound but not meaning (e.g. "table" becomes "cable"; "telephone" becomes "television"). In fact, there appears to be a tendency for phonemic paraphasias to become assimilated to another real word when there is one in the speaker's language that is phonologically close to the target. A special class of phonosemantic blends are those in which the erroneous word shares both sound and meaning with the target (e.g., "broom" becomes "brush"). These errors differ from malapropisms in that the person using a malapropism does not appreciate the inappropriateness of the word used. The aphasic, given the opportunity, would usually distinguish the meaning of the target word from the paraphasic one.

Neologistic Paraphasia

Neologistic paraphasia is the production of a nonsense word or words, usually without recognition of error (e.g. "table" becomes "tilto"). Most instances of neologistic paraphasia occur in the context of severely disorganized speech, in which it is difficult to discern whether any individual neologism took the place of a particular intended word. Neologisms are often obtained from Wernicke's aphasics during attempts at picture naming. In these instances, of course, the target is known.

The examiner who is attempting to categorize response errors may be forced into arbitrary decisions that have little to do with the process behind the patient's error. As discussed in Chapter 4, this is a consideration in distinguishing between articulatory errors and phonemic paraphasias. It is a particular problem on the borderline between phonemic paraphasias and neologisms. In some instances—particularly in the case of conduction aphasics—phonemic paraphasias appear to represent a disorder in the sequential organization of phoneme or syllable-sized segments of a word whose basic phonological framework has been retrieved. Consider the case of a patient who attempted to name "zodiac," but uttered "zokiad" on each of multiple attempts to correct himself. When only a fragment of the phonology of the target word is retrieved to guide the output, one may obtain "vord" for "valve" or "postocus" for "octopus." Either of these might be classed as a neologism because so little of the intended word can be identified in them. At the extreme are totally confabulated nonsense words (e.g., "rickus") that have no resemblance to anything the patient might have intended. Such neologisms may also appear as recurring intrusions in the patient's conversation.

RESPONSE TO PHONEMIC PRIMING

Patients who fail to retrieve a concept name on request are often aided by having the first sounds of the word provided by the examiner. This form of prompting, called "phonemic cuing" or "phonemic priming," is very informative for the examiner. Further, it may allow the patient an opportunity to succeed before moving on to another task and so avoid the frustration of failure. Response to such prompting sometimes takes the form of a reflex-like and instantaneous completion of the fragment given, without the patient repeating the onset of the word. In other instances, the patient retrieves the entire word with some effort after hearing the cue.

Failure to benefit from phonemic priming also takes diverse forms. Some patients complete the provided fragment with another word that fits the stem, but is unrelated to the target. For example, in priming for the picture "camel," the examiner may offer "ca . . . " and the patient may complete it as "camera." Some patients are brought no closer to the phonology of the target word than they were before being helped.

As we interpret the responses to phonemic priming in various types of aphasia, we must bear in mind that it entails a number of converging mechanisms. One of these is word recognition. The spoken fragment activates, from past experience, one or more words that begin with the given sound. Another mechanism is the word production system, which may be set into operation almost automatically on being primed with a first sound. Both of these are mediated by auditory perceptual processes. Finally, phonemic priming depends on the patient's appreciation that the prompting that he or she is offered is related to the effort to retrieve a particular word.

Successful use of phonemic priming indicates some integrity of function in each of these areas. Failure may indicate that auditory perceptual processes are deficient, or else that long standing associations to word phonology are so damaged that traces can no longer be reconstituted. Completion of the prime with an irrelevant word may signal that the patient cannot maintain the "set" to restrict his or her responses to words that are semantically appropriate to the stimulus picture.

ANOMIA IN NONFLUENT APHASIC PATIENTS

Free conversation

At all stages of recovery, there is a relative preponderance of substantive words over words that provide the grammatical matrix of sentences. A transcript from a severe Broca's aphasic exemplifies this speech pattern:

> **Examiner:** What brought you to the hospital?
> **Patient:** Yeah . . . Wednesday, . . . Paul and dad . . . Hospital . . . yeah . . . doctors, two. . . . an' teeth.

In this exchange, the patient was trying to explain that his father had brought him into the hospital on Wednesday to have some work done on his teeth. The sample is typical of the severely agrammatic patient, in the absence of any word combinations and of any grammatical morphemes other than "and." The patient refers to himself by his name, apparently unable to use the pronoun "I." Because his speech consists largely of common and proper nouns, in what sense can we consider him anomic?

In fact, like most patients of this type, Paul's vocabulary is extremely sparse. He can retrieve laboriously a bare minimum of the key words to convey an intended message. Given a test of picture naming, he can produce only the most common object names (e.g., house, bed, and pencil), while failing such words as "scissors," "flower," and "comb." His conversational speech includes very few verbs. In the preceding sample, he omits the word "came" in the obligatory context "Paul and dad— hospital."

Verbs are lacking, not only in sentence contexts, but in picture naming tasks carried out by agrammatic patients. This characteristic of agrammatic speech will be developed in the discussion on category specific dissociations in naming.

Motor Articulatory Factors

Because motor articulatory difficulties are prominent in Broca's aphasics and in other nonfluent patients, it has been suggested that the word retrieval process has proceeded up to the point of articulatory realization, but is blocked at that final stage. Luria (1970) for example, proposes that the ability of Broca's aphasics to benefit from phonemic priming indicates that they have the "acoustic image" of the words and that consequently their production errors represent difficulties of articulatory realization, rather than errors of semantic substitution.

To be sure, nonfluent aphasics are more likely than other aphasics to block on the formation of the initial sound and are often aided by phonemic priming. Indeed, Goodglass and Stuss (1979) suggested that the degree of response to phonemic priming is an index of how profoundly impaired the word retrieval process is, irrespective of the type of aphasia. In the nonfluent aphasic, the ability to reconstitute word sounds on hearing a cue is often relatively intact in spite of severe output difficulties. It is rare to find a patient, however, who does not have persistent retrieval difficulties on some relatively common words, even after phonemic priming. Using such responsiveness as an index of severity of word retrieval damage, there are Broca's aphasics and other nonfluent patients who have an anomia that is more severe than one observes in most patients with "anomic aphasia."

There are many instances in which a nonfluent patient's articulatory distortions give convincing evidence that most or all of the phonological representation of a word has been retrieved, yet the oral production is barely intelligible. Urging the patient to try again, several times, often results in successively more accurate production. That is, each repetition appears to make an additional contribution to refreshing the motor articulatory memory. Providing a complete model of the word for repetition has a similar effect, but even after such repetition, further practice with the word results in additional facilitation. Such instances suggest that motor articulatory memory may be dissociated from phonological retrieval.

Among Broca's aphasics with agrammatism, there is sometimes a remarkable disparity between good success on picture naming and extremely disabling anomia during free conversation. One such patient, a woman who had suffered a stroke involving pre- and postcentral gyri with deep extension, presented classic telegraphic speech production and excellent auditory comprehension. Her conversation was marked by constant frustration because she could retrieve very few substantive words to convey her ideas. Yet, on a picture naming test, she demonstrated a near normal vocabulary, with prompt responses to some difficult items and no trace of hesitancy on easier ones. The disparity between her confrontation naming and her access to lexical items during conversation was attributed to the hypothesis that the combined processing load of forming sentences and supplying the vocabulary to fill them was much more disruptive than the latter operation by itself.

Recall of Written Words

A feature commonly observed, but not exclusive to nonfluent aphasics, is the partial preservation of written word-finding in the presence of anomia to confrontation naming. These patients may insist on reaching for a pencil to write their responses the moment they become aware of a retrieval block. In many instances, the result is only partially correct, retaining the beginning, the ending, and some structurally prominent letter features. However, occasional Broca's aphasics who fail in oral naming have a high success rate in writing their responses.

Can the retention of oral spelling be taken as evidence that the patient really "knows" the word, but is simply blocked at the level of articulatory implementation? Whereas this may be the pattern in some patients, Friederici, Schonle, and Goodglass (1981) obtained evidence that for many Broca's aphasics, written naming results from direct activation of a visual graphemic code, independent of oral phonology. They found that

Broca's aphasics were, on average, superior in written over oral responses to a 30-picture naming test. For those who had superior written performance, visually and semantically determined errors predominated. For example, the picture "toboggan" was written as "snow" (a semantically motivated paragraphia); the picture of "raft" was spelled "PAFT" (visually determined). The subgroup of Broca's aphasics who named aloud correctly more often than they spelled correctly were also more likely to make phonologically determined writing errors (e.g., "anker" for "anchor"; Friederici *et al.*, 1981). A comparison group of Wernicke's aphasics performed correctly about equally in oral and written naming.

The work of Frederici *et al.* supports a "dual coding" hypothesis. Namely, that the picture to be named may activate two independent channels of representation: a phonological one, mediating oral responses, and a visuo-graphomotor one, mediating written responses. When the phonological channel is blocked, written responses may be superior and the errors made may reflect no influence of phonological access. That is, the oral naming failures of these patients are at a deeper level than that of articulatory implementation. They recover no inkling of the sound of the target word. For the other subgroup of patients, writing may be considered to be "parasitic" spoken phonology.

ANOMIA IN FLUENT APHASIA

Free Conversation

The severity of anomia in fluent aphasics spans the range from very slight impairment to total failure, overlapping the range of impairments observed in patients with nonfluent disorders. The clinical appearance of the deficit, however, is very different, and differs in characteristic ways among the subtypes of fluent aphasics: that is, Wernicke's, conduction, anomic, and transcortical sensory aphasia.

Common to all the fluent aphasics is the contrast between the patient's facility in initiating the grammatical framework for sentences and the striking inability to retrieve the information—carrying words—nouns, verbs, and adjectives. From the speech of these patients, it is clear that anomia is not a loss of access to all vocabulary because the words that have a primarily grammatical function in free conversation are unaffected. Pronouns, prepositions, copulas, and auxiliary and modal verbs are readily available to the fluent, anomic patient, as are many high frequency nouns and verbs that enter into expressions of time (e.g., "the other day") and expressions of basic activities (e.g., "went to work").

Confronted with the repeated inability to retrieve essential words, fluent aphasics fall back on a number of possible strategies at the point of failure. These include:

1. Uncompensated blocking with exclamations of frustration. For example:

"I gave him a . . . Oh God! I know it! I can't . . . Why can't I say it?"

2. Substitutions of vague or indefinite words, such as "thing" or "something" in lieu of nouns or "do it" in lieu of verbs. A typical passage from one patient with Wernicke's aphasia was

"Haven't been around there at all since we got into this time here, anything about her . . . only because we had to do that, and then she got back with it . . ."

3. Circumlocutions describing the appearance or function of the target concept. For example:

"I lost my . . . I keep my money in it."

4. Substitutions of erroneous words or neologisms. Green's (1969) jargon aphasic patient produced the following sequence when explaining that his vision was poor:

"See, my rekfid is . . . are bad. Oh, may cathopes noe too good. Well, my gupa wasn't too good."

Patients with anomic aphasia are most prone to use circumlocutions and indefinite words, rarely producing neologisms or other paraphasias. These strategies are apparent in the following transcript from a young man who suffered an embolus affecting the posterior speech zone after open-heart surgery for an aortic valve replacement.

    E: Tell me what you experienced at the beginning of your illness.
    P: I had a . . . one or two or three . . . there's one . . . I had a . . . I know the exact part of it. (Patient is attempting a circumlocution for "aortic valve" by referring to it as being one of two or three similar structures.)
    E: You're pointing to the operation on your chest.
    P: Yes . . . I had a vord . . . a lord . . . a . . . a . . . it was repla . . . it came back.
    E: A valve?
    P: Yes, of the / æore / . . . the . . . the . . . there are three or four different things that they could have in mind.

> E: And it was after that operation . . .
> P: Yes, about a day later. I was under watchamacall it . . . under . .
> E: Anesthesia?
> P: No . . . where they put you, just two or three people . . . You stay there for a couple of days.
> E: In the intensive care unit?
> P: Right . . . at that time I got this . . . s . . .

As is evident from the circumlocutions attempted by this patient, he has sufficient semantic appreciation of his target concepts to attempt definitions of them. On occasion, he retrieves a fragment of the phonology of his target and may be led to an inappropriate completion (valve becomes "vord . . . lord"; aorta becomes / æore/), but he is acutely aware of these errors, once they are emitted. In this respect, he approaches the error type characteristic of conduction aphasia (see the following and Chapter 8).

The free conversation of Wernicke's aphasics is replete with errors of word use, but they are often embedded in sentence structures that are so far afield from a discernible topic that it is difficult to classify them as substitutions for a presumed target. In the following sample (from Jones and Wepman, 1965), a patient describes the scene on TAT card 2: a young woman standing with books in her arms, portrayed in a farm scene with family members engaged in farm labor.

> "Well, all I know is, somebody is clipping the kreples and some wha, someone here on the kureping arm, . . . why I don't know."

One of the author's own jargon aphasics responded to the question, "How are you today?" as follows:

> "I feel very well. My hearing, writing been doing well. Things that I couldn't hear from. In other words, I used to be able to work cigarettes I didn't know how. . . . Chesterfeela, for 20 years I can write it."

The free conversation of conduction aphasics presents a very different pattern of word retrieval problems—one in which it is usually clear what word is being attempted—both from the sentence context and from the recognizable approximations that the patient produces. In the following extract, a patient with conduction aphasia is engaged in an opening conversation:

> (Well how are you feeling Mr. K.?) Well, I was a little tight earlier . . .
> One word . . . toyce . . . toy . . . tensh . . . (tense?) tench . . .

Another patient, describing the "Cookie Theft" picture of the Boston Diagnostic Aphasia Examination, is trying to report that a boy is falling off a stool; then, that water is overflowing from a sink.

"He's falling off the t . . . t . . . t . . . Anyhow, the mother is t . . . t . . . she's. . . . The water is falling over the fink . . . fink . . . stink . . . sink . . . .

Picture Naming

Whereas free conversation maximizes the differences in word-retrieval behavior among types of aphasics, the task of picture naming is a great leveler. Free conversation allows the fluent aphasic to create a sentence context of high frequency words that may escape semantic constraints and allow the generation of a jargon composed of real words or neologisms. This has led to the generalization that Wernicke's aphasics make more semantic paraphasias than Broca's aphasics.

The picture naming task has come to be the standard procedure for both clinical assessment and research on word retreival. It places all subjects on a more equal footing: confronted with a specific stimulus, they are constrained to supply a name for it. The proportions of semantic and phonemic paraphasias are similar for all types of aphasics, according to the data of Kohn and Goodglass (1985). Rambling, off-target comments are still produced by some Wernicke's aphasics. These are patients who do not perceive the picture as an item to be labeled, but rather as a stimulus for a tangential commentary.

TWO FORMS OF PHONEMIC PARAPHASIA

It has been noted earlier that phonemic paraphasias always involve partial activation of word phonology. It is important, from both a clinical and theoretical viewpoint, to distinguish between phonemic paraphasias that are anchored in a stable framework and those that are products of a transient and unstable state of phonological activation.

The behavioral basis for the distinction that is made here is in the character of successive attempts at self-correction in the picture naming task. A predominance of stably anchored phonemic paraphasias is typically observed in conduction aphasia, whereas fleeting phonological resemblances to target words are more common in Wernicke's aphasia. The diagnostic distinction, of course, entails an anatomic distinction. Furthermore, we consider these discrete varieties of paraphasia to result from disruptions in different phases of the word retrieval process.

Examples of stable paraphasia:

TARGET WORD	RESPONSE
dart	cart . . . part . . . chart
broom	broo . . . croo . . . broom
scroll	scrip . . . screwl . . . scrit . . . roll it up . . . sholl . . . scroll.
bench	fence . . . park bence . . . bench
pinwheel	Pan . . . P E A . . . peanwheel. pinwill . . . penwhale . . . pinfin . . . no pinwheel.

Characteristic of stably anchored paraphasias are the following:

1. Phonemic paraphasias are a dominant error type in these patients.
2. There is considerable variability as to the structure of the errors of any one patient. In some instances, only a single sound may be transposed or deleted; in others, there may be intrusions of large extraneous segments.
3. Patients' behavior suggests that they have "found" the word; patients often display intense effort, with repeated stabs at self-correction.
4. Successive attempts may correct one error and introduce a different one, but they do not wander progressively from the target.
5. Phonemic priming rarely helps because the patient usually produces the initial sound without assistance.

Kohn's (1984) analysis of the paraphasias of conduction aphasia leads her to characterize them as "postlexical." This term refers to a model in which a particular lexical entry has been contacted and that the breakdown is at the stage of organizing the phonological sequence for motor execution.

Contrast these errors with the shifting and unstable phonemic paraphasia of Wernicke's aphasics. We use the term "unstable" in the sense that a partial sound match with the intended word may be detected in one attempt, but disappears in the next. The clinical characteristics of these errors are the following:

1. They occur as one of multiple types of paraphasic errors by the same patient; among these are partial or complete neologisms and verbal paraphasias.
2. Patients who make these paraphasias occasionally make multiple self-corrective attempts, but also let many erroneous utterances go uncorrected.

3. Successive self-corrective attempts, when they occur, are more likely to lose their phonological resemblance to the target word than to maintain it.

4. Patients are often unaware of uttering the correct word in a series of attempts.

Unstable phonological paraphasia arises in an early phase of the word retrieval process, in contrast to the other form of paraphasia that has been characterized as "postlexical."

TWO-WAY FAILURES OF WORD KNOWLEDGE

Some patients with fluent but anomic speech have a striking failure in grasping the meaning of words provided for them. Characteristically, they repeat the given word over and over, but cannot attach it to a referent. This phenomenon, referred to by Luria (1970) as "alienation of word meaning," is observed in transcortical sensory aphasics, whose lesion lies at the temporo-occipital junction (Luria, 1970; Alexander *et al.*, 1989). We may speculate that this zone and its subjacent white matter contains the pathways through which visual, tactile, and auditory aspects of objects gain access to the language zone. Patients with extensive lesions in this area are often agnosic in several sensory modalities (Alexander *et al.*, 1989).

CATEGORY-SPECIFIC PHENOMENA IN NAMING

It is common to find aphasic patients whose naming difficulty is exceptionally severe in a particular word category, or else for whom a particular word category is well preserved, in comparison to their general level of naming ability. Category specific dissociations are even more widespread in lexical comprehension than in lexical production, and it seems compelling to infer that a common principle applies in both situations. As observed in the opening paragraph of this chapter, a given category (e.g., letters of the alphabet) may be regularly observed to be deviantly well preserved in naming, but selectively impaired for comprehension. Such opposite effects in production and comprehension rule out explanations in terms of word frequency, size of set, or prior experience with the word category.

Goodglass *et al.*, (1966) reported the first systematic study of the most common lexical dissociations in aphasia. They found that the naming of letters was most often an exceptionally easy category for aphasics, whereas the naming of unselected objects was most often the hardest category. Goodglass *et al.* (1986) confirmed this observation and found, in addition, that the categories of colors and body parts are also often exceptionally well retained. These dissociations are much more frequently observed in fluent than in nonfluent aphasic patients.

It is less common to observe word categories that are selectively *impaired* for name production than those that are preserved. Hart, Berndt, and Caramazza (1985) described a patient who recovered from aphasia in all respects except for the inability to name fruits and vegetables. Similar difficulties have been described for the naming of animals (Hart and Gordon, 1988). The first level of explanation is to propose that the brain's lexicon is organized by categories; however, this is no more than a description of the phenomenon and leads to a dead end. For one thing, there are innumerable ways in which objects may be categorized, but so far only two semantic classes have been found in which naming is selectively damaged, and only in rare instances. Another unusual and equally puzzling form of selective anomia is that affecting proper nouns. Semenza and Zettin's (1989) patient could not retrieve the name for any person, country, city, monument, and so on, although he could identify them from pictures by describing their characteristics (e.g., a famous actor) and he could select them from multiple pictures on hearing their names. He could also provide a list of men's or women's names, as long as there was no requirement of matching the name with an individual. One clue to the nature of his disorder is that he could not form new arbitrary associations between pairs of words. Thus, one could generalize his difficulty as one of retrieving words that refer to unique objects or that have an arbitrary link to other unique words.

VERBS VERSUS NOUNS

We have previously noted that verbs are commonly deleted from the agrammatic sentences of Broca's aphasics in free discourse. Investigations of the naming of isolated verbs, through the presentation of pictured actions, reveal that here, too, agrammatic patients have a higher failure rate on verbs than on nouns (Kohn, 1989; Miceli *et al.*, 1984). It has been speculated that this deficiency is, in some way, tied to the fact that the verb carries a strong load of syntactic implications that may make it vulnerable to agrammatism. However, Bates and Chen (1991) have recently shown that Chinese agrammatics are similarly deficient in producing verbs, even though verbs in Chinese have no morphological marking. The fact that verbs are difficult for agrammatic speakers, even as isolated pictures, does not support the view that the syntactic function of the verb is the source of the difficulty for agrammatic speakers.

In contrast to agrammatic Broca's aphasics, individuals with a purely anomic aphasia perform far better on naming pictured actions than in naming objects (Zingeser and Berndt, 1990). Yet, the association of verb superiority with anomia and of noun superiority with agrammatic aphasia is not without exceptions. Zingeser and Berndt (1990) showed that selective difficulties for nouns versus verbs may be dissociated from their expected relationship to aphasia type. Thus the noun/verb dissociation joins other category-specific lexical retrieval dissociations in search of a satisfactory explanation. The receptive aspect of category-specific dissociations will be reviewed in Chapter 7 on auditory comprehension.

MODALITY-SPECIFIC ANOMIA

The great bulk of observations of naming disorders give no suggestion that anomia is related to the sensory modality through which the stimulus is presented. However, the fact that clear-cut instances have been described in which patients failed to name objects presented through a particular sense modality led several investigators to study this relationship in series of patients. Spreen, Benton, and Van Allen (1966) compared 21 patients who had anomic aphasia with respect to naming by touch and naming by visual confrontation. They found that only five were superior either in tactile over visual presentation, or visual over tactile stimulation. The remaining 16 showed no difference between sense modalities of stimulation. Goodglass, Barton, and Kaplan (1968) compared naming to olfaction, touch, vision, and sound, finding that only 2 of 12 subjects showed a significant dissociation between sensory modalities. They concluded that with few exceptions, regardless of the sensory modality through which an object is experienced, the activation of its name is mediated by a concept that is modality independent.

Optic Aphasia

The rare instances in which an object can be recognized, but not named on visual presentation are well documented and were first described by Freund (1889) using the term "optic aphasia." In these cases, evidence of recognition is that the patient can pantomime the use of a stimulus object or give a verbal account of its features, without being able to name it. Bauer and Rubens (1985) suggest that the distinction between visual agnosia and optic aphasia is not a reliable one. Rather, they report that patients who are unable to recognize what they see, may evolve to a state in which they can describe or pantomime the use of seen objects, but still cannot name them. Although the fine localization that distinguishes optic aphasia from visual agnosia has not been delineated, the lesions involved are always at the fringe of the visual association areas of the occipital lobe, such that they may interrupt the outflow of information from visual to language areas.

Callosal Disconnection Anomias

The most clear cut and dramatic modality-specific naming disorders are those resulting from the interruption of fibers that carry visual or tactile information from the right hemisphere to the language zones of the left hemisphere. Geschwind and Kaplan's (1962) patient could correctly manipulate such objects as scissors and comb with his left hand, but could not name them until they were placed in his right hand. Gazzaniga, Bogen, and Sperry's (1965) callosectomized subjects could name any object that was briefly flashed in their right visual field, but denied having seen those that were flashed in the left.

MODELS OF NAMING

The assessment of naming disorders is almost invariably based on naming to visual (pictorial) confrontation. Theorists agree that in this condition, the retrieval of the phonological form of a concept name is initiated by some features of the visual stimulus that identify it as a known object with a unique configuration of semantic properties. At this point, theories of visual confrontation naming diverge into *serial stage* models and *parallel processing* models.

In normal discourse, however, the activation of concept names is not initiated by pictures. In fact, only a minority of the concepts whose names we produce are picturable at all. Some are actions, abstract nouns, adjectives, or adverbs. If picture naming and concept naming in free discourse share a common process, it must begin with the activation of a configuration of semantic property representations that are best satisfied by either a unique phonological string (i.e., a word) or by a small set of possible candidate strings.

But the generation of words in free discourse is subject to many more dynamically interacting influences than is the case for confrontation naming. For one, the preceding verbal context exercises word associational influences. Thus, in the context, "The pitcher threw the...," the utterance "ball" is so overdetermined that the activation of the concept of "a ball" is redundant, and may play little role in the generation of the phonological form "ball." Furthermore, evidence from slips of the tongue indicates that two or more word forms that are destined for slots downstream in a sentence may be activated concurrently, so that a word that is in readiness may be uttered prematurely in the slot intended for another one. This would result, for example in the production, "Put the pot on that lid" for "Put the lid on that pot."

For these and other reasons, the much more constrained task of visual confrontation naming is the basic paradigm used for creating and testing models of word retrieval, even though it can be applied only to picturable objects.

SERIAL STAGE MODELS

The traditional modeling approach regards object naming as the outcome of a series of operations, each of which must be completed in turn, with the output of each stage passed along to the next. Stage models may either be conceived in purely psychological terms or else assigned to anatomical structures in the brain. For example, consider one of the most clearly elaborated contemporary models of staged psychological processes: that of Levelt (1989).

In this schema, the perception of a picture or object to be named gives rise to a complex of semantic features associated with the object. Among these features is a "core" characteristic which unequivocally distinguishes the concept of this object from other semantically or visually similar objects. The next stage of processing is the activation of the unique word concept that satisfies the activated semantic properties. This word concept is referred to in Levelt's model as the "lemma." Other theorists (e.g., Dell, 1986) use the term "word node" for the same construct. The lemma does not itself have any phonological properties—it represents the sense that one has a word available that precisely matches the required semantic configuration, as well as the syntactic restrictions that are entailed (e.g., if animate, it may take verbs of possession, sensation, mental state, and so on).

Normally, only a single lemma is chosen, although in rare instances competing lemmas result in competing phonology. Errors in lemma selection may result from competition between similar concepts or from verbal association between lemmas.

Once a lemma is selected, it uniquely addresses one entry in the phonological lexicon, a store of phonogical word forms, and this entry is then realized, syllable by syllable, as a phonetic plan for articulation. The phonetic plan is then transferred to the motor implementation system. Experimental evidence obtained by Sternberg *et al.* (1978) indicates that in single word naming, the phonetic plan is completed before articulation begins; the longer the planned word, the longer the latency to voice onset. Hence, an articulatory buffer, or temporary storage mechanism, is postulated so that as the beginning of a word is realized in articulation, the rest of it can be held in readiness.

This type of serial stage psycholinguistic model is most readily translated into a serial stage anatomical model, such as that of Geschwind (1969). Geschwind proposes that when an object is to be named, visual form recognition is mediated in the occipital lobe and transferred to the region of the left angular gyrus, where the concept is generated. The phonological form is then activated in Wernicke's area and transmitted via the arcuate fasciculus to Broca's area, where it is converted to a motor plan that is then implemented via the motor cortex. The correspondence between the psycholinguistic and anatomical models is illustrated in Fig. 5.1.

A psycholinguistic model that postulates that words and their syllable and segmental constituents are stored and retrieved from a lexicon as needed can be adapted successfully to an account of many types of normal speech errors, or "slips of the tongue" (Levelt, 1989). For example:

Word choice errors may result from the misselection of a word node that has been activated by a close associate to the target concept ("comb" becomes "brush").

Word choice errors may result from the activation of a word node linked by verbal association to the target word ("comb" becomes "hair").

Phonological segments or even whole morphemes may be transposed from one slot to another or interchanged ("feel like playing" becomes "peel like flaying"; cited by Levelt, 1989, from Shattuck-Hufnagel, 1982).

The anatomical model also has *prima facie* support from well-known clinical observations. For example, optic aphasia, as described earlier, supports the reality of the first step in the anatomic sequence; that is, the step from visual association cortex to the language zone. Geschwind's attribution of a central role in naming to the left angular gyrus is based on both anatomic and clinical grounds. Anatomically, this zone appears to serve as a convergence area for connections from auditory, visual, and tactile association areas. Geschwind argued that the development of this convergence area in humans makes it possible for us to assign names to concepts—a capacity lacking in any subhuman forms. On the clinical side, the angular gyrus is one of the sites in which a lesion may produce

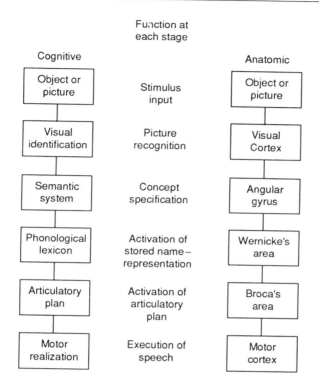

Figure 5.1. Parallels between cognitive and anatomic serial stage models of object naming.

a pure anomic aphasia, without impairment of auditory comprehension.

The assignment of auditory word forms to Wernicke's area has been a popular notion, originating with Wernicke himself. Luria (1970), too, notes that lesions of this zone result in the disorganization of the sound representation of words, along with severe name retrieval difficulty. The role of the arculate fasciculus as the transmission pathway between Wernicke's area and Broca's area can be traced historically to Lichtheim's model (1884), where such a connection was seen as essential for the act of repeating a heard word. Geschwind argued from anatomical data that patients with conduction aphasia had lesions deep to the supramarginal gyrus that were along the path of the arcuate fasciculus. Finally, the attribution of the motor implementation stage of Broca's area is a simple extension of the well-known observation that articulation is the speech function most specifically affected by injury to the anterior speech zone.

Yet, a closer examination of the evidence from the naming failures of aphasic patients indicates that both the psycholinguistic stage model and its anatomical counterpart are considerably oversimplified. On the anatomic side, the stage model would require that aphasics with lesions anterior to (or downstream from) Wernicke's area should have tacit knowledge of the phonology of words that they are attempting to name, even when they cannot implement the articulation. This is simply not the case. Goodglass *et al.* (1976) found that Broca's aphasics were not significantly better than chance in identifying the first sound or the number of syllables of a target word. Conduction aphasics, who were superior to all other subgroups, could do so for only one-third of the targets that they failed to name. Nor is there evidence that patients with angular gyrus lesions either have more impaired word retrieval or more impaired conceptualization than those with anterior speech zone lesions.

On the psycholinguistic side, it is apparent that the word production errors of aphasic cannot be accounted for by a model predicated on the activation of just those phonological segments that correspond to a particular lexical entry. In the following examples of partial phonological retrieval, we see that neither syllable sequence nor internal syllable structure need be honored. The patient may begin with any salient phonological feature of the target word and add phonological associates from left to right, or right to left. Segments incorporated into the utterance obey English phonotactic rules, but may be totally unrelated to the target.

TARGET PICTURE	RESPONSE
whistle	tris . . .chi . . .trisle . . .sissle . . .twiss
mask	nas . . .nasp . . .nap
mask (second patient)	fask . . .fac- fan . . .fan . . .face . . .fisk
harmonica	con . . .caca . . .commat . . .mon . . .no!
rhinoceros	reenosaurns . . .ryahoceros

The following examples of word choice errors have superficial resemblance to semantic slips of the tongue; that is, it is usually possible to discern a semantic link to the target. However, they are not accidental exchanges, because the correct alternative is not available to the aphasic speaker; furthermore, the associative link is often much more remote than would be plausible in a "normal" slip of the tongue.

TARGET PICTURE	RESPONSE
tongs	choppers
visor	a sunrise lid
pinwheel	a flower . . .it's a toy . . .a daisy

These errors from aphasic patients appear to expose the workings of lexical phonological retrieval at an earlier level in its unfolding than is tapped by slips of the tongue from normal speakers. They suggest that word phonology is assembled around an initial precurser, usually including the stressed vowel and often a conspicuous consonant cluster as well (e.g., "con" for "harmonica" "kella" for "helicopter"). Contamination with semantically associated morphemes is frequent even in primarily phonogically dominated errors ("renosaurns" for "rhinoceros"; "face" and its variants contaminated with "mask").

AN ATTEMPT AT INTEGRATION

While accepting the positive contributions of the sequential staged models—both anatomic and psycholinguistic as working hypotheses—it is apparent that they paint a deceptively neat picture. It does not seem likely that the brain's solution for the naming process includes either strictly sequential localized stages or stores of word forms or syllables. Contemporary neural network models of the parallel processing type (e.g., McClelland and Rumelhart, 1986) suggest a way of recasting the concept of name retrieval that may dispense with such traditional constructs as the lexicon.

The author and colleagues (Goodglass *et al.*, 1991) have proposed a model (Fig. 5.2) for picture naming that is more open to accommodating the preceding types of aphasic naming errors, without diminishing its adaptability to normal slips of the tongue. Although the model is explicitly framed in terms of the naming of visually presented objects, it can, in principle, be adapted to concept name retrieval in free discourse.

In this model, as the structural features of a familiar object emerge from the early visual processing of a picture, activation spreads into three tracks:

1. *A very rapid and poorly differentiated activation of a broad range of semantic properties of the perceived object.* Evidence for such activation is the enhancement of recognizability of words associated to a preceding picture; that is, words that share some of its semantic properties. Goodglass *et al.* (1991) detected such enhancement for the recognition of written words, 100 msec after a semantically related priming picture. Levelt *et al.* (1991) detected early enhancement in the recognition of spoken words after a semantically related picture.

In the author's view, this activation serves the biological role of rapidly alerting the individual to significant connotations in incoming stimuli. But in the word retrieval process, it serves as a "spoiler," rather than as

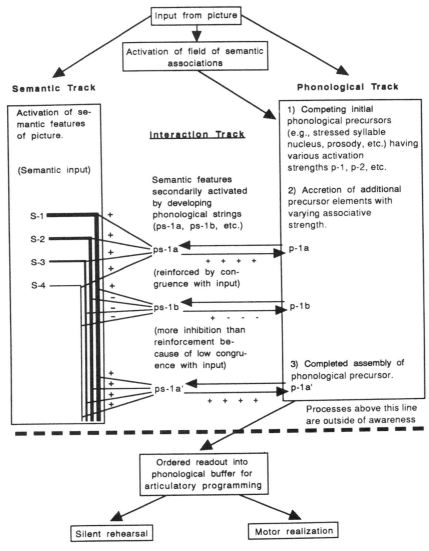

Figure 5.2.   A proposed spreading activation model of picture naming. In this schema a continuously developing process is portrayed as though it is broken down into successive steps. Specifically, we assume that perceptual analysis of the object picture is accompanied by continuously developing activation of semantic features of the object and activation of corresponding phonology.

Initial competing phonological precurser elements are labeled p-1, p-2, etc. As they activate additional associated phonological elements, the resulting competing clusters are represented as p-1a, p-1b, p-2a, etc. (Only p-1a and p-1b are shown.) Each developing cluster of phonological features activates semantic features (ps 1-a, ps-1b) that an early stage of word access—spoiler, because it can be suggested that this broad activation is the source of semantically based errors that have the opportunity to emerge when the more focused aspects of word retrieval (components 2 and 3) are dysfunctional.

2. *The "semantic track."* Activation of semantic properties specific to the target object. In the diagram (Fig. 5.2), this component is termed "semantic input." It is the reference criterion from which developing phonological strings receive either reinforcement or inhibition (see component 4).

3. *The "phonological track."* Activation of the earliest phonological precursor(s) of the target word as immediate associate(s) to the earliest specification of visual object identity. The first activations may involve precursors of more than one possible response word, resulting in an early competition between candidates. Phonological precursors of off-target responses may also be spun off from the broad semantic activation described as component 1.

The earliest phonological precursors are presumed most often to include the syllable nucleus (initial consonant plus vowel) of the stressed syllable. The word onset, even when it is not the stressed syllable, also appears to have an advantage as the element most likely to lead to successful completion of a word (Kohn *et al.*, 1987). In this model, we refer to the activity assigned to the right-hand column as the "phonological track." This corresponds to our presumption that the first phonological elements to be activated accrete both preceding and following phonological elements that have occurred with them in the speaker's past experience of speech production. The activation strength of an initial phonological precursor is presumed to depend on the frequency and the exclusivity of its concurrence with the eliciting picture or semantic content. The phonological track, then, is conceived as a collection of developing phonological groupings, in competition with each other, beginning with one or more initial precursor. The core of the name retrieval process is described as component 4, the "interaction track." This component is the locus of interaction between candidate groupings of phonological elements and the semantic input provided by the picture

---

receive reinforcement or inhibition (marked + or −) through congruence or lack of congruence with input semantic features (S1, S2, etc.). This reinforcement or inhibition is fed back to the developing phonological precursors (feedback is symbolized by the lower of the two-way arrows). In this diagram, only p-1a is assumed to gain the reinforcement to go on to completion as p-1a'.

Temporal relationships between phonological elements are assumed to be coded, but not represented in real time in the precursor stage (above heavy dotted line), but this coding is converted to real time in the readout.

(component 2). Such interaction results in reinforcement of semantically congruent and inhibition of noncongruent phonological groupings.

The following are two more characteristics of the activity of the phonological track: (a) The initial phonological activation need not be limited to a syllable nucleus. If the activation is strong enough, it may involve a number of salient phonological features of the target word, or even a whole word. In such instances, our model is not very different from a model that postulates a store of preformed lexical forms. (b) Phonological activity is in a coded form that is not accessible to consciousness. Even though this activity is to be converted downstream to articulatory instructions and corresponding auditory imagery, it is not yet experienced as an auditory representation. In our conception, the representations of phonological precursers may well be unordered in real time, but carry coded information concerning phonological order. For example, syllables that are coded as word-final and word-initial may be in an activated state at the same time in the same cluster in the phonological track.

4. The "interaction track." While the assembly of phonological groupings is in progress, partially assembled, competing candidate groupings are passing activation along to their own semantic associates. These secondarily activated semantic associates, in turn, receive reinforcement or inhibition from the original semantic input, depending on whether they match or conflict with it. This reinforcement or inhibition is passed on to the phonological cluster that gave rise to the secondary semantic activation. In most cases, semantically noncongruent phonological clusters are eliminated early, and the optimal response reaches threshold for readout into a rehearsal buffer. If no phonological cluster has reached threshold after about 1500 msec, the speaker becomes aware of a word-finding delay.

The completion of the assembly of the phonological precurser cluster, or the awareness that no response is available, marks the access to awareness of the product of the interaction track. Goodglass, Theurkauf, and Wingfield (1984) reported evidence that 1500 msec marked a transition between normal "automatic" word finding and the awareness of prolonged effort, without success up to that point. Our view, expressed in the studies by Kohn *et al.* (1987) and Goodglass, Wingfield, and Wayland (1989) is that the interaction track continues its work as long as the individual remains in the set to name the stimulus, and continues to be inaccessible to consciousness. Although the speaker may make conscious efforts to hasten word retrieval by bringing associations to mind, our evidence is that most such efforts have only an illusory effect. The time to word retrieval is unpredictable in cases of prolonged search; once the retrieval threshold is attained, it is completed in milliseconds, and the desired word (or name) subjectively pops into mind out of the blue.

For the normal speaker, when the preconscious phase of word retrieval is complete, the word enters a rehearsal buffer to be read into the motor realization system or played out in subvocal rehearsal. This is the first conscious experience of the word as an auditory representation. We have proposed that precurser phonology is a temporally unordered cluster of elements. The chief reason for this proposal is that precurser phonology would consume an inordinate amount of time if it were deployed in real time, from left to right. But this proposal means that the temporal coding of the phonological elements is read into a real time representation in the rehearsal buffer. This is one transition which may be a source of errors in sound ordering. The next source of errors is in the conversion to motor articulatory instructions. Both of these error sites are "postlexical" in the sense referred to earlier in this chapter. They are likely to be the points at which normal slips of the tongue and some of the phonological errors of conduction aphasics enter the speech stream.

To be sure, this is a highly conjectural model. Its significance in this context is that it shows that it is possible to conceive of a word being regenerated on each occasion of its use, thus dispensing with the notion of a lexicon of preformed words. We argued earlier that the errors encountered in aphasia appeared to be incompatible with such a lexicon. In this model, the interaction track is the highly vulnerable filtering apparatus that normally suppresses mismatches of any sort between phonological elements and the intended semantic message. The phonological track may be the source of both phonological and semantic paraphasias, any of which may survive to realization if the interaction track is dysfunctional, even if the input semantic track is intact.

Chapter **6**

Disorders of Syntax and Morphology

Syntax refers to the collection of devices evolved in natural languages for representing the almost endless variety of relationships among words that a speaker can use to convey information, questions, orders, and emotional states. Syntax includes the use of word order and highly standardized conventions for grouping and marking relationships between thought units. Relationships are marked through the use of free-standing grammatical operators, appended markers, or other rule-governed modifications in the phonological structure of lexical terms that specify their relationship to other terms. The system of rules for the modifications of word forms to signify their relationships to other words in the sentence is the "morphology" of the language. Morphology, therefore, is intimately related to syntax and, in some circumstances, is understood to be included by that term.

Why such an abstractly formulated definition of syntax in a volume on aphasia? The reason is that it is necessary at the outset to dispel the popular assumption that syntax represents an undifferentiated psychological capacity that can be damaged or spared as a unit in various forms of aphasia. Careful analysis of the impairments in sentence usage by aphasics shows, for example, that the use of word order is resistant to damage both in the production and interpretation of sentence meanings. For English speakers, it is natural to assume that the first noun or pronoun is the subject (or actor) and that the noun or pronoun following the verb is the object of the action (or patient). Word order is a conspicuous feature of a sentence and may dominate its interpretation, even when small grammatical morphemes (is, -ed, and by in the sentence "The horse is kicked by the dog") impose the reverse assignment of the roles of actor and patient.

In English, the subject-verb-object (SVO) word order is the basic or "canonical" sequence. This particular canonical sequence is shared by many languages, but not by all. Japanese, for example, is an SOV language. In some languages, the animacy or inanimacy of a noun may have a compelling role in determining which term is the subject. In such languages, it is clear that semantics is tightly bound up with syntax. Bates and her co-workers (Bates *et al.*, 1991; Tzeng *et al.*, 1991; Vaid and Pandit, 1991) have shown that the expectations that differ between speakers of various languages persist after a person is aphasic. In the case of individuals who are bilingual, the expectations of meaning interpretations that are derived from word order or from noun animacy may result in different interpretations in the two languages of the same patient, depending on which language she or he is tested in.

Speakers of a minimally inflected language, like English, are hardly aware of such syntactic variables as the case of a noun or pronoun or the mood or aspect of a verb, unless they have studied a foreign language in which these subtle differences in grammatical function are obligatorily marked. Grammatical relationships that are indicated by a case marking preposition in one language may be signaled by a morphological change in a noun in another language, or else not marked at all. For example, in English, verbs like "to order," "to instruct," or "to obey," take a direct object ("He ordered the child to clean his room"); in other western languages they take an indirect object (e.g., French: "Il a demandé à l'enfant de nettoyer sa chambre").

There are much deeper differences among the languages of the world with respect to relationships that must be marked in some but that are ignored in others. For example, gender differences among common nouns is unknown in English, but must be correctly expressed in many other languages. On the other hand, the Germanic and Romance languages use definite and indefinite articles which are absent from Russian, Chinese, and many other languages and which create obstacles for learning their use by speakers of those languages.

Considerations about the nature of syntactic operations in the production and comprehension of connected speech are central to the interpretation of the phenomenon of agrammatism in aphasia.

AGRAMMATISM—CLINICAL PRESENTATION

From the early nineteenth century, when attention began to be paid to the peculiarly linguistic aspects of aphasic output disorders, a distinctive form of linguistic breakdown was noted. The earliest description of agrammatism that we have found is that cited by Tissot, Mounin, and Lhermitte (1973), attributed to an 1819 work by Deleuze: The patient "used exclusively the infinitive of verbs and used no pronouns. For example, she said, 'Souhaiter bonjour, rester, mari venir.' (Wish [infinitive] good day; stay [inf.]; husband come [inf.]). She produced absolutely no conjugated verb."

Deleuze's summary characterization of this speech pattern underwent little change in the next century. For example, Alajouanine (1968) defines agrammatism in the following terms:

Agrammatism is hard to define other than by the essential fact which the patient's speech makes evident; reduction of the sentence to its skeleton, relative abundance of substantives, almost invariable use of verbs in the infinitive, with suppression of the small words and loss of grammatical differentiation of tense, gender, number, as well as of subordination; the richer a language is in distinctions of these types, the more glaring agrammatism will appear and it will grow still more apparent as recovery of access to vocabulary takes place (whence the impression that agrammatism seems to increase in severity in the course of reeducation). This agrammatic difficulty is seen also in oral reading and in writing to dictation (p. 84).

PSEUDOAGRAMMATISM

In the following examples, the sparsity of grammatical morphemes in relation to the nouns and principal verbs is obvious because the patients quoted are producing enough speech to create grammatically obligatory contexts for the omitted forms. But in the earliest stage of recovery from nonfluent aphasia, one usually hears only single-word utterances, laboriously retrieved and produced in response to questions. For example, "What happened to you?" Patient: "'troke ... stroke." It is not to be assumed that the patient's failure to respond "I had a stroke" is an instance of agrammatism. At this stage, we prefer to use the term "pseudoagrammatism," considering these one-word responses to be similar to the holophrastic sentences of very young children. (The term "pseudoagrammatism" was first applied by Pick (1913) to the speech of the severely retarded.) Pseudoagrammatism may evolve, with recovery, either toward fully grammatical or toward prototypically agrammatic speech.

Agrammatism

As patients' access to lexical words improves, they begin to convey information by either stringing one-word sentences together or by multiword utterances in which the absence of obligatory grammatical morphemes becomes apparent, as does the primitive nature of the syntactic juxtapositions. The following dialogue is a sample of such totally agrammatic output from one of the author's patients.

> E: Can you tell me about why you came back to the hospital?
> P: Yes . . . eh . . . Monday . . . eh . . . dad . . . Peter Hogan and dad . . . hospital.
> Er . . . two . . . er . . . doctors . . . and . . . er . . . thirty minutes . . . and . . . er . . . yes . . . hospital. And . . . er . . . Wednesday . . . Wednesday. Nine o'clock. And . . . er . . . Thursday, ten o'clock . . . doctors . . . two . . . two . . . doctors . . . and . . . er . . . teeth . . . fine.
> E: Not exactly your teeth . . . your g-
> P: Gum . . . gum . . .
> E: What did they do to them?
> P: And er . . . doctor and girl . . . and er . . . and er gum . . .

Myerson's analysis (Myerson and Goodglass, 1972) of this patient's grammatical repertory showed that it consisted of the following:

1. An utterance may consist of a Noun Phrase *or* a Verb Phrase, either one optionally followed by an adverb, *or* of an adverb alone.
2. Up to two utterances may be linked by "and," but by no other conjunction.
3. A Verb Phrase consists of a verb stem plus an optional *ing* plus an optional particle. Thus, an example of maximum verb stem expansion is "falling down." Alternatively, a Verb Phrase may consist of a predicate adjective, without expression of the copula.
4. Adverbs may be in the form "one day" or as place names without prepositions. Adverbs of time may consist of a Noun Phrase of measure, optionally followed by an adverb (e.g., four years ago).
5. Noun Phrases consist of a noun optionally preceded by a cardinal number. Nouns are not preceded by an article, but they are pluralized as required by a preceding number. The indefinite article is used after a noun of measure, as in "five hundred tons a day."

A sample from one of Luria's (1970) patients shows severe agrammatism in a patient who has recovered considerable vocabulary. In telling about a recent movie, he says:

"Odessa! a swindler! down there . . . to study . . . the sea . . . (gesture of diving) . . . into . . . a diver! Armenia . . . a ship . . . went . . . oh! Batum! a girl . . . ah! Policeman . . . ah . . . I know! . . . cashier! . . . money . . . ah! . . . cigarettes . . . I know . . . this guy," etc.

Telegraphic Speech

With further recovery from agrammatism, word groupings and simple sentences appear, scattered among agrammatic forms. Commonly, verb + object combinations appear before subject + verb combinations. Even when all the main elements of an SVO sentence appear, some grammatical deletions may persist—particularly deletions of articles, auxiliary verbs, and prepositions. Sentences with a deleted main verb ("Joan and I . . . coffee") may continue to appear. This stage of partially recovered agrammatism is referred to as "telegraphic speech" because of its resemblance to the elliptical constructions used for economy of words in a telegram.

VARIANTS OF AGRAMMATISM: PROBLEMS OF DEFINITION

We have called attention at the beginning of this chapter to the fact that the manifestations of agrammatism differ from language to language. Yet even within a single language, the details of grammatical aberrations may vary from patient to patient. These variations make it extremely difficult to provide a firm descriptive definition of the disorder that can be unambiguously applied. This has provoked particular conflict among theoretical neurolinguists seeking a definition that can be formulated in terms of specific linguistic operations.

DEFICIENCY IN MORPHOLOGY OR SYNTAX?

The prototypical form of agrammatism entails both omissions of grammatical functors and a breakdown of sentence structure into groupings that rarely exceed three or four syntactically related words. Agrammatism is so regularly associated with nonfluency of speech output that it is often cited as one of the defining features of nonfluency. Geschwind likened the pattern of fluent, but morphologically defective, speech to a caricature of "cigar-store Indian" talk and felt that it was indicative of a malingered speech defect. Nevertheless, fluent output, with characteristically agrammatic misuse or deletions of morphology, has been described by knowledgeable observers. A particularly amusing incident in the author's own experience involved a patient who spoke in complete, but morphologically defective sentences, characterized by the omission of verb inflections and constant substitution of the strong form "me" of the first person pronoun in place of "I." After one of innumerable corrections by his speech therapist, he exclaimed:

"I! I! Everybody tell me 'I'! But me forget!"

Other cases of fluently produced, structurally complete sentences with agrammatic errors of morphology were described by Miceli *et al.* (1983).

Tissot, Mounin, and Lhermitte (1973), in a study of 19 French-speaking agrammatic aphasics, observed that many of their patients appeared to suffer from either primarily syntactic or primarily morphological forms of agrammatism. Those with primarily syntactic disorders produced fragmented sentence structures, but within phrasal word groups the use of articles, pronouns, and prepositions was predominantly normal. Those with primarily morphological deficiencies produced SVO sentences, but deleted pronouns, prepositions, and auxiliary verbs. Their patients could not be considered to have a purely morphological agrammatism (as could those of Miceli *et al.*) or a purely syntactic agrammatism. For example, the substitution of infinitives for finite inflected verb forms was observed in both types of agrammatic patients.

OTHER VARIATIONS IN LINGUISTIC SYMPTOMATOLOGY

Except in the cases of the most severely agrammatic patients, there are few constructions and morphological forms that are not available on occasion, within simple (nonembedded) sentences. Gleason *et al.* (1975) found that their agrammatic subjects produced correct output on at least one of their efforts in each of ten constructions. Gleason (unpublished) found that although there is an overall hierarchy of difficulty for the production of morphological forms by English speaking agrammatic aphasics, this is not constant across patients. For example, some individuals usually delete articles but not the plural *s* marker; others do the reverse. Miceli *et al.* (1989) found that there is so much variability from patient to patient in the structures that are failed by agrammatic speakers (in Italian) that it is futile to attempt a definition of this disorder in terms of specific linguistic structures that are affected. There is, however, general concurrence as to a number of prototypical features that create a "family resemblance" among patients who are judged to be clinically agrammatic—at least among speakers of English and the European languages in which the phenomenon was first described, French, German, Russian, and Italian. The variations in symptomatology to be found in other languages will be developed later in this chapter.

PARAGRAMMATISM

The difficulty in characterizing the "true" underlying deficit in agrammatism is highlighted by attempts to contrast and distinguish it from "paragrammatism." In their clinical presentation, prototypical instances of these two disorders make a very different impression on the listener. In contrast to the nonfluent, dysprosodic output of the agrammatic, the patient with paragrammatism usually speaks at a normal or hyperfluent rate, with natural speech prosody. In spite of the presence of inappropriately chosen or neologistic words, there is no lack of morphology—that is, articles, prepositions, auxiliary verbs, and noun and verb inflections fall into place just as effortlessly as in the speech of a normal person. Whereas the variety and complexity of sentence structures is reduced on average, some patients produce long sentences with embedded constructions and sentences that begin with a subordinate clause. This is not to say that paragrammatic speakers do not also omit and substitute grammatical morphemes. Beyond errors with the "little words" of grammar, they also produce forms in which the syntactic structure is incoherent and aimless, with nouns appearing in verb slots and vice versa. (See the extract of paragrammatic speech quoted in Chapter 5.)

The fact that both agrammatism and paragrammatism affect the same language domain led to the use of the terms "expressive agrammatism" and "receptive agrammatism"—the latter applied to the fluent form because of its typical association with receptive (Wernicke's) aphasia. The term "paragrammatism" was proposed by Kleist (1913) and has persisted.

Nevertheless, not all writers agree that there is a fundamental difference in the syntactic capacity of paragrammatic as compared to agrammatic patients. In particular, they reject the view that paragrammatic speech indicates the preservation of syntactic skills that have been lost by agrammatics. For example, Heeschen (1985) argued that these contrasting speech output patterns were an artifact of different adaptive strategies available to fluent and nonfluent patients in an unconstrained speech situation. Specifically, Heeschen believed that agrammatics use a strategy of avoidance; that is, they delete rather than produce erroneous forms.

As a test of this hypothesis, he subjected a group of paragrammatic aphasics and a group of agrammatics to the task of describing simple subject-action-object pictures in complete sentences. He found that in this experimental constraint the proportion of grammatical morphemes produced by agrammatics increased over the proportion that they produced in spontaneous speech so that it was similar to that produced spontaneously by paragrammatics. However, this increase in proportion of grammatical morphemes by agrammatics was totally accounted for by the increase in errors. In short, Heeschen found a way to make agrammatic patients resemble paragrammatics by obliging them to attempt morphological forms that they did not produce correctly and that they tended to avoid in free conversation.

Although Heeschen correctly argues that the underlying syntactic deficit cannot be directly inferred from unconstrained speech, it is not possible to accept his experimental results as negating other clinical observations. For example, minimally constrained narrative or free conversation allows paragrammatic patients the opportunity to freely use subordinating constructions and verb morphology that are unlikely to be elicited in the highly constrained sentence creation task that was used in Heeschen's study—constructions that can almost never be elicited from agrammatics under any conditions. Thus, the highly constrained picture description task may itself create an artifactual leveling of performance.

The difficulty of capturing the difference between agrammatic and nonagrammatic aphasic speech through constrained elicitation techniques is also illustrated by Goodglass and Mayer's (1958) effort. They required their subjects to repeat sentences of progressive length and grammatical complexity. They found that the most discriminating errors of the agrammatics are those based on a molar analysis of sentence patterns that reflect a tendency to fall back on the most habituated and simple constructions. These included (1) the use of stereotyped but inappropriate sentence openers; (2) the loss of subordination and coordination between clauses; and (3) loss of the inverted interrogative word order. Omissions of grammatical morphemes were only marginally more frequent for the agrammatics. These patients actually had more inappropriately inserted or substituted grammatical morphemes than did nonagrammatics. Clearly, there are no grounds for considering an omission of a grammatical morpheme to be an agrammatic error and a substitution of one to be a paragrammatic error, as has been the practice in recent studies.

EXPRESSIVE/RECEPTIVE AGRAMMATISM: EARLY RESEARCH

Although agrammatism was initially described as a speech output disorder, it did not escape the conjecture of Salomon (1914) that it might have a receptive counterpart. He had this possibility in mind when he required an agrammatic patient to make grammaticality judgments, offering his patient sentences that either conformed to or violated German grammar. On the basis of his patient's failures in these judgments of grammaticality, Salomon concluded that receptive agrammatism might regularly coexist with expressive agrammatism. Salomon's observations were followed by those of Forster (1919) and Isserlin (1922). Forster's agrammatic subject had intact comprehension of grammatical structures; Isserlin's three agrammatic patients showed comprehension of grammar ranging from virtually intact to severely defective. Isserlin's conclusion, shared by others of his era and by Ombredane (1951), was that receptive difficulties in the comprehension of syntax are autonomous from agrammatism, they may be found in agrammatic patients, but are more regularly observed in those with sensory (Wernicke's) aphasia. The author agrees with the opinion of Tissot *et al.* that the failure to distinguish between well-formed and ungrammatical speech is a commonplace and undiscriminating feature of the most severe cases of aphasia—cases that include many patients who are agrammatic, as well as those who are not.

SPEECH, WRITING, REPETITION, AND ORAL READING

Most patients who are severely agrammatic in their speech production are similarly impaired in their writing (if they can write), and in their oral repetition. Goodglass and Hunter (1970) found that their agrammatic patient had more fragmented syntax in his writing than in his free narrative. They attributed this difference to the facilitation of syntax provided by the speed and prosody of speech, even nonfluent, agrammatic speech. However, other observers (e.g., Isserlin, 1922; Pick, 1931), insist that patients with agrammatism usually write in more grammatically complete form because the stability of the written production and the opportunity to think through and correct efforts relieve the urgency and time pressure of oral communication. There is no shortage of reports in the literature of patients who are agrammatic in speech but who write normally. This was the case in the two Italian-speaking patients described by Miceli *et al.* (1983) and in the case of a Japanese agrammatic described by Sasanuma, Akio, and Kubota (1990).

Partial or total disappearance of agrammatism when the patient is given a model to repeat is also commonly observed. This was the case with Isserlin's (1922) first patient, both in repetition and in reporting orally what he had read. Goodglass and Mayer's patients, however, and the patient described by Goodglass, Fodor, and Schulhoff (1967) were tested with repetition tasks and clearly displayed their syntactic deficits under those conditions. Opportunities to compare speech and writing in agrammatic patients are limited by the fact that many of these patients are too severely agraphic to justify such comparisons.

Oral reading is also subject to specific deficits that sometimes make a comparison with speech production questionable. In particular, the problem of deep dyslexia may coexist with agrammatism. In this disorder, patients may be unable to read aloud the free grammatical morphemes of the language, whether presented as isolated words or in connected text.

They also ignore or substitute bound morphemes (verb inflections) and derivational affixes. The mechanism by which grammatical morphemes are particularly affected in deep dyslexia is different from that which makes them the target of errors in agrammatism. Nevertheless, the oral reading of a deep dyslexic patient sounds agrammatic and may lead to the incorrect conclusion that agrammatism is equally expressed in free conversation and oral reading.

Unfortunately, systematic comparisons of oral reading and free conversation of agrammatic patients are not common in the literature. The English speaking agrammatic patients described in the work by Menn and Obler (1990) were almost free of agrammatism in oral reading of connected text. This was interpreted as indicating that these agrammatic patients needed only to have the grammatical morphemes supplied for them in order to produce organized sentences with adequate prosody. The counterpart of this explanation is that given the impossibility of spontaneously accessing the essential grammatical morphemes, the patient adopts a form of expression (i.e., agrammatism) in which she can maximize her communicative effectiveness using those words that are available to her.

On the surface, the appearance of agrammatism in speech but not in writing would appear to argue for a disorder that exclusively affects the oral production of grammatical words. But the fact that it also commonly affects both of these output modalities would support a view that assumes an impairment affecting an underlying fund of grammatical knowledge. On the other hand, implicit in many writers' interpretations is the assumption that the agrammatic is not deficient in his or her underlying knowledge of syntax, but is making a strategic adaptation to a particular output problem. In the next section, we will consider some of the theoretical efforts at understanding the mechanisms of this disorder and the experimental work that supports these efforts.

EXPLANATORY THEORY AND RESEARCH

Agrammatism as Economy of Effort

A number of authors have offered the view that the agrammatic style emerges as an adaptation to the patient's difficulty in producing speech. Because of this difficulty, the agrammatic goes directly to the terms that convey the most information. Pick (1923) suggested the German term "Notsprache" (emergency speech) to describe the tendency to eliminate all redundant words under the stress of an impaired speech system— whether due to aphasia or other factors, such as limited mastery of the language. Pick's concept of economy of effort reappears in contemporary neurolinguistic theory in the form of Heeschen's formulation (described earlier) and Kolk's formulation.

Kolk *et al.* (1985) argue that agrammatism does not represent the loss of syntactic knowledge or ability, but rather a slowing of the process of computing the structures to be used or of retrieving the specific grammatical morphemes involved. The recourse to agrammatic forms of expression represents a decision made by the patient as to a strategy he or she may use to adapt to this difficulty. An alternative might be to speak very slowly, in simplified, but complete grammatical forms. However, difficulties with short-term memory for partially computed utterances may make it impossible to complete a message without an inordinate number of fresh starts. The patient quickly learns that the telegraphic style is more efficient because it allows shorter syntactic strings and hence a shorter load on short-term memory. Note that the chief difference between Kolk's formulation and that of Pick (i.e., "Notsprache") lies in Kolk's emphasis on the voluntary strategic choice entailed in agrammatism and Pick's implication that the patient is following a biological principle of economy of effort. For both of these authors, the fact that the form of expression changes with the nature of the communicative situation is evidence against a loss of knowledge. Both of them cite written expression as one form that is not as tolerant of omissions and errors as is oral discourse.

Kolk, like Heeschen, presents evidence that agrammatic speech cannot be defined by reference to omissions of grammatical morphemes; rather, there are correct and incorrect forms of agrammatism. In Heeschen's example, the agrammatic patient, attempting the sentence *"Der schöne Mann putzt die Schuhe"* (The handsome man shines the shoes), would not reduce it to *"Schön Mann putzen Schuh"* (Handsome man shine shoe) as though he were following the rule of deleting articles, noun and adjective inflections, and substituting infinitives for finite verbs. The correct agrammatic form would be *"Schöner Mann schuhe putzen"*; that is, there are certain morpho-syntactic regularities that are extremely resistant to agrammatism in German. One of these requires that the infinitive form of the verb appear at the end of the sentence. The agrammatic patient, in replacing the present tense inflection with an infinitive, is then required to reorder the words in the message to comply with a strong word order rule.

Hofstede and Kolk (1989), examined the use of agrammatic speech by normals. They found that agrammatic speech is commonly adopted by native speakers of a language when they are attempting to give explanations to foreigners with limited comprehension. Transcribing the speech of Dutch interviewers speaking with immigrant workers, they found that virtually every form of agrammatic utterance was represented in the simplified communications of the interviewers. Just as the adoption of the agrammatic style is a conscious strategy for the normal in this circumstance, Kolk argues that it is also a conscious strategy for the patient.

An important feature of Kolk's argument that should be appreciated bears on the point in the generation of the message at which the patient's decision takes effect. For Kolk, this takes place at the point of prelinguistic formulation of the conceptual content to be incorporated in the message. For example, anticipating that the incorporation of subject + verb + object may exceed his or her computational and short-term memory capacity, the agrammatic patient plans an utterance that will specify only subject and object, assuming that the specification of the verb is redundant and can be inferred by the listener from the context. He or she may later decide that the verb should have been specified and add it as a supplementary one-word string (e.g., "Donkey . . . man . . . kicking"). Kolk's formulation is given in the context of Garrett's model (1975) of sentence generation. For Kolk *et al.* (1985) a sentence structure system (SSS) automatically applies the rules of syntax to whatever input it receives from the message generation stage. The normal English speaker's presentence message will include specifications that are normally encoded in a fully grammatical sentence. These may include the notion as to whether a particular noun has been referred to earlier (determining the use of a definite versus indefinite article) and information as to the time of an action (to be encoded grammatically as verb tense). The deletion of these specifications from the preverbal message formulation makes it impossible for the SSS to produce a grammatical sentence, but this is a matter of indifference to that system, which is automatic and nonjudgmental. The system turns out an utterance that applies grammatical rules to the extent that they can be imposed on the specified content. Thus, word order is preserved even when (as in Heeschen's example) it follows a language-specific rule.

Loss of the Relational Use of Words

In 1956, Jakobson presented his view on the polarity between "similarity disorder" and "contiguity disorder" in language use (see Chapter 2). Jakobson saw agrammatism in terms of a much more fundamental change than the omission of grammatical morphemes. Contiguity disorder entailed a loss of the sense of relationship between words that was reflected in an inability to use the syntactic devices that denote such relationships. Agrammatism represented a shift toward the use of words as purely nominal concepts, strung together with minimal syntactic marking. This, in Jakobson's view, accounted for the agrammatic's abandonment of inflected verb forms for the infinitive, and for their substitution of the nominative case of nouns for oblique cases in inflected languages. Verb inflection marks the agreement in number and person between verb and subject, but the concept of subject–verb relationships is dissolved for the patient with contiguity disorder. The verbal infinitive serves as a name for the action, conveying the concept of the verb without marking it with any syntactic ties to other words.

In Jakobson's reasoning, there was a hierarchy of vulnerability of syntactic relationships and of their respective marking devices, whether of a morphological or syntactic nature. Luria (1970) fully espoused Jakobson's approach, but referred to the basic defect of agrammatism as a loss of "predication." Like Jakobson, he saw agrammatic patients as using words in their nominative sense—that is, as a list of separate labels of concepts. He relates the dearth of verbs in the speech of these patients to the predicative role of the verb in a message. Compare this formulation to that of Kolk. They are similar in that both see the agrammatic patient as abandoning the reference to certain types of relationships between words. They differ in that Luria accounts for it as a loss of the capacity to convey these relationships in language, whereas Kolk holds that the simplified language is a deliberate adaptation made for the sake of economy of time and effort—some patients can shift voluntarily into and out of the agrammatic register, depending on how they perceive the pragmatics of the situation.

At the same time, Luria evokes Vigotsky's concept of "inner speech" in his account of agrammatism. For Vigotsky (1934), inner speech was a postulated silent stage of sentence formulation that mediated between the preverbal intent to convey a message and the development of a fully elaborated sentence frame. Inner speech has a simplified, elliptical syntax, as though it were intended for oneself. Lacking inner speech, the agrammatic cannot make the transition from concepts of individual words to formal syntax.[1]

Goodglass, Fodor, and Schulhoff (1967) offered a partial account of agrammatic symptoms from a totally different viewpoint, one that relates the threshold for initiation of an utterance to the "saliency" of available words in the message. "Saliency" is defined roughly as a combined effect of semantic significance and word stress. According to this proposal,

---

[1]One cannot escape the similarity between the notion of inner speech as a step toward sentence formulation and the stages in the evolution from an intent to a sentence as described by Lordat (1843), later by Pick (1913), and again by Garrett (1975).

unstressed functors are elements of low saliency that cannot serve to initiate speech. The agrammatic speaker is therefore likely to delete initial functors and start with a lexically full word, such as a noun (which also carries some stress in the sentence). Functors that immediately follow the stressed word are more likely to be produced because they do not have the burden of initiating the utterance. Their proposal was illustrated with the results of extensive testing with a single, severely agrammatic patient, using the task of repeating short sentences, where stress and position of grammatical functors were systematically varied. Goodglass *et al.* found that their patient systematically deleted unstressed articles, copulas, or modals in the initial position as in

The door is open → Door is open.
Can John dance? → John dance?

But he regularly produced opening stressed words, whether nouns or functors, and unstressed functors in the second position, as in

Can't he dance → correct.
Open the door → correct.

In their 1968 article, Goodglass *et al.* did not attempt to explain the full range of agrammatic symptoms. Yet, the notion that semantically "empty" words are less accessible for utterance may be extended to provide a fuller account of agrammatism. In the absence of functors, over-learned patterns of syntactic organization are disrupted and the patient is forced to construct utterances that are necessarily simplified and agrammatic. This account, like that of Kolk, entails adaptation to a limitation. However, the origin of the adaptation is not assigned to a reduction of the content of the intended message (as in Kolk's model) but to an incapacity to utter necessary elements that confronts the patient as he or she begins to speak.

Agrammatism as a Central Disturbance of Linguistic Processing Rules: The Syntactic Deficit Hypothesis

Jakobson's contribution represented the first attempt to relate specific symptomatology in aphasia to a theoretically defined linguistic operation. Yet Jakobson's formulation dealt with speech output only. He did not conceptualize "contiguity disorder" as having a receptive aspect. In adopting Jakobson's view, Luria, too, emphasized the output aspect of impaired predication. Yet he later (1970) made provision for a role for inner speech in the comprehension of sentences when he suggested that the listener must condense a heard sentence in inner speech in order to deal with its syntax. The loss of inner speech could then be offered as an explanation of the impaired comprehension of syntax that may be found in agrammatic patients. This comment is given only in passing. Luria's principal concern with receptive disturbances of syntactic processing has nothing to do with agrammatism, nor does it have an expressive counterpart. It is the logico-grammatical disorder to be found in his syntactic aphasics. This will be elaborated in a later section.

The assumption of parallelism between production and receptive processing of syntax that emerged in the 1970s was much more rigorously rooted in linguistic theory than any earlier conjectures, such as those of Salomon or Luria. The parallelism of the 1970s was clearly an expression of the spirit of Chomskyan generative linguistics. This approach holds that there are strict computational rules that must be followed to create a well-formed sentence from the conceptual elements in the "deep structure." These rules exist as "knowledge representations" and govern both the production and the interpretation of sentences in any modality: speech, listening, reading or writing. It was a natural presumption that agrammatism represented one of two possibilities, either the degradation (or loss) of certain rule representations or a performance deficit affecting production that did not affect the knowledge of the rules.

An influential study was carried out by Zurif, Caramazza, and Myerson (1972), showing that agrammatic patients performed randomly when required to show which words in a sentence were most closely linked to each other. The patients failed when the relationships within the sentence could only be inferred through grammatical decoding (as in "The friend John invited was late"), but the patients had no difficulty in dealing with sentences in which the relationships were totally fixed by word meaning (as in "The cake mother baked was tasty"). Because the tests were carried out in the graphic modality, Zurif *et al.* inferred that the patient's agrammatism entailed a loss of access to grammatical rule representations in receptive as well as expressive processing. There followed a number of studies in this vein (e.g., Saffran, Schwartz, and Marin, 1980) that were limited to agrammatic patients and that equated their deficits in syntactic decoding to their agrammatism. Agrammatic patients were said to have "asyntactic comprehension."

Within the framework of central processing disorder, a number of explanatory principles were offered. Kean (1977) suggested that the disorder was mistakenly considered one of syntax, but was better conceived as a disorder of phonology. Kean referred to the fact that the grammatical morphemes that are omitted have no role in the assignment of word stress in the sentence, hence they do not qualify as phonological words. Agrammatism, then, would be defined as the inability to deal with morphemes that are not phonological words. (Note the similarity to the model of Goodglass *et al.* with respect to the role assigned to word stress.) A totally different suggestion was offered by Bradley, Garrett, and Zurif (1980). They found that normal subjects appeared to be able to use a rapid acting mechanism to distinguish grammatical functors from lexical words, but that agrammatic patients had no access to this special purpose mechanism. Hence their processing of grammatical morphemes was slow and could not support the rapid access to these elements that was essential for normal syntactic processing.

Another account of agrammatism was developed by Grodzinsky (1990) on the basis of Chomsky's (1981) Government and Binding theory. In Chomsky's theory, syntactic structures that depart from the canonical position of agent preceding and object following a verb leave a trace (t) in the original position of the noun or pronoun that has been moved. In order to interpret a passive sentence correctly, one must connect the thematic role of the displaced object with its trace. For example in the sentence "The man was kicked by the horse," there is a trace of the real object (man) immediately after the verb: The man was kicked (t) by the horse. Grodzinsky's postulate is that the agrammatic aphasic is unable to appreciate the co-reference of "the man" and (t), and hence the patient is reduced to chance levels in determining whether "man" is the real subject or the real object of the verb "kicked."

The flaw that affected almost all the investigations that were motivated by the syntactic deficit hypothesis (and similar central rule representation notions) is that they examined only agrammatic patients and not those with grammatically fluent speech output. There is ample evidence that difficulties in the interpretation of sentences, such as passives, that depart from the canonical word order are common among aphasics, irrespective of whether they speak agrammatically or not (Lesser, 1978; Goodglass and Menn, 1985; Martin and Blossom-Stach, 1986; Goodglass, Christiansen, and Gallagher, in press; see also reviews of the problem by Schwartz, Linebarger, and Saffran, 1985; Martin *et al.*, 1989; Berndt, 1991). It is the author's position that agrammatism is a disorder of speech production, that problems in the interpretation of sentences appear as often among fluent aphasics as among agrammatics. The failures of fluent aphasics can be shown to be at the level of syntactic decoding and not merely a result of impaired lexical comprehension (Naeser *et al.* 1987a,b).

LOGICO-GRAMMATICAL DISORDERS

There are many converging factors that determine the ease or difficulty with which incoming, grammatically organized messages can be processed. Some sentences can be processed from left to right, as the words are perceived. For example, in the sentence "Ten men, dressed in soldiers' uniforms, held up the train as it was emerging from the tunnel," the successive lexical items can be unambiguously semantically decoded as they are perceived. The meaning of the sentence can be derived from the semantics of the key words, from left to right, without backtracking in auditory memory. However, if we consider a sentence like "Flying the plane was one of the first women to be employed as a pilot by the airline," it is apparent that the first phrase has to be replayed mentally part way through the sentence in order to make sense of it. Impairment of auditory working memory may make it difficult or impossible to follow sentences that cannot be unambiguously decoded from left to right. Sentence length and complexity of embedding are among the factors that understandably make sentences difficult for aphasic patients to interpret.

Luria (1970) called attention to another type of syntactic comprehension problem that he referred to as an impairment of logico-grammatical relationships. These are failures to interpret a semantically reversible relationship between two terms when the direction of the relationship is signaled only by a case-marking grammatical morpheme, or by word order. This problem is illustrated by the relationship of possession involving two animate nouns such as "father's sister" or the contrast between agent and object in the sentence "Touch (or "point to") the comb with the pencil." The aphasic patient, when asked if "my father's sister" is a man or a woman may answer randomly, unable to grasp how the possessive marker, 's, fixes the relationship between those terms. Given the command to point to the comb with the pencil, he or she is most apt to pick up the comb and use it as the implement, under the assumption that the first object mentioned is the one to be handled. The frequency with which we observe complete failure on tasks of this type is astonishing to one who assumes that they are short, easy expressions. In retrospect, we can say that fixing the direction of a reversible relationship is an extremely heavy load on an inconspicuous grammatical morpheme, and one that is exquisitely sensitive to the effects of aphasia. Relationships that depend on the interpretation of locative prepositions (in front of/in back of; over/under) or prepositions of time (before/after) are somewhat less fragile, possibly because of the semantic content of these prepositions.

Luria considered the impairment of logico-grammatical relationships to be the hallmark of the syndrome of semantic aphasia, a form of fluent aphasia associated with parietal lobe injury and with difficulty in grasping spatial and quantitative relationships. In our experience, these difficulties are found equally in patients with frontal and temporal lesions, consistently sparing only those who have recovered to a mild level. It may be that Luria was impressed by the fact that his semantic aphasics failed on these items in spite of their minimal impairment in vocabulary access, productive syntax, or auditory comprehension.

CROSS-LINGUISTIC STUDIES OF AGRAMMATISM

In 1951, Ombredane, speaking of agrammatism, wrote, "In any case, the proportion and the complexity of these diverse means of expression are not the same in all languages, and as a result, the nature and the degree of aphasic phenomena must differ according to the language used. A comparative study of aphasia among patients speaking languages of differing structures confronts future researchers as a fruitful task." This task was finally undertaken by Menn and Obler, and the results, based on the collaboration of clinician–linguist teams in 14 countries, was published in 1990. Among the languages studied were some with different canonical word orders from the familiar SVO (Japanese SOV), some without a prescribed word order (Polish and Finnish), some that dispense with many free grammatical morphemes, replacing them by bound morphemes (Finnish), and other radical variations from the type of grammatical rules that are familiar to speakers of English and the major Germanic and Romance languages of western Europe. The findings from this study confirm the universality of some of the features of agrammatism noted in the literature, but also reveal that others vary in a rational way as a function of the syntax of different languages. To summarize the most salient findings:

1. All patients with agrammatism show a markedly reduced variety of syntactic forms, with a short span of words of utterance structures.

2. Free grammatical morphemes are much more subject to omission than to substitution.

3. Exempt from omission are those grammatical particles that do not play a role in the internal phrase structure, but are discourse controlled. These include initial conjunctions (such as "and") and clause final particles such as, in Japanese, the emphatic particle "*yo*," the question-marking particle "ka," and the confirmation-seeking particle "ne." The last of these functions like a tag question in English (e.g., "Didn't he?" and "Isn't it?"), but unlike a tag question, the particle requires no agreement with any word in the preceding clause.

4. Bound morphemes (verb and noun declensions) are more likely to be substituted than deleted. These substitutions are not random but come from within the same declensional paradigm—often a form that carries less semantic specificity and serves as a sort of default form. However, as Menn and Obler point out there is no strict directional hierarchy of

substitutability of one form for another. The same patient, for example, may substitute a singular for a plural and a plural for a singular at different points. One observation concerning substitutions of bound morphemes is significant. There are more substitutions of inflections of verbs that have extensive paradigms (i.e., many inflectional forms) than those that have only a few (like English regular verbs). It is as if the more declensional forms that are available to choose from, the finer and more vulnerable are the relational distinctions that must be discerned and retained in recovering the required form.

5. Agrammatic speakers of languages that have a canonical word order display a strong inclination to maintaining that order, even at the expense of grammaticality. This is seen in English in the patients' inability to use the passive or the inverted verb–subject order of yes–no questions (e.g., "Is the door open?")

Menn and Obler also point out that in languages that use case marking on nouns, the deletion of a main verb does not prevent the appropriate case marking from being applied to the object noun. Similarly, Grodzinsky (1990) observes that the object noun may be used in conjunction with an uninflected or infinitival verb form. Both of these observations would contradict the Jakobsonian (and Lurian) proposal that verbs are used in a nominal, nonpredicative sense by agrammatics. It is also contrary to the attribution of impaired verb access by agrammatics to the fact that verbs always have a syntactic implication that make them difficult for agrammatic patients to cope with. The problem of the dissociation between verb accessibility and noun accessibility is thus relegated to the general area of category-specific dissociations in lexical production and lexical comprehension that is discussed in Chapter 7.

It is appropriate to conclude with the general (though tentative) characterization of agrammatism offered by Menn and Obler on the basis of their cross-linguistic comparisons. Their account avoids the reductionism of many earlier theories and specifically places the disorder in the realm of language output functions. First, they suggest that the patients are impaired in their ability to compute the specifications of grammatical morphemes that mark relationships within the sentence. This computational load falls more heavily on morphemes that relate two or more words within the clause (e.g., the possessive marker) than it does on those that are locally determined (e.g., the article). Underspecified grammatical morphemes are omitted (if free standing) or substituted (if bound). Grammatical morphemes that do not require syntactic computation, such as clause final particles in Japanese, are unaffected.

The second component of agrammatism is a markedly reduced span of positional planning space that prevents patients from dealing with word order relationships among multiword thought units and reduces them to minimal-sized clauses. Word order, per se, though it is an important syntactic device, is not impaired in agrammatism.

Within this framework there is room for variation in symptoms as a result of individual patients' strategies. The difference between this view and that of Kolk, is that Kolk assigns the strategic decision to a stage of message formulation that precedes the syntax computation process. In the author's view, the clinical evidence is too variable to permit a choice between these positions. Moreover, there are ample observational data that are not subsumed by either of these theoretical positions. The most insistent of these data is the inability of severely agrammatic patients to *repeat* even three- or four-word phrases that require the use of a noncanonical word order or that involve beginning an utterance with an unstressed grammatical morpheme. Because the operation of repetition would appear to relieve patients of syntactic computation demands, an account that is couched only in computational terms ignores an important aspect of agrammatic production. Although a totally comprehensive theory of agrammatism is still not at hand, current descriptions of agrammatic phenomena give a more coherent story than those of 50 years ago.

Chapter 7

Disorders of Auditory Comprehension

INTRODUCTION

It is rare to examine an aphasic patient who comprehends spoken language with normal speed and accuracy at the level of sentences and vocabulary of everyday complexity. The factors that contribute to reduced comprehension are multiple and interacting. Any attempt to reduce them to one or a few principles can only result in a more or less approximate description of the clinical phenomena. Thus, we offer an account here that comes close to, but does not completely explain how auditory comprehension may suffer following aphasia of various types. We will touch on the role of speech–sound discrimination, on the attachment of meaning to auditorily perceived words, on the processing of sentences, and on the role played by attention, short-term auditory memory, and cognition.

It is good to keep in mind from the outset that some of these factors (e.g., speech–sound and word meaning recognition) may be selectively impaired as a result of focal lesions, and may contribute to clearly defined aphasic syndromes. Other factors, such as attentional and short-term auditory memory problems are more difficult to isolate, plus they interact with the first two factors mentioned. Overlying all of these are situational variables—notably the personal relevance and emotional significance of the subject matter of communication. In aphasia, these latter factors may totally determine whether comprehension will be effective or not.

IMPAIRMENTS IN THE PROCESSING OF SPEECH SOUNDS

The study of normal speech perception shows that there is a subtle and complex relationship between the perception of sound per se and the perception of speech sounds. Even when speech sounds are taken out of the context of real words and presented in isolation, the ability to discriminate them from other speech sounds engages an auditory mechanism that is specialized for speech. Research carried out by Liberman and his associates at Haskins Laboratory (Liberman *et al.*, 1967) suggests that speech perception differs from perception of other sounds in a number of characteristic ways. One of these is "categorical perception." This term refers to the fact that normal listeners are extraordinarily sensitive to slight changes in the acoustic signal at the boundary point between two similar sounds. For example, the most important cue to the difference between a voiced and unvoiced consonant (as in *ba* versus *pa*; *da* versus *ta*) is the amount of time between the release of the closure of the vocal tract and the beginning of vocal cord vibration for the following vowel. When this interval, called the voice onset time (VOT), is shorter than 30 msec, the consonant will be heard as voiced (e.g., *ba*). However, when the VOT is longer than 30 msec, it will be perceived as unvoiced (*pa*). When listeners are asked to make same–different judgments between two presentations of a consonant–vowel combination that differ only by a few milliseconds in VOT, they are unable to perceive a difference if both presentations are either shorter than or longer than 30 msec. However, when the two presentations straddle the critical value of 30 msec, listeners are convinced that they hear the two different consonants—the one voiced, the other unvoiced.

A second feature of speech sound processing is that it is left hemisphere controlled. That is, when competing speech sounds are presented to the two ears in a dichotic listening format, the sounds reported from the right ear are more often correct than those from the left ear (Shankweiler and Studdert-Kennedy, 1967). No other category of sound has been found to show a similar left hemisphere dominance. Many nonspeech sounds (melodies; environmental noises) are preferentially processed in the right hemisphere; others are unlateralized.

PURE WORD-DEAFNESS

Studies of patients with severe aphasic speech comprehension disorders have revealed only one type of patient for whom there is a suggestive relation between loss of language comprehension and disruption of basic mechanisms for the perception of speech sounds. These are patients with pure word-deafness. Yet, the data for two word-deaf patients who have been carefully studied (Miceli, 1982; Auerbach *et al.*, 1982) are somewhat inconsistent and fail to give convincing evidence of a causative relation between failures on tests of categorical perception and difficulties of speech comprehension.

Pure word-deafness is a clinically uncommon condition in which speed comprehension is severely or completely disrupted, while all other aspects of language—speaking, reading, and writing—remain intact. it was first given its currently used label by Kussmaul (1887). Although audiometric testing usually shows normal hearing levels, the patient acts as if hard of hearing and frequently makes comments like "I can't hear you." Partial comprehension of words always reflects misperception of sounds—never a semantically based error of word comprehension, as would be most typical in Wernicke's aphasia. Most cases reported have had bilateral temporal lobe lesions, although unilateral left temporal lobe lesions have also been found to result in pure word-deafness. Auerbach *et al.* (1982) believe that there are subtle differences in the pattern of sound discrimination between unilateral and bilateral lesion cases. Both Auerbach and Miceli found that their patients made many errors in identifying and discriminating stop consonants when presented in combination with the vowel *a* (e.g., *ba*, *ta* and *ga*). Discrimination of place of articulation was much more difficult than distinguishing a voiced from an unvoiced consonant. Yet, Auerbach's patient responded accurately to changes in the acoustic parameters for voicing and for place of articulation when tested with synthetic consonant vowel stimuli. He also showed the boundary effect in a test of categorical perception of VOT intervals, although far less markedly than a normal control. Miceli's patient differed from Auerbach's chiefly in her failure to identify place of articulation (*ba* versus *da* versus *ga*), when the acoustic parameter for this discrimination was varied along a continuum. Both patients were no longer able to recognize melodies or to sing. Miceli's patient had a marked auditory agnosia for environmental noises, but Auerbach's was only slightly impaired in this regard.

A very different picture emerges on the examination by Denes and Semenza (1975) of a patient who had an equally severe loss of speech comprehension, and who was equally intact in all other aspects of language. This individual was thought to have suffered a unilateral left hemisphere stroke, on the basis of electroencephalograph findings, although his brain scan did not reveal a lesion. Denes and Semenza's patient was just as poor as the bilateral cases in discriminating and identifying consonants, but his errors were randomly distributed, without regard to place versus voicing distinctions or to whether sounds differed in both place and voice. He could sing, but could not identify familiar melodies, even those that he had just sung. He could match environmental sounds with pictures of the source that produced them, but was unable to name the source when tested without pictures present. This rare phenomenon, "acoustic anomia," may be understood if one postulates an anatomical disconnection between the auditory processing zone and the language system.

It is notable that all of these patients retained the ability to recognize vowels. Because vowels are relatively long in duration, whereas stop consonants depend on the processing of very rapidly changing acoustic signals, it is plausible that pure word-deafness is particularly disruptive for discriminations based on short acoustic events, as argued by Auerbach. In this connection, it is notable that these patients are able to count taps or clicks only when they are presented very slowly. Albert and Bear (1974) reported a patient with pure word-deafness whose comprehension of speech was greatly enhanced by slowing the rate of presentation.

There is no doubt that pure word-deafness, more than any other disorder in the spectrum of aphasia, entails a breakdown of speech sound perception at an elementary level. Yet this breakdown is not complete, as vowels, continuant consonants, distinctions of voicing, and a certain percentage of place of articulation discriminations continue to be made. Impaired comprehension of connected speech can be attributed, in part, to a slowing of the processing of speech input. however, the impairment in comprehension of single words appears disproportionate to the impairment of individual speech sounds. It seems inescapable that this disorder entails a loss of the ability to integrate auditory speech patterns beyond the level of individual sounds.

Anatomical accounts of pure word-deafness (Geschwind, 1965) revolve on the integrity of Wernicke's area on the left, but its isolation from both ipsilateral and contralateral auditory input. This can be caused, in bilateral lesions, by destruction of Heschl's gyrus or its connections on the right and similar destruction on the left. The auditory radiations, carrying information from the lateral geniculate body to Heschl's gyrus through the temporal isthmus, are commonly compromised by subcortical lesions. For word-deafness from a unilateral lesion, one would also expect interruption of the subcortical fibers that emerge from the corpus callosum, carrying auditory information from the right hemisphere. In theory, it is the integrity of Wernicke's area that permits all other language functions to proceed normally. One puzzle is why word-deafness is not seen more frequently in cases with extensive left subcortical lesions affecting both the left temporal isthmus and auditory pathways from the corpus callosum. It is possible that this disorder can appear only when the Wernicke's area homologue in the right hemisphere is totally unable to process word meanings from auditory input. Such total absence of rudimentary language comprehension in the right hemisphere may be exceptional and account in part for the rarity of severe word-deafness.

SPEECH SOUND PERCEPTION IN APHASIA

The strongest proponent for a connection between speech sound perception and word meaning recognition in aphasia was A. R. Luria (1970). For Luria, a disorder of "phonemic hearing" results from left temporal lobe lesions and accounts for the breakdown in the access to word semantics in acoustic sensory (Wernicke's) aphasia. Luria uses the term "phonemic" in the sense of contemporary linguistic usage: that is, the classification of an acoustic pattern by a listener as a particular member of the sound repertory of his language. Unlike Auerbach *et al.* (1982), who saw the problem of pure word-deafness as an acoustic processing breakdown at a "prephonemic" level, Luria does not implicate elementary acoustic perceptual processing. It should be emphasized that Luria is discussing the mechanism for impaired meaning comprehension in what we call Wernicke's aphasia, and not in pure word-deafness. The experimental evidence on which Luria relies involves tasks of distinguishing a change between stop consonants in a series of consonant–vowel presentations or correctly producing a series of alternating consonants in such a series. It is unclear how a failure of discrimination of individual sounds results in confusions along semantic lines (rather than phonemic misperceptions).

Blumstein, Baker, and Goodglass (1977a) and Baker, Blumstein, and Goodglass (1981) objected to Luria's account on the grounds of both clinical observation and everyday experience. Clinically, it is common for Wernicke's aphasics to repeat a test word after the examiner and still fail to comprehend it. Further, it is rare for these patients to misinterpret a word as though it were another word with a similar sound. Errors in word recognition are almost always along semantic, rather than phonological lines. This would be difficult to explain on the basis of inaccurate sound perception. From everyday experience we know that connected speech has so much redundancy that conversations over a telephone with poor sound quality can be quite effective even though many individual consonants are poorly perceived.

Blumstein *et al.* required subjects to make same–different judgments between pairs of spoken words with minimal phonological contrasts (e.g., pear versus bear; pin versus tin). Real words and nonsense words were used. The subjects were Broca's aphasics, Wernicke's aphasics, mixed nonfluent aphasics, and a mixed group of fluent aphasics without temporal lobe involvement. Mixed nonfluent aphasics made the most errors in phoneme discrimination and Broca's aphasics the fewest errors. Wernicke's aphasics, though the most impaired in auditory comprehension by a significant margin, were not significantly different from the nonfluent aphasics in their discrimination scores; in fact, they were numerically slightly superior to them. All groups made more discrimination errors on nonwords than on real words.

In a follow-up study, Baker *et al.* (1981) repeated the preceding auditory same–different discrimination test along with two additional tasks, administered to Broca's and Wernicke's aphasics. In the second task, the auditory presentation of an object name was followed by a picture of either the same object or of one that had a minimal phonological difference in its name (e.g., pear (spoken), bear (picture)]. In the third task, the spoken name was followed by a multiple choice of four pictures: the target (e.g., pear), a semantic distractor (e.g., grapes), a phonological distractor (bear), and a semantic associate of the phonological distractor (wolf). As before, Wernicke's aphasics made more errors than Broca's aphasics. However, three reasons argued against attributing their performance to a primarily phonemic discrimination deficit. First, error rates were much higher when semantic mediation was required (Experiments 2 and 3) than when a phonemic discrimination alone was to be made. Second, in Experiment 3, the preponderance of errors were semantically, rather than phonologically based. The semantic preponderance was more marked for Wernicke's than Broca's aphasics. Third, Wernicke's aphasics rarely chose the distractor that was a semantic associate of the phonological distractor. If their errors had been due to a phonological misinterpretation of the spoken stimulus, they should frequently have been led to the choice of a semantic associate of this word, just as they often chose a semantic associate of the actual spoken stimulus. The fact that these choices did not occur casts further doubt on the interpretation that their failures are simply a failure of phonemic discrimination.

In support of Luria's view, however, is the fact that there was an interaction between phonological and semantic difficulty. The more difficult the phonological discrimination, the greater the likelihood of a semantically based error. Conversely, when semantic mediation was required (Experiments 2 and 3), the number of phonological errors as well as the number of semantic errors increased, both for Broca's and for Wernicke's aphasics. Thus, contrary to our *a priori* reasoning, a phonological discrimination load may contribute to semantically based misinterpretations.

COMPREHENSION OF WORD MEANING: LEXICAL SEMANTICS

Most of our understanding of disorders of word meaning comprehension derives from tasks in which the patient selects, from multiple choice, an object named orally by the examiner. There are great disparities among aphasic patients in their level of competence on this task. Patients with lesions in the pre-Rolandic cortical areas show relatively little impairment. Those with lesions of Wernicke's area in the superior temporal gyrus are, at least initially, severely impaired. It was on this basis that Wernicke and subsequent neurologists attributed to Wernicke's area the function of storing the memories for words and their meanings. As we have noted earlier, severe difficulties in word comprehension may also arise from subcortical lesions involving the temporal isthmus that interrupt the input to Wernicke's area from the medial geniculate body of the left thalamus. Even more complete isolation of Wernicke's area from auditory information may occur when the lesion also interrupts the fibers carrying information from the right hemisphere homologue of Wernicke's area, that emerge from the corpus callosum, posterior to the body of the left lateral ventricle.

CHARACTERISTICS OF IMPAIRED WORD COMPREHENSION

Because word comprehension is most commonly tested by having the patient point to a named object or word, failure to perform correctly cannot be taken as evidence that no meaning association has taken place in the patient's mind. Failure to point may be due to an apraxia for the purposeful action of pointing, to failure to grasp what the examiner expects, or to wandering attention. Alternative modes of testing comprehension are all open to problems specific to the test procedure. For example, asking questions about a named concept (e.g., "Is an elephant an animal?" or "Is a spoon to write with?") depend on eliciting a reliable yes–no response and on the comprehension of the entire question. No means has yet been devised for directly probing the inner state that results from hearing a word. Yet the simple pointing technique can be used with reasonable assurance of its validity if the patient responds correctly on words that can plausibly be considered easier than those on which he or she fails. Similarly, if the error in pointing response reflects partial, but inadequate comprehension of the stimulus word, it may be assumed to be a valid indicator. This would be the case, for example, if the patient pointed to his shoulder when asked to show his elbow.

Another fundamental fact that has become evident is that a word meaning cannot be regarded as a unitary bit of knowledge that is either available to the patient or lost. The response to a spoken word may be manifest at any or all of a number of levels. At the highest level is a one-to-one appreciation of the precise semantics of the stimulus. That is, in a multiple choice pointing task, the patient will select the named object from a multiple-choice set of objects of the same category. When precise comprehension is impaired, the patient may still grasp the category or connotation of the spoken object, so that he or she may turn to the appropriate category of objects if there are several categories available. Once in the appropriate category, the patient's selection of a specific response item may be random. For example, the test card that we regularly use allows a choice of response from a group of colors, numbers, or common objects. Given the name of a color to find, the patient almost never looks among the objects or numbers, but may choose an incorrect color. Similarly, when a patient is asked to locate parts of his or her own body, the most likely type of confusion is the substitution of one major joint for another, for example, pointing to "elbow" when given the word "knee" (Semenza and Goodglass, 1985). Parenthetically, it should be observed that the ability to select an object picture from a set of objects of diverse categories (e.g., "bear" from among a bear, a flower, a window, and a bottle) is not evidence that the patient specifically comprehends the word "bear." One needs to know whether this patient could distinguish between bear, wolf, lion, and tiger—that is, words that share connotation (fierceness) and category (wild animals).

Should we regard the selection of response to the precise referent of the named object as a refinement of the more general response to category or connotation? The author's interpretation of these observations is that there are two different types of semantic activation involved. The response to connotation is much more robust in the face of brain damage. It may persist when the patient appears to have totally lost the sense of the specific referent for the spoken word. The persistence of partial comprehension at the level of connotation or category is the typical error response observed in the examination of Wernicke's aphasics, as well as of patients with mixed productive and receptive features. It is not observed in patients with word-deafness, however.

There are other phenomena observed in aphasic patients that indicate the possibility of motor or autonomic system responses to words that the patient cannot identify. The most easily demonstrable of these is the motor response to the name of a body part when the patient has been asked to point to the named location. Given the stimulus "show me your chin," the patient may instantly bring his hand up to the level of his face and grope around, sometimes repeating to himself "chin . . . chin" as he tries to find the part that he does not quite understand. If then required to show his foot, he may immediately glance downward, but make only a vague reaching gesture toward his leg. In these instances, the body part name has elicited a positional response.

Milberg and Blumstein (1981) have used the primed lexical decision technique to show that response to meaning category is preserved in Wernicke's aphasics, even though these patients are unable to demonstrate specific comprehension of the name of the stimulus object. In this technique, the subject is required to make a rapid judgment as to whether a written letter string (or a spoken stimulus) is a real English word or whether it is a nonword. These presentations are primed immediately in advance by the presentation of a word that is semantically related, or else unrelated to the target stimulus. Wernicke's aphasics, like normal individuals, were significantly faster in making a positive lexical decision about test words that were primed by a related word, than about those that were preceded by an unrelated word. Paradoxically, Broca's aphasics did not show such differential priming effects, even though the Broca's aphasics were much more successful in demonstrating that they could identify the spoken words by pointing to their corresponding objects.

These observations suggest that the semantic system that mediates one-to-one identification of a referent may be different from that which mediates a response to its category or to an associated object. In the view of Milberg and Blumstein, the latter type of response is automated, whereas the former is volitional.

CONTEXT-EMBEDDED WORD COMPREHENSION

Some words that in isolation elicit no evidence of recognition, or only a global, category-related response are promptly and accurately responded to in an action context. The most regularly demonstrable instance of this behavior is the normal response to the request "Shut your eyes" by patients who, having a dense comprehension disorder, have been unable to point to their eyes on request. Similar dissociation of comprehension between isolated words and action context-embedded words may be found for both familiar requests, such as "Let me see your tongue," and unfamiliar requests, such as "Rub your ear."

The examples given have all involved body parts. But the phenomenon of context-embedded comprehension can also involve nonbody objects. For example, patients with global comprehension impairment usually respond promptly to the request "Move your chair a little closer" or "Turn your chair toward me."

These phenomena have important implications for word comprehension, not only by aphasic patients but in normal conversation as well. It is tempting to assume that the concept of "chair" or "eye" or "ear" is fully activated by contextual embedding. It is more likely that these words are grasped only in the narrow sense of their relevance to the action. What the patient responded to was the total command and the aspect of the object that made it relevant to the requested action. Relating to the representation of concepts in the brain and the realization of specific instantiations of a concept, Damasio (1989) writes, "the range of representations that form the basis for a concept varies from individual to individual, depending on the acquaintance with the object . . . the value of the object to the perceiver, and so on. No less importantly, the range of representations varies from instantiation to instantiation, within the same individual and even representations of the same type vary from instantiation to instantiation. . . . The process is influenced by the surrounding context, the state of mind and soma of the perceiver, and by the modified experience that repeated instantiations produce." To this view, with which the author entirely concurs, the author would add that the concept is a conglomerate of processes, some of which are much more resistant than others to the effects of damage to the language apparatus of the brain.

CATEGORY-SPECIFIC DISSOCIATIONS

In our discussion of category-specific dissociations of word retrieval, in Chapter 5, we pointed out that these dissociations in naming were closely related to similar dissociations in word comprehension. This relationship between input and output modalities is complex. In some cases, it appears to be reciprocal; that is, some word categories that are commonly vulnerable to selective impairment (e.g., body part names and letter names) are found to be selectively preserved for production in otherwise anomic patients (Goodglass *et al.*, 1986). It is rare that a particular word category is vulnerable to deficiencies in both production and auditory comprehension. Such parallel impairments have been described in the case of body parts in a single case report by Dennis (1976) and in the case of colors, in association with pure alexia, by Geschwind and Fusillo (1966).

The first formal study of category specific dissociations by Goodglass *et al.* (1966) was motivated by our observation of how frequently a near total failure to grasp body part names was observed in patients with disorders of auditory comprehension who were nevertheless able to identify other categories of objects reasonably well. The 1966 study revealed that letters of the alphabet was the category most frequently impaired in auditory comprehension and the most frequently selectively preserved in naming tasks. Common objects showed the reverse effect; they were usually well identified in response to their names, but suffered more from anomic production failures than any of the word categories tested.

A case study reported by Goodglass and Budin (1988) described the testing of a patient who showed a severe form of selective failure of auditory comprehension for the categories of body parts, colors, numbers, and letters, although his comprehension of every other word category was virtually flawless. This case was remarkable chiefly because of the excellence of the patient's auditory comprehension in all but the affected categories. The case was important in other respects as well. The patient had extremely well preserved word-reading ability and instantly identified any color, body part, or number that was presented to him in writing.

The fact that normal responses were available on written presentation is clear evidence that these comprehension failures are specific to the auditory modality. The patient had no disorder of body image. The integrity of body image in most patients who failed to identify body part names was already demonstrated by Semenza and Goodglass (1985) and was later confirmed in a study by Benedet and Goodglass (1989). A further bit of evidence from Goodglass and Budin's patient confirmed the specificity of his disorder to the particular words that designated body parts. When asked to point to the location of articles of clothing (such as belt, collar, socks, and sleeve), he showed little difficulty, either on his own body or on the drawing of a mannequin.

The fact that selective word comprehension difficulty was confined to the auditory modality was brought home dramatically because of this patient's excellent word reading ability. Such selectivity can always be demonstrated in patients who are not alexic. In fact, there has never been a report of a category-specific comprehension impairment in reading in an aphasic patient.

While category-specific dissociations of word comprehension almost always involve selective impairment, selective preservation of auditory word comprehension is most frequently observed in the case of geographic place names, an observation that is particularly dramatic in patients with global aphasia. This observation occurs in the task of identifying locations on an outline map of the United States and includes city names (Boston, Chicago, Miami), geographic features (Mississippi River), and large entities (Mexico, Canada, Atlantic Ocean). It was first reported in print by Wapner and Gardner (1979), and contrasted with the structurally similar task of identifying body parts by Goodglass and Butters (1989).

Until 1973, category-specific dissociations of naming or word comprehension in aphasics were described only with reference to the small number of tightly cohesive categories that we have just mentioned. In that year, Yamadori and Albert described what they referred to as "word category aphasia" in an anomic patient, who was unable to point to named objects if they were large, man-made objects in the room. His failures included words such as "chair" and "wall." He had no difficulty with identifying small manipulable objects, but he was unable to identify body parts that were named for him.

Warrington and her associates (Warrington and Shallice, 1984; Warrington and McCarthy, 1983; Warrington and McCarthy, 1987) contributed a large series of case observations that went beyond the report of Yamadori and Albert. Their initial observations led them to consider animacy/inanimacy as the factor that determined success or failure in comprehension. For example, Warrington and Shallice's postencephalitic patients could not identify animals, foods, or flowers, but did well with small manipulable objects. Warrington and McCarthy's (1983) aphasic patient showed the reverse dissociation as she failed to select pictures of common household objects from their spoken names, but performed surprisingly well in identifying different flowers, foods, and animals. In their later (1987) review of this problem, Warrington and McCarthy proposed that the dichotomy between primarily functionally conceived and primarily visually conceived objects may be a more adequate account of the basis for semantic dissociations. They point out that man-made objects are conceptualized chiefly through their function, whereas animals and other animate objects are known chiefly through their physical properties—especially form. They suggest that the sensory channels through which objects are experienced may be differently weighted as a function of their contribution to the knowledge of the objects' essential features. This may provide a link to lesion-specific effects, on one hand, and to common psychological categorization on the other.

The broad semantic groupings studied by Warrington and her colleagues may represent a different dissociative mechanism from the close-knit semantic categories studied by Goodglass and his associates. It may be notable that Goodglass' observations are specific to aphasics and are restricted to the auditory receptive modality. Those of Warrington are more frequently seen in post-encephalitic patients, although they also occur in aphasics. Furthermore, in patients who had sufficient speech to be tested for their ability to define the target concepts, Warrington and associates found parallel failures in giving definitions to the failures that existed in word comprehension. Up to now, there has been little evidence of a specific anatomic basis for one type of dissociation versus another in word comprehension.

COMPREHENSION AT THE MESSAGE LEVEL

In the examination of severely impaired aphasic patients, the examiner is often surprised by the alacrity with which a patient correctly confirms

or corrects comments concerning recent events related to his or her illness, and comments referring to family, work, or living situation. This
impression that the patient has little disturbance of auditory comprehension may suddenly be reversed on beginning formal testing and finding
that the patient is unable to point to any named object or to answer the
simplest yes–no questions concerning factual knowledge. The influence
of what we have, in the Boston University Aphasic Center, termed as
"comprehension in a real life context" is one of the important variables
in auditory message processing.

"Real life" communications tend to be short and syntactically simple.
The factor of syntactic complexity has been touched on in Chapter 6 on
disorders of syntax and morphology, as it bears on auditory comprehension. Additional aspects of sentence structure affecting receptive processing will be discussed in this section.

"REAL LIFE" CONTEXT AND COMMUNICATION

"Real life context" as applied to verbal interaction with aphasics is a
term improvised by a number of investigators (H. Goodglass, M. L. Albert, and N. H. Estabrooks) at the Boston University Aphasia Center to
subsume a number of features that were thought to be best summarized
by that term. These features and examples of illustrative verbalizations
that have elicited appropriate responses are the following:

1. Emotional impact - warnings or admonishments about personal presentation ("There's a smudge on your cheek"; "Your fly is open").
2. Situationally relevant action request ("Bring me some water from
   the sink, in that cup").
3. Personally relevant factual question/comment ("You have four
   kids?") (patient rejects and corrects by showing two fingers).

It is clear that the terms "real life"" context or the currently popular
"ecologically valid" communication are, at best, descriptive and lack explanatory power to account for the persistence of auditory comprehension of messages of the foregoing types.

COMPREHENSION OF "AXIAL" COMMANDS

It was Geschwind (1965) who pointed out the robustness in auditory
comprehension of commands involving midline or "axial" structures.
Among these are such commands as "Stand up," "Turn around," "Take

a bow," and "Look up." The dissociation of comprehension of axial commands from profound auditory comprehension failure for other content, including very simple limb commands, is most striking in some patients with Wernicke's aphasia. What is particularly puzzling in this phenomenon is that the context of an axial command may carry with it an appropriate response to specific nouns or verbs. We have commonly demonstrated that patients can perform accurately when asked to "Stand like a boxer" or when instructed "Let me see how you dance." Moreover, it is possible to elicit multistep performances, such as "Take two steps backward, turn around, and sit down again."

The key element in Geschwind's proposed explanation is that the movements involved are bilaterally innervated, using nonpyramidal pathways. The response to axial commands may therefore be mediated by mechanisms other than the route from Wernicke's area to the left hemisphere motor association areas that is thought to mediate limb commands. Residual language comprehension function in the right temporal lobe may play a role. Variability among individuals in right hemisphere language capacity may account for why axial commands are dramatically preserved in some patients, but not all.

SENTENCE STRUCTURE AND COMPREHENSION

In Chapter 6, we touched on some syntactic factors that make sentences easy or difficult to process auditorily. In particular, we noted that when the powerful cue of word order was in conflict with the marking signaled by bound or free grammatical morphemes, patients might respond randomly or even interpret a sentence completely on the basis of word order cues. We also noted that when the semantics of the informational words in the sentence allowed only one plausible interpretation, patients usually responded correctly. It has been shown that aphasic speakers of a highly inflected language, like German, are more attuned to using noun or verb inflections to interpret syntactic functions of words in a sentence than are English speakers. However, even German-speaking patients are more swayed by expectations dictated by canonical word order than they are by inflection, so they are apt to err when a noncanonical order is used.

There are other considerations, in addition to word order and sensitivity to grammatical morphemes, that affect sentence processing by aphasic patients. One of these is maintaining the relationship between subject and verb when they are separated by an embedded clause. For example, when given a sentence like "The boy who called the cop ran after the thief," the aphasic patient may interpret it as saying that the cop ran after the thief. Such a misinterpretation is less likely, as Goodglass *et al.* (1979) pointed out, if the message is expanded into two independent clauses as in "The boy called the cop and the boy ran after the thief." The sentence as originally given interposes another plausible subject, "cop," before the verb "ran." Furthermore, that noun immediately precedes the verb and, following the "minimal distance" heuristic is likely to be perceived as the subject of the verb. In addition, real world knowledge makes it just as likely that the cop ran after the thief as that the boy did. To the normal listener, the relative pronoun "who," following a noun, is a strong signal that the main clause verb for that noun subject is to be expected downstream in the sentence. Maintaining such syntactic expectations across intervening words is a particularly challenging cognitive load for the aphasic subject.

Chapter 8

Disorders of Repetition

INTRODUCTION

Although the ability to repeat from a spoken model may appear unrelated to normal communicative activity, the status of this ability has proven to be an important diagnostic indicator in the typology of the aphasias, insofar as it may be selectively damaged or selectively preserved in certain patients. As we have noted earlier (see Chapter 2), the repetition mechanism plays an important role in the typology derived from the Wernicke-Lichtheim model. A disproportionate impairment of repetition was thought to be the hallmark of conduction aphasia, whereas a disproportionate preservation of repetition was the major feature of the transcortical aphasias.

Logic, as well as clinical observation, supports the assumption that repetition of a spoken model requires, on the one hand, adequate auditory perception of speech and, on the other hand, preservation of the mechanisms of articulation. In this chapter, we review the clinical symptomatology of impaired and preserved repetition and reconsider the anatomic and psychological basis for normal and disordered performance.

THE PLACE OF REPETITION IN NORMAL SPEECH

The ability to imitate speech sounds and, ultimately, words and sentences is thought to develop during the babbling period of the preverbal infant. Even before the infant begins to model sounds produced by others, its spontaneous vocal play brings about the sense of correspondence between phonatory and articulatory gestures and their acoustic product, as perceived auditorily. Though we have little understanding of how this learning takes place on a neural level, it is certain that humans are endowed with a system that is exquisitely prepared to acquire these correspondences in a fashion that is automatic, requiring only the intention to verbalize to set it in motion. It is presumably on the basis of this initial experience with spontaneous verbalization that the infant is then able to imitate the sounds of its language, as heard from the speech of its mother and other speakers.

The path from babbling to veridical imitation and accurate articulation is, of course, not a straight line. Some sounds are generally more easily acquired than others, but this order of acquisition, as Menn (1981) points out, is only probabalistic across children, with much variation among individuals. Before mastering the phonology of the language, even for imitation, children must get past the period in which errors of articulation are imposed by either intrinsic features of the immature phonological apparatus or else by such cognitive influences as overgeneralization of articulatory rules. The course of acquisition of adult speech-modeling capacity is also marked by a period during which the child may have a single output pattern for two or more different sounds and has yet to discriminate the differences between the heard model and his or her own production. Such familiar error types as " 'tory" for "story" and "lellow" for "yellow," illustrate only two of many common error patterns. A detailed discussion of the maturation of phonological control is out of place here, but excellent reviews can be found in Ferguson and Garnica (1973), Menn (1979), and Studdert-Kennedy (1978).

Even when accurate imitation at the word level is mastered, the ability to repeat phrases and sentences is influenced by the development of verbal short-term memory and syntax. The retention of a sentence for repetition reflects the interaction between short-term phonological storage and the encoding of word meanings, and of syntactic patterns as they are perceived in the spoken model. Sentences of more than a few words are not repeated by pure parroting but are reconstituted, in part through the aid of the subject's knowledge of sentence structure and of the meaning of the message and, in part, through veridical phonological short-term memory.

Whereas much of the preceding may seem self-evident, it is easy to forget when confronted with some of the apparently paradoxical performances of aphasic patients—For example, the limitation of repetition span to one or two disconnected words in a patient who may be able to repeat a five- or six-word string in the form of an organized sentence.

REPETITION IMPAIRMENTS AND SPONTANEOUS OUTPUT

For most aphasic patients, the repetition task elicits performances that are generally similar in quality and degree of impairment to their spontaneous or conversational speech. This is true for patients with articulatory impairment associated with Broca's aphasia, with global aphasia, and with anterior subcortical aphasias characterized by impaired articulation. It is most especially true for patients having the almost purely articulatory disorder termed "aphemia."

Repetition in Broca's Aphasia

Patients with Broca's aphasia and similar restrictions of speech output can usually produce somewhat more speech through repetition than they can without such a model. At the one-word level, these patients can repeat words that they have not been able to retrieve spontaneously, although their word repetition is still limited by articulatory difficulties and they break down in attempting to repeat long or phonetically complex words. Providing a model for repetition often assists them in improving their articulation of words that present articulatory problems without such assistance.

Given phrases and sentences to repeat, their limitations in speech planning span, in articulation, in syntax, and in short-term memory quickly come into evidence. A model for repetition usually elicits more output than they have available spontaneously, but the margin of advantage is small. We will contrast the output of a patient with a moderately severe agrammatic Broca's aphasia under conditions of free narrative and in repetition.

Free narrative

The patient is describing the "Cookie Theft" scene from the Boston Diagnostic Aphasia Examination: A boy is reaching into a cupboard for a cookie jar while his stool is beginning to tip over. His sister is standing near him reaching up for a cookie.

"Cookie . . . Okay, . . . the cookie jar . . . and the kid is a . . . uh . . . Stool . . . bump . . . the skool . . . skool . . . uh . . . hurt . . . and girl . . . I don't know . . ."

Repetition

MODEL	REPETITION
Come in	Come bin
Have a seat	Have a seat
Take off your coat	Coat . . . no coat . . . hat . . . coat.
Do you want a drink?	Do da drinkarink . . . drink . . .

Just a cup of coffee.	Copt a coffee . . . coffee . . . copt a coffee
Is it still raining outside?	Raining outside?
They don't make them like they used to.	Like usedyou . . . uh . . . make 'em like da used to.
It's not whether you win or lose, but how you play the game.	Is . . . lot . . . no whether to lose . . . ren . . . and lose, but how to play the game.

Although the limitations of this man's agrammatism are conspicuous, particularly in his inability to repeat the grammatical functors at the beginning of a question, there are instances in which he goes far beyond his spontaneous speech capacity, both in the number of uninterrupted words in a string and in his use of grammatical functors ("how to play the game"). Such improvement as a result of a model is not seen in patients with profound articulatory impairments nor in patients who have aphemia. That is, it appears that a model for repetition is least effective in relieving difficulties that are at or close to the elementary motor control level; they are *most* effective in facilitating processes at a higher level of cognitive processing, such as word retrieval or the framing of sentences.

Repetition in Wernicke's Aphasia

Repetition by Wernicke's aphasics generally reflects the degree and type of impairment heard in their conversational and responsive speech. It suffers from their impairment in semantically processing the spoken model for reproduction. Unlike transcortical aphasics, who have remarkably well preserved phonological short-term memory, Wernicke's aphasics, at best, retain only fragments of the veridical phonology of the model, which may emerge during their attempts to repeat. Repetition by Wernicke's aphasics also suffers from a breakdown in the phonological assembly process—particularly in the automatic monitoring and guidance of developing phonological strings before they reach the motor output system. This failure allows many wordlike units that have bits of the target phonology mixed with paraphasic intrusions to attain motor realization. Because many Wernicke's aphasics are profoundly anomic, in addition to having reduced auditory short-term memory, they have particular difficulty in retaining, for repetition, lexical items beyond the first word or two of a multiword model.

The feature that pervades the repetition of Wernicke's aphasics, as it does their spontaneous and responsive speech, is the propensity for paraphasic intrusions of well articulated, but extraneous syllables, words, or phrases. There is, as yet, no complete and satisfactory explanation of how these intrusions are generated. One can only assume that the same mechanism is at work in their attempts at repetition as in their free speech. At a descriptive level, one can say that they have easy access to the production of phonological sequences, whether appropriate to the target or not, and to morpho-syntactic sequences, appropriate or not, often coupled with disinhibition of speech production and absence of self-monitoring. The manifestations of these features in repetition attempts is usually on par with their evidence in conversation.

Repetition of single words by these patients is usually much superior to their attempts at multiword utterances. A characteristic error is what we have labeled "augmentation," that is, appending an extra syllable or two to a word, usually one that forms another real word or compound word, with the model as the beginning. For example:

MODEL FOR REPETITION	RESPONSE
black	blackboard
shoe	Shoelace

Other examples of repetition by patients with Wernicke's aphasia:

MODEL FOR REPETITION	RESPONSE
He parks the car.	He park . . . he came with the car. He came with his car.
It goes between two others.	It went two cars . . . between the cars.

SELECTIVE DIFFICULTY WITH REPETITION

In the two preceding sections we have reviewed different forms of impairment in repetition in which the deficit in repetition resembled the deficit in conversational speech, both in quality and severity. The special status of repetition as an aspect of aphasia, however, arises from the disorders in which repetition is selectively impaired—where the failure of repetition is not explained by either impaired comprehension or impaired motor speech implementation. In these instances, we may suppose that the lesion has damaged the substrate for the system that has been perfected in the early years of childhood for making speech output correspond to a heard model. Yet, there is controversy, both as to the nature of the disorder in these cases and as to the site of causative lesions.

CONDUCTION APHASIA

According to Lichtheim's (1884) elaboration of Wernicke's earlier schema, interruption of the pathway between the auditory speech center and the motor output center should result in a failure of repetition. Because such an interruption could occur without impairment of either of the two centers themselves, Lichtheim predicted that patients should be found who had unimpaired comprehension and facile speech output, yet were unable to repeat what they heard. This was his anatomical account of conduction aphasia—a disorder that was predicted on a logical basis before it had been described clinically.

In the clinical presentation of conduction aphasia, the selective defect of repetition may be a salient and impressive feature, or it may be a relatively minor symptom, detected by its qualitative characteristics rather than by its severity. Equally central as a feature of this disorder is the frequent appearance of phonemic paraphasia—during free conversation, during attempts to name pictures, and during repetition. Unlike the patient with Wernicke's aphasia, patients with conduction aphasia are usually acutely aware of the inaccuracy of their production and make repeated attempts at self-correction. As they do so, they may correct one portion of the target while introducing a new error elsewhere, sometimes wandering further afield and sometimes approaching closer to or even succeeding in saying the desired word. For example one patient attempting to name a picture of a whistle produced "tris ... chi ... trissle ... sissle ... twiss ... ciss." On a different day, he offered "whistles ... spin ... twissle ... siss," overlooking and not benefiting from his first almost correct production. For the picture of "pretzel," he produced "trep ... tretzle ... trethle ... tredfle ... ki." What is particularly notable in this behavior is the stability of the phonological skeleton around which the various attempts revolve and its resistance to decay in the face of interference from a succession of attempts. When offered alternative pronunciations of the target by the examiner, these patients are invariably accurate in rejecting those that are even minimally inaccurate and endorsing those that are correct.

In repetition of words, conduction aphasics show difficulties in the selection and sequencing of phonemes for production, with resulting output that is very similar to their difficulties in picture naming. On the one-word level, their success in repetition is closely correlated with the length and phonological complexity of the test word. Whereas patients with the most severe repetition problems may fail on common one-syllable words, it is much more common to find that short words are easily repeated but those with even minimal phonological complexity become hopelessly tangled.

The repetition of phrases or sentences is usually much more difficult and may produce failures in patients who have little difficulty with single words. Here too, the degree of familiarity of the phrase makes the difference between smooth performance and complete failure.

Aside from articulatory problems that arise when the patient becomes enmeshed in self-corrective efforts, the delivery of conduction aphasics is phonologically facile and syntactically organized. They are "fluent" aphasics in the sense that much of their production in free conversation or narrative is in the form of syntactically organized runs of words that may allow long phrases or sentences without interruption. However, conduction aphasia rarely occurs without some disorder of syntax and some anomia; that is, scattered among their well-organized sentences are instances of tangled syntax and even agrammatic omissions. Word-finding difficulty may further disrupt their output. In their free conversation, it is often striking that phonemic planning problems arise when patients are attempting to produce nouns or major verbs, whereas the grammatical words are unaffected. That is, the characteristic production difficulty of the conduction aphasic emerges at the point of maximum information.

The foregoing summary of clinical features of conduction aphasia sheds doubt on the notion that it is primarily a disorder of repetition, and even more doubt on the anatomic interpretation of a disconnection of an auditory language center from a motor speech planning center. Let us consider some of the alternative notions.

PSYCHOLINGUISTIC ACCOUNTS OF CONDUCTION APHASIA

Dubois *et al.* (1964) offered one of the earliest interpretations of conduction aphasia in terms of information processing, on the basis of experimental data. They had patients with conduction aphasia attempt to repeat nonsense words of varying syllabic length and real words similarly varied in length. They found that the difficulty in repeating nonsense words increased directly with the number of syllables; whereas in the case of real words, syllabic count was not predictive of item difficulty. They interpreted this result as indicating that difficulty in implementing a phonological sequence depended on the degree of uncertainty of the phonological information to be encoded at the start of each syllable. In the case of nonsense words, the uncertainty was multiplied as each new syllable appeared; in the case of real words, uncertainty was maximal at word onset, but decreased during successive syllables.

Dubois *et al.* used this principle to explain why conduction aphasics were deficient in supplying opposites that used a negating prefix (like versus dislike) as compared to those that involved different roots (open versus close). In their analysis, words that used a negating prefix confronted the speaker with a high-information decision at the end of the prefix as well as preceding it. Those words that used a lexical opposite had only one point of high information—at the beginning of the word. They contrasted this effect found in conduction aphasics with the opposite effect observed in anomic aphasics. The anomics had great difficulty in accessing a new lexical form, but had no difficulty combining a negating affix with a word that was supplied for them.

The interpretation by Dubois *et al.*, however, is difficult to reconcile with the findings of Pate, Saffran and Martin (1987), as cited by Berndt (1989). The latter investigators found that when an identical phonological string was spoken as a single word (e.g., "murderous") it was more difficult to repeat than when it represented two words ("murder us"). That is, Pate *et al.* found that the number of syllables within a single word was highly predictive of the repetition difficulty faced by conduction aphasics. The example just given involved the use of an affix (*-ous*). It is not clear whether increasing the length of a word by affixation entails a different processing load from a similar syllable count in a monomorphemic word. In any case, it seems clear that difficulty with repetition, per se, is not a sufficient definition of conduction aphasia.

Geschwind, in his clinical demonstrations often pointed out that conduction aphasics have extraordinary difficulty in repeating sentences that consist largely of grammatical functors—pronouns, prepositions, and low-information verbs (e.g., "Why did she do it to him?"). He introduced the test phrase "No ifs, ands, or buts" as a password that was sure to be failed by any conduction aphasic. In subsequent years, we have observed numbers of conduction aphasics who had extraordinary difficulty in sequencing the words of functor-loaded sentences, but systematic data collection failed to confirm the reliability of this feature in unselected patients with conduction aphasia.

SHORT-TERM AUDITORY MEMORY DEFICIT

In 1969, Warrington and Shallice described a patient with a residual aphasia of 11 years standing that had resulted from a left parieto-occipital skull fracture. Although his aphasic disability at the time of the study was relatively mild, he had a severe impairment in repetition span for strings of words or letters. His span for similar strings presented visually was considerably better than his auditory span. Warrington and Shallice suggested that this case might represent a pure form of conduction aphasia that could be attributed to a deficit in auditory short-term memory.

Because auditory memory impairment had never before been offered as an explanation for conduction aphasia, this proposal drew considerable criticism. Indeed, because the authors concentrated on the reporting of performance on strings of unrelated words, there was little in the case description to convince the reader that the patient displayed the standard clinical features of conduction aphasia. Two more cases were reported by Warrington, Logue, and Pratt (1972) in which there was a similar severe deficit in repetition associated with a marked reduction in auditory, but not visual, short-term memory. Both of these cases had parietal lobe injuries. One of the patients was described as having no expressive language impairment, whereas the other was halting and circumlocutory. Again, clinical description of the language impairment is too scanty to judge whether either of these patients resembled conduction aphasics in the character of their production errors.

One response to the proposals of Warrington and associates, was a case report by Strub and Gardner (1974) of a conduction aphasic who shared some of the auditory memory deficits described in the foregoing three cases, but who also gave evidence that his production deficit could not be explained by the memory impairment. Strub and Gardner argued that the disorder was in the realm of language production, and not in memory. Nevertheless, further studies of auditory memory function in conduction aphasics (e.g., Tzortzis and Albert, 1974) found that their conduction aphasics had deficiencies in auditory memory, the role of which in repetition failure had to be considered. In our own clinical examination of conduction aphasics we have invariably noted impairments in auditory span. Yet, we agree with Strub and Gardner that these do not give a sufficient account of the impairment in phonological sequencing for production that is apparent both in naming and in repetition. A particularly telling argument is the persistence of the auditory trace that permits conduction aphasics to continue self-corrective attempts at a target word and to identify it correctly from multiple choice after these interfering efforts, while continuing to fail in their reproduction of the word.

The term "reproduction conduction aphasia" has been suggested as a way to refer to the classical form of the disorder in which phonological production problems go well beyond what could be accounted for by an auditory memory impairment. Most reports concur in finding that these patients are as impaired in oral reading and in naming as they are in repeating.

Kohn (1984), contrasting the phonemic paraphasias of conduction aphasics with those made by Broca's and Wernicke's aphasics, emphasizes the consistent phonological link between the successive attempts of conduction aphasics and the target word. She considers most of these failures in production to be "postlexical"—that is, arising at a point when the abstract phonological representation of the word has been achieved, but prior to its motor realization. She suggests a stage of "prearticulatory programming" as the point of breakdown. Kohn's interpretation is not unlike that of Dubois *et al.* (1964) in placing the breakdown at a late stage of production.

PARAPHRASING

In milder cases of conduction aphasia, the repetition of short sentences is feasible, but usually includes errors. A characteristic type of error involves paraphrasing while retaining the meaning of the model sentence. For example, given the model "The plane is about to land," the patient may repeat "The plane is going to land." Paraphrasing is much more likely to involve changes in grammatical functors than in significant lexical items. Impairment of auditory short-term memory may offer an explanation for these effects. Grammatical functors can be expected to bear the brunt of short-term memory deficits because during the on-line decoding and storage of the model sentence, the semantic value of the lexical terms serves as a strong aid in retrieving their phonology. The grammatical functors, however, provide no word-by-word semantic information to aid in verbatim recall.

DEEP DYSPHASIA: A RARE REPETITION DISORDER

Michel and Andreewsky (1983) described a patient who characteristically failed in repetition by substituting semantically related words for the model provided by the examiner. Among the errors cited by the authors are

STIMULUS	RESPONSE
balloon	kite
beggar	tramp
kernel	shell
independence	elections

Repetition was more likely to be accurate for concrete than for abstract nouns and better for nouns and adjectives than for verbs. When verbs were repeated, they were in the infinitive, rather than in any finite form that may have been provided. The patient was completely unable to repeat grammatical functors or nonwords. When giving semantic substitutions, as in the preceding examples, he was usually convinced that he was repeating what he heard, although he could be led to express uncertainty if pressed by the examiner.

The authors suggested the term "deep dysphasia" to describe this pattern of repetition failures because of the close parallel between this pattern and the one observed in the oral word-reading failures of patients with "deep dyslexia." In both instances, there is a "part of speech effect" (nouns are superior to verbs which are superior to grammatical functors) and a complete inability to deal with pronounceable nonwords. Also, in both instances the pattern of failure suggests almost total failure of phonological input in guiding word production and an overreliance on an imperfectly functioning semantic route to word retrieval.

Michel and Andreewsky's patient had an unusual pattern of language deficits. His auditory comprehension was impaired and his speech production displayed a mix of features of fluent and agrammatic aphasia: impaired naming, frequent literal paraphasias, and a tendency to use agrammatic constructions in speech production. A remarkable feature was this patient's virtually intact reading comprehension and relatively well preserved ability to write—particularly to write words that he could not produce in speech. An example of the dissociation between oral and written language is that he could not match any of four very common irregular verbs, spoken orally, to their written forms in a multiple choice list. Yet he wrote the infinitive form of each of the verbs alongside the corresponding form on the page of test stimuli to demonstrate his comprehension of the written words.

A patient (SM) with a very similar pattern of semantic substitutions in word and sentence repetition tasks was studied by Katz and Goodglass (1990). He resembled Michel and Andreewsky's patient in the part-of-speech effect in his repetition failures, including the near total failure in repeating grammatical functors and nonwords. Like their patient, SM complained of having almost instantly lost the trace of the sound of a word he was given for repetition, although he retained its meaning. He was severely impaired in object name retrieval, making about the same proportion and type of semantic misnamings on picture confrontation as he did in repetition. Further, like the patient of Michel and Andreewsky, SM read with comprehension at a rate considerably better than he could understand orally. His oral reading was virtually flawless, both in speed and accuracy. Unlike the patient described by Michel and Andreewsky, SM read orally without slowness or phonological impairment.

Katz and Goodglass attributed SM's repetition impairment to the combination of his immediate loss of phonological short-term memory and his deficient ability to name on the basis of semantic activation. That is, it was reasoned that on hearing a word for repetition, SM decoded its semantics while almost immediately losing the phonology from short-term memory. This left him in the subjective state that he described as knowing what had been said, but having forgotten what the word was. Repetition for him meant renaming the concept that he retained, without any guidance from a partial phonological trace. In this renaming, he was subject to the same difficulties that he encountered in any picture naming task—that is, the propensity to semantic paraphasic substitutions.

Although the combinations of deficits that were found both in SM and in Michel and Andreewsky's patient is rare, these cases are useful in clarifying the boundary conditions of conduction aphasia. These patients had common characteristics that are not found in conduction aphasia: (1) both had temporal lobe lesions and impairment in word comprehension; (2) both had fairly good oral reading, that of SM was virtually perfect; and (3) their repetition failures consisted predominantly of semantic substitutions and often retained no trace of the target phonology. Unlike conduction aphasics, they did not make repeated, phonologically guided efforts at self-correction. In comparison with models of conduction aphasia, the disruption of deep dysphasia appears to be at an earlier, prelexical processing stage.

Other variants of deep dysphasia have been reported. For example, the case of Howard and Franklin (1988), MK, made semantic errors in repetition that appeared to be due to impaired access to meaning through input phonology. His short-term auditory retention was not sufficiently impaired to account for his erroneous repetition on the basis of a loss of the phonological trace. Thus, while experimental investigations indicated that the patient did not lose the phonological trace of what he had heard, this information was overridden by the conflicting semantic misinterpretation of the stimulus words. Like the other cases cited, MK's success in repetition was a function of the semantic properties of the stimuli presented: words superior to nonwords, lexical terms superior to functors, and concrete nouns superior to abstract ones.

TRANSCORTICAL MOTOR APHASIA

The syndrome of marked impoverishment of spontaneous speech with a normal ability to repeat words and sentences and preserved auditory comprehension is known under the term "transcortical motor aphasia" by writers who follow the classical taxonomy of the Lichtheim model (1884); it corresponds closely to the symptomatology of Luria's (1970) "frontal dynamic aphasia."

The inability of these patients to organize a response in conversation is well illustrated by a quotation by Freedman, Alexander, and Naeser (1984) from a patient of theirs who was trying to give an account of the Cookie Theft scene (previously described):

"Well it's . . . trouble with this . . . I can't tell . . . having trouble"

It is typical for patients to begin with a discourse-opening formula, such as "Well, I . . .," and then to block or to swear in frustration. Without external stimulation, it is rare for them to make any effort to speak. A subgroup of patients of this type are quite successful in giving one-word or very short answers to questions requiring a brief informational response. Typically, these patients do very well in picture naming or in providing simple factual information. However, this capacity cannot be offered as a universal trait of transcortical motor aphasics. Many patients who meet the principal criteria are severely impaired in naming. They tend to respond well to phonemic priming when they fail to name a picture, but they are also prone to offer an incorrect completion for the stem provided.

Repetition of words and sentences ranges from far superior to other speech efforts, to being indistinguishable from normal. In repetition, these patients display normal articulation, normal reproduction of syntax—regardless of its complexity, and good retention of the vocabulary used in the model provided. Other aspects of language use are variable from patient to patient. Such variability is reported for oral reading and reading comprehension. Writing is always described as impaired.

In describing the difficulties of patients with frontal dynamic aphasia, Luria places the emphasis on the loss of spontaneity of thought processes that is reflected in their inability to think of anything to say. Even when given a picture situation to describe, they cannot organize the sequence of the ideas that they might convey. Instead, they perseverate by repeating elements of a sentence they have just used. For Luria, this disorder is on the border between an impairment of thinking and one of language. The preservation of repetition is mentioned in passing, as part of case descriptions, but it is not as central to Luria's concept of frontal dynamic aphasia as it is to the classical syndrome of transcortical motor aphasia.

LOCALIZATION OF TRANSCORTICAL MOTOR APHASIA

Benson (1979), following Geschwind's teaching, grouped the aphasic syndromes in two anatomic groups: those caused by perisylvian lesions, in which repetition was impaired, and those caused by border zone lesions, in which repetition was spared. The border zone lesions are in the zone where the vascular territory of the middle cerebral artery merges with that of the anterior cerebral artery anteriorly, and with the territory of the posterior cerebral artery, caudally. In the case of transcortical motor aphasia, it is the anterior borderzone that is affected.

The lesion is typically just anterior or superior to Broca's area, generally involving subcortical structures. In their study of 15 patients with variants of this disorder, Freedman *et al.* (1984) found that the "common feature" of the patients lesions was damage to a subcortical site just lateral and anterior to the frontal horn of the left lateral ventricle. In some instances, the left supplementary motor area was involved.

Lesions of the supplementary motor area often result initially in muteness, which shortly abates, but leaves the patient with a severe difficulty in initiating speech. Freedman *et al.* suggest that lesions either in the supplementary motor area or along its outflow path, which passes anteriolaterally to the frontal horn, may effectively deprive the cortical speech zones of input from the limbic system that is needed for inititating speech.

TRANSCORTICAL SENSORY APHASIA

When posterior portions of the border zone territory are affected, auditory language processing and word retrieval are affected, while repetition continues to be well preserved. In the syndrome of transcortical sensory aphasia, speech output may be uninhibited and paraphasic, often with profound anomia. Some patients with this syndrome have a remarkable preservation of oral reading skills, but their reading is without comprehension. Similarly, their remarkably intact repetition may also be devoid of comprehension.

The clinical picture of transcortical sensory aphasia includes some interesting features that are seen occasionally in the motor transcortical form. One is the tendency of the patient to repeat back part of what he or she has been asked. This repetition has some of the quality of echoing, but it is not involuntary and occurs only in the context of social interchange. This tendency also expresses itself in the patient incorporating some or all of his interlocutor's words in framing his answer.

Studies probing the limits of patients' accuracy in verbatim repetition have shown that these patients almost invariably correct grammatical errors in the model provided, but they do not amend semantically nonsensical word choice. Thus, when asked to repeat "The boy hung him coat in the icebox," the patient's response would be "The boy hung his coat in the icebox." Many patients with transcortical aphasia are surprisingly successful in repeating nonsense words or words spoken in a foreign language. That is, some of their repetition may be based purely on phonological recoding, without support by lexical processes. Of course, real words and meaningful sentences permit the repetition span to be much greater, as it would be in normals.

Preserved repetition skills also go hand in hand with a preserved ability to recite memorized passages. Typically, a patient with transcortical aphasia (motor or sensory) can recite the Lord's Prayer on request, with little or no assistance.

ISOLATION OF THE SPEECH AREA

A unique case of preserved repetition of speech in the absence of all other communicative interaction was described by Geschwind, Quadfasel, and Segarra (1968). This case was that of a young woman who had suffered massive cerebral damage from carbon monoxide poisoning. She was incapable of any response indicating comprehension of speech or of producing any communicative utterance. She did not interact socially in any way that would permit demonstration of preserved cognitive function, but accepted feeding and nursing care. Yet, on being addressed, she sometimes echoed questions or responded with the stereotyped phrase "So can daddy." More remarkably, given the beginning of a familiar song or verse, she continued it. For example, when provided with "Ask me no questions," she completed it with "I'll tell you no lies." The fact that this was not confined to old overlearned patterns was evidenced by her learning new commercial jingles and popular tunes that she heard repeatedly on the radio that was kept going by her bedside. Her delivery was parrot-like and did not appear to be addressed to any person. With time, her condition deteriorated and she declined to a virtually vegetative state.

Upon autopsy, she was found to have massive and symmetrical hemispheric destruction sparing the auditory system, and Broca's and Wernicke's areas, along with their connecting fiber tracts. There was destruction of tissue surrounding the central perisylvian speech zone, both cortically and subcortically. Thus it could be assumed that auditory input to her language zone had no access to any other brain activity.

This case provided considerable support for the view that the anatomic basis for repetition is in the core of the perisylvian zone, comprising Wernicke's area, Broca's area, and their interconnections. Repetition in this case, however, was more akin to parrot-like echoing of parts of questions than like the voluntary repetition of words or sentences that is seen in patients with transcortial aphasia—motor or sensory. The preservation of the ability to learn new jingles after a few hearings and the general preservation of overlearned sequences is the most salient language-related observation. Because the patient was incapable of any purposeful interaction, perhaps true voluntary repetition could not have been expected.

Mixed transcortical aphasias, involving multiple lesions in both anterior and posterior parts of the border zone territory are not unusual. They are commonly the result of impaired blood flow in the internal carotid artery, which places at risk the entire periphery of the area irrigated by the middle cerebral artery.

SUMMARY

The investigation of selective impairments of repetition and selective preservation of this capacity have clarified some of the functional relationships at work in speech production and comprehension. To begin with, it is clear that an impairment of short-term auditory verbal memory of any sort must affect repetition, even though it may have only minor impact on the comprehension of connected speech. Thus, the cases described by Warrington and Shallice (1969) and by Warrington, Logue, and Pratt (1972) demonstrate that severe restrictions of short-term auditory verbal memory may result from left parietal lobe lesions. The accounts of these cases go little further than to show that such memory impairment prevents the retention of auditorily presented word lists. But the cases that Michel and Andreewsky (1983) and Katz and Goodglass (1990) termed "deep dysphasia" exemplify an apparently much more profound disturbance of auditory retention. In these cases, the phonological trace lasted only long enough for semantic interpretation to be completed and was then unavailable to the patient. We cannot say whether these "deep dysphasics" simply had a more severe form of verbal short-term memory deficit than the patients described by Warrington and her associates. The fact that the "deep dysphasics" produced repetitions that had only a semantic and no phonological relation to the stimulus raises the possibility that failure of word retention may not be identical with failure of the auditory phonological trace. Warrington's patients all had parietal lobe lesions. Those of Michel and Andreewsky, and of Katz and Goodglass had temporal lobe lesions with initially severely impaired auditory comprehension. The difference in lesion sites lends plausibility to the notion that the auditory retention failures in the two types of patients involved subtly different levels of auditory processing.

The severely impaired repetition of the "deep dysphasics" suggests that a purely semantic route to repetition cannot be adequate. That is, if the individual recalls only the meaning and not the sound of what he or she has just heard, the attempt to supply a name for that meaning is just as apt to be wrong as correct. But this inference is tempered by the fact that the patient of Katz and Goodglass had similar name retrieval problems in picture naming. Clearly, the mechanism proposed for the semantic repetition errors of Katz and Goodglass' patient, SM, cannot account for those of MK, the patient of Howard and Franklin, which appeared to involve an earlier aspect of input processing. That is, MK semantically misidentified the words that he heard, and then offered these misinterpretations in repetition. In contrast to SM, his ability to name to confrontation was only slightly affected.

Short-term auditory verbal memory has been found to be impaired in patients classified as conduction aphasics, but this impairment is neither sufficiently severe, nor sufficiently related to their specific symptomatology to serve as an explanation of their failures. The distinctive characteristics of these patients are observed not only in repetition, but also in naming and in free conversation. They occur in single-word production, which is well within the memory span of these patients. They appear to involve the transition from a relatively stable phonological representation to the implementation of motor speech. The phonological representation arises either from an auditorily presented model for repetition, or from a concept whose phonological code has been partially or fully retrieved by the patient and is being held in a short-term buffer memory. It is in the readout of this code into a real-time motor plan that production fails, with characteristic errors of phonological sequencing, omissions, and substitutions that are described as "phonemic paraphasias." The attribution of this breakdown to a disconnection between the auditory language zone and the motor speech control zone, as proposed by Wernicke (1874) and Lichtheim (1884), and more recently by Geschwind (1965), no longer seems viable. A processing disorder involving cortical tissue in the perisylvian region has recently been proposed (Damasio and Damasio, 1989) in opposition to the earlier notion that there is a disconnection in white matter between Wernicke's and Broca's areas.

From the selective preservation of repetition, we learn that repetition may be divorced from semantic processing, though it cannot be divorced from auditory memory. There is considerable clinico-pathological evidence, particularly the Geschwind *et al.* (1968) case of isolation of the speech area, that preservation of the Broca-Wernicke area complex may be the sufficient condition for retention of the ability to repeat—at least in echoic fashion. Of course the identification of the central perisylvian zone as containing the neural substrate for repetition is not equivalent to endorsing the notion that the breakdown of repetition is based on a disconnection between auditory and motor language centers.

Chapter 9

Disorders of Reading

The normally hearing child learns to read through the medium of previously acquired spoken language, particularly through the auditory representation of words and sounds. Reading, at least during its acquisition, appears to consist of associating a graphic code to already familiar auditory patterns of syllables, words, and word groupings. It would not be farfetched to suppose that the neural substrate for reading is built on and includes at least part of the neural substrate for understanding speech. The consequence of such an assumption would be that an impairment in the comprehension of speech is accompanied by a parallel impairment in reading.

In the great majority of aphasic patients, this expectation is supported in a rough way. That is, patients who have a severe compromise of auditory language comprehension, such as global aphasics and Wernicke's aphasics, usually have correspondingly severe impairments in associating written words to their sounds or their meanings—often even in recognizing letters by name or in matching letters across forms of script or print. We shall refer to this generalized loss of meaning and sound associations to written symbols as "aphasic alexia," that is, alexia that appears to be secondary to loss of oral language. Aphasic alexia may cover the full spectrum of severity. When the patient has some residual reading comprehension, one can usually demonstrate that the reading disability has many analogies to impairments of auditory comprehension, such as word frequency effects, differences among parts of speech, and relative robustness of connotative comprehension as compared to specific denotation. These will be described in further detail.

However, the attribution of aphasic alexia to the impairment of the auditory language system is a highly imperfect principle. For one thing, reading impairments of a similar nature are found in aphasics of many types, including those with primarily speech output disorders, such as Broca's aphasics. Reading impairments in Broca's aphasia are usually mild, but may be severe in cases of deep-going lesions. On the other hand, Wernicke's aphasics sometimes retain considerable functional reading ability. Hécaen (1969) reported that Wernicke's aphasics whose lesions did not extend posteriorly beyond the Sylvian fissure had relatively preserved reading ability. The more the lesion extended posteriorly, encroaching on the region of the angular gyrus, the more severe the alexia. As we have noted earlier (Chapter 3), angular gyrus lesions can produce severe impairments of written language—in both reading and writing—with relatively mild impairment of speech output or comprehension. For this reason, the angular gyrus region has been regarded as mediating the associations between input received from the visual association areas of the occipital lobe and the auditory language system.

In recent years, a great deal of attention has been centered on forms of reading disorder that can be described as "dissociative alexias." Although these constitute a small proportion of the neurologically based acquired reading disorders, they are of extreme theoretical importance and have contributed both to an understanding of normal reading processes and to understanding how these are implemented by the brain. One subset of these "dissociative" alexias have a very distinct anatomical basis. These include "alexia with agraphia," associated with angular gyrus lesions, and "alexia without agraphia" (also called "pure alexia" or "letter-by-letter reading"). The other subset involves selective dissociations of particular cognitive components of reading for which there is no clear anatomical basis. These include "deep dyslexia," "phonological dyslexia," and "surface dyslexia." The three latter forms of disorder are all primarily manifested in oral reading. In our review of the reading process, it is vital to distinguish oral reading from reading comprehension. Oral reading may be intact when comprehension is nil (as in some patients with transcortical sensory aphasia), whereas errors in oral reading may mask adequate comprehension.

THE COGNITIVE BASIS FOR READING

In order to deal with the dissociations among cognitive operations in reading it is necessary to give some consideration to the multiple and interacting character of these operations. In an alphabetic language, like English, the multiplicity of these interactions is maximized. Many people assume that we read by associating each letter in a written word with its corresponding sound, stringing these sounds together, and then recognizing the meaning of the assembled word. Most children learn to read through "phonics"—the skill of rapidly assembling the sounds of a letter string to reconstruct the phonological representation of a word. In fact, the normally competent English reader can sound out in this way pseudo-words that he or she has never seen (e.g., "ztixo"). Moreover, there would be a high level of agreement among individuals as to how this pseudo-word should sound. This mode of recoding letters into sounds is termed "grapho-phonemic correspondence." It is a strategy that is universally applied by readers of English in arriving at a pronunciation (sometimes incorrect) of foreign names. Obviously, grapho-phonemic correspondence rules are of little use in pronouncing irregular words (e.g., sure, sugar, cough, colonel, or yacht), or abbreviations (e.g., Mr., Mrs., lbs, NY). Yet, irregular words and abbreviations are seemingly read aloud with as little hesitation as are regularly spelled words. Thus, these phenomena of normal reading show that word phonology may be activated directly by a familiar letter string, totally bypassing letter-to-sound conversion which would only lead to an incorrect production.

The principle of grapho-phoneme conversion, although necessary in initially learning to read through the phonic method and for deciphering unusual foreign names, may be superfluous to the normal reader when faced with an unfamiliar English word or name. A number of theoreticians (Glushko, 1979; Henderson, 1982) propose that a pronounceable nonword receives its phonology through the activation of known words that share some of its letter sequences—a process that suggests pronunciation by analogy.

From what has been said so far about reading, one might assume that the meaning of the written word is accessed only after it is sounded, either in oral reading or in silent rehearsal. If this were the case, it would be impossible to carry out silent reading at the speed that a normal reader does so; it would also be impossible to distinguish between the meanings of homophones with different spellings (e.g., him versus hymn; our versus hour).

Thus we see that reasoning only from the everyday experiences of normal reading, there are at least three routes available from the written word to oral reading with comprehension: that of grapheme–phoneme conversion, whole-word activation of phonology, and direct access from the written word to its semantics. This abridged list does not include reading unfamiliar words by analogy with known ones, nor does it consider whether words that are interpreted semantically, directly from print, are accessed phonologically at the same time, or whether phonological access consists of naming the semantic concept that has already been attained.

The foregoing analysis is most relevant to word-by-word reading. The oral reading of connected text entails a number of further complications, among them, the fact that the reader has silently scanned well beyond the word that he is uttering at any moment. The amount of lead in silent reading (the eye-voice span) can be determined by blocking the reader's vision as he is saying a particular word and measuring how many more words of the text he can produce. A further issue arises in silent reading, which can be carried out more than twice as quickly as oral reading (Gibson and Levin, 1975). This concerns the nature of the subjective experience where the words are heard rapidly "in the head" during silent reading. We do not know how this inner experience of "hearing" one's silent reading relates to the overt realization of written word phonology. These problems of oral and silent reading of connected text surely have a bearing on the performance of aphasics with mild and residual reading difficulties, but they are outside the scope of this chapter.

The alternative, interactive paths from print to sound and meaning, comes into the foreground when we are confronted with cases of deep dyslexia, phonological dyslexia, and surface dyslexia—the forms of dyslexia involving dissociations between these cognitive components. For insight into anatomic disconnection disorders of reading, it is necessary to refer back to the anatomy of visual input to the language system, which was reviewed in Chapter 3.

APHASIC ALEXIA: CLINICAL AND PSYCHOLINGUISTIC FEATURES

Symbol Recognition

Even global aphasic patients who have no useful comprehension or production of oral or written language can usually match letters or short words across types of script, for example, upper case cursive versus lower case print—this, in spite of their failure to select letters from a written multiple choice on oral request. For most patients, the identity of letters as familiar entities that may appear in varied physical form is maintained, even though there is no longer a verbal label attached to them. The recognition of numbers may follow a different course from the recognition of letters. It is often better preserved. Patients who cannot identify letters from their name are often more successful with numbers. When they are not, they can usually match written digits with the corresponding number of fingers held up by the examiner. That is, written numbers are more likely to retain a conceptual value when letters have only an identity as familiar visual entities. It is often instructive to confront a patient with Roman numerals, which may be recognized as well as the corresponding Arabic number. It is possible for patients to select Roman numerals from multiple choice but to be unable to select the same symbols by their letter names.

Lexical Processing in Reading

The severely impaired aphasic patient is likely to fail if asked to find the name of an animal (e.g., "cow") in a short list of animal names or to find the name of a flower (e.g., "tulip") among a number of familiar flower names. In contrast, when the word "tulip" or "cow" appears in a list of words from diverse categories, the patient's success rate may approach 100%. This common observation is merely another demonstration, in the sphere of word reading of a phenomenon that is already familiar in the sphere of auditory word comprehension. The "meaning" carried by a written word is not an indivisible concept, but one having multiple layers that may be differently affected by aphasia. The most robust component of the concept is the connotation which is shared by all members of its category (e.g., flowers versus animals). Patients whose lexical semantic processing is impaired may still be able to distinguish from each other words from different connotative categories. A much more fragile level of comprehension is the ability to distinguish among members of the same category—particularly those sharing a strong connotative quality. For example, within the category of animals, tame domesticated ones (cows, sheep, and goats) would be more confused with each other than with a fierce animal or a reptile.

Many patients with aphasic alexia show an advantage in the understanding or oral reading of words the semantic qualities of which are intensified by either an emotional load or by strong picturability. For example, Landis, Graves, and Goodglass (1982) found that emotionally loaded words (e.g., love, kill, stab) were more successfully read aloud (60.6% correct) than either concrete nouns (e.g., boat, bird, coat—50.8% correct) or abstract, nonemotional words (time, fact, half,—40.2% correct) when all word groups were matched for frequency. Each of these trials was statistically significant. That is, concreteness effect, as well as the emotionality effect, influenced the readability of the stimulus words. Ten of the 22 aphasic patients studied produced one or more semantic paralexias in reading the 36 stimulus words. Subsequent analysis (Landis *et al.*, 1983) revealed that these 10 subjects had the largest left hemisphere lesions in the population and were therefore most likely to be using right hemisphere processing. The occurrence of semantic paralexias, however, was not an index of the severity of impairment in word reading.

Because patients with aphasic alexia show some effects of word semantics in their ability to read aloud and comprehend words, it might be supposed that they do poorly in reading grammatical morphemes such as prepositions that have only case-marking functions and little semantic content. The disadvantage for grammatical morphemes is slight or absent in most patients when they are either required to select these words from multiple choice on oral presentation or to read them aloud. They are probably read through the medium of whole word phonology, which is highly overlearned in these high frequency words. Patients with aphasic alexia are also found to use letter-to-sound cues in order to select non-sense words from a multiple choice array. They are naturally more likely to observe letter-to-sound correspondence at the beginning of such non-sense words than to detect differences between nonsense words that have the same initial sounds.

Sentence Comprehension in Aphasic Alexia

Written sentence comprehension by aphasic patients has not been sub-jected to psycholinguistic analysis. Any such analysis that attempted to go beyond an overall score would be extremely difficult. The interpreta-tion of connected text involves the integration of cues of many types, all subject to inference by the reader. Primary among the cues available are inferences drawn from the semantics of the lexical items in a sentence. For example, given the sentence frame "Birds build . . ." and a multiple choice of "nests," "fly," "eggs," and "walls," any one of the first three terms might be chosen on the basis of their semantic relationship to the word "birds," but only the first combines the semantic constraints (or real world knowledge) of both the subject and the verb. The ability to in-terpret correctly the meaning of grammatical or morphological elements in written text appears, from our observations, to differ in much the same way as it does in spoken sentences. The most difficult task in our mor-phosyntactic reading battery was judging number only from the pres-ence or absence of the final *s* in the third person singular of the verb. Next in order of difficulty were the recognition of the possessive-marking fi-nal *s* and the interpretation of subject–object roles in the passive case. The easiest discrimination was plural marking by the final *s*. Next easiest was the interpretation of gender and number denoted by possessive adjec-tives. There is little to indicate that the relative difficulty of these mor-phosyntactic forms in silent reading varies among types of aphasics when there is a control for the severity of the patient's impairment in lex-ical comprehension.

DISSOCIATIVE ALEXIAS

Alexia with Agraphia

Dejerine (1891) first described the loss of reading and writing ability, without involvement of spoken language, associated with a lesion of the angular gyrus of the left cerebral hemisphere. Alexia with agraphia following angular gyrus injury may be accompanied by anomic aphasia as the most prominent impairment. These cases are among the most infrequent forms of selective written language disorders and have not been subjected to careful neuropsychological study.

Alexia without Agraphia

The first anatomically supported case of "pure alexia" with retention of writing ability was also described by Dejerine (1892). (See Chapter 3 for a review of the anatomical mechanism.) The prototypical severe form of this disorder involves the inability to recognize words or letters, and consequently a complete inability to read. For some patients, the recognition of numbers is spared, while letters are either inconsistently recognized or totally failed. One striking feature in the performance of these patients is the ability to write normally but not to read back what they have recently written. These patients typically can understand words orally spelled for them as rapidly as a normal individual, and can read by touch words whose letters are formed for them on the palm of their hand or on a finger tip. These observations make it appear convincing that their alexia is due to a complete loss of visual input to the language system, while access through auditory or tactile channels reveals intact knowledge about the written form of words.

Total inability to recognize written symbols, however, is not the rule in pure alexia. Commonly, these patients can recognize and name most letters as well as many high frequency words. They usually adopt the strategy of spelling out written words to themselves, letter by letter. Hence, they are often referred to in the current literature as "letter-by-letter readers." Letter by letter reading is an imperfect strategy because occasionally letters are misread and because the memory load in long words is too great for patients to decode them correctly.

As letter-by-letter readers recover, their success in word recognition is inversely related to word length, suggesting that they have progressed from identifying one at a time with their fingers to identifying them more rapidly, but still one at a time, by visual scanning. Friedman and Alexander (1984) argued that a general elevation of thresholds for the recognition of familiar forms is responsible for restricting these patients to dealing with one letter at a time. A similar elevation in exposure time requirements was found for form recognition in pictures.

Some patients with this disorder have been shown to respond to connotative semantic features of words at exposures that were much too short for the word to have been recognized explicitly (Coslett and Saffran (1989), cited by Behrman *et al.*, 1990). There is sufficient variation from patient to patient so that one must be cautious about stating generalities about the underlying deficit in pure alexia. For example, Behrman, Black, and Bub (1990) found no evidence that their patient was responsive to semantic features of words that were exposed too briefly for her to read letter by letter.

The standard anatomical account for the mechanism of pure alexia leaves a paradox unexplained. If the disorder is caused by the disconnection of visual input from the right cerebral cortex from the language zone of the left hemisphere, why does this disconnection not similarly affect the naming of objects? That is, why does it not always produce an "optic aphasia"? This question was considered by Geschwind and Fusillo (1966) who suggested that the reason lies in the location of callosal pathways from right to left brain association areas that are available for objects, versus those available for written words. In Geschwind's view, the written word, as perceived by the right visual cortex, is a purely visual stimulus, with no associations outside of the visual domain. Objects, however, on recognition in the right hemisphere activate associations in various modalities through which they have been experienced, for example, tactile, olfactory, sensorimotor, or affective. Interhemispheric pathways from many brain structures are therefore available to have these associations shared between the hemispheres and therefore activate verbal labels, just as if they had originated in the left hemisphere.

Color naming and color name comprehension are commonly impaired in patients with pure alexia. This was the case in the report of pure alexia by Geschwind and Fusillo (1966). Geschwind proposed the same account for color aphasia as he had for word blindness. Namely, that colors, being purely visual experiences, are represented only in the visual association areas, just as letters are, and can therefore reach the language zone only via the splenium of the corpus callosum. Splenial damage along with destruction of the left visual cortex therefore cuts off color information from the left hemisphere, just as it does written word information.

Although this account is plausible, standing by itself, it does not explain why color name disorders are present in some pure alexic patients but not in others. Damasio and Damasio (1983) looked for anatomic markers for the presence and absence of color name aphasia in patients with pure alexia. They found that this disorder is present only when certain anatomic requirements are met: there must be a right hemianopia along with damage to both the left lingual gyrus and the left hippocampal area.

DYSLEXIAS DUE TO COGNITIVE DISSOCIATIONS

We have noted earlier that patients with aphasic alexia need not have an absolutely uniform breakdown in all aspects of reading—that semantic properties of words result in a bias to better performance with nouns over grammatical functors, and with emotionally loaded or highly picturable words over neutral, abstract words. However, as long as patients retain the ability to use whole-word phonological associations and to apply some graphophonemic conversion principles in reading, the effects of semantic word properties are not conspicuous. In the patients to be considered here, however, severe difficulties in matching familiar letter groupings to phonological patterns result in highly paradoxical performances.

DEEP DYSLEXIA

The syndrome of deep dyslexia was first described by Marshall and Newcombe (1973). The two most salient features of this disorder appear in oral reading: frequent substitution of a semantically related word (i.e., semantic paralexias) for the written stimulus and the inability to read aloud grammatical functors, which are either entirely skipped over or misread with a different and often unrelated functor. Similar patterns of oral reading errors appear when the patient attempts connected text and when word lists are presented for reading. The semantic paralexias frequently have no structural or phonological resemblance to the stimulus. For example, "accident" might be misread as "tragedy." However, misreadings based on spelling resemblance are also common.

An example of a possible reading of a sentence by a patient with deep dyslexia is

> (Stimulus) The waiter brought some syrup for his pancakes.
> (Reading) "Servant bring . . .honey . . .the waffle."

The immediate impression from these errors is that the patient derives some meaning directly from the written word, leading him to supply a word with a related meaning, but the sound equivalent of the stimulus totally escapes him. Detailed analyses of the pattern of success and failure of deep dyslexics confirms these impressions, but they also add another dimension to the definition of the problem. The data that emerge from error analysis lead to the following fuller account of this disorder.

Nouns are read more accurately than verbs and adjectives.
Grammatical functors are omitted or substituted with other functors.
Semantically based substitutions are made for words of any form: nouns, verbs, adjectives, or adverbs.
Inflectional and derivational affixes are often omitted or substituted.

Verbs are often nominalized.

There is no advantage for short words or regularly spelled words over long or irregularly spelled words.

The following examples of oral reading errors are selected from the appendix or Coltheart, Patterson, and Marshall (1980).

Semantic substitutions:

Nouns:	turtle → crocodile	cone → ice cream
	edition → journal	night → sleep
	product → factory	colonel → uniform
Verbs:	admit → event	drove → car
	excavate → hole	bring → towards
	shining → sun	guessed → query
Functors:	had → of	where → whither
	the → is	down → under
	under → in	instead → because

Visual errors:

bush → brush	decree → degree
signal → single	ceremony → cemetary
gain → grain	shape → sharp

Although all of the foregoing features of deep dyslexia are observed in oral reading, simple tests of written word discrimination provide further evidence of the virtually complete absence of the activation of phonological associations to either letters, letter groupings, or whole words.

Patients cannot match homophonous real words; that is, given the word "colonel" they cannot select "kernel" from a group of words as matching it in sound.

Patients cannot match pseudohomophones; that is, given the word "cough," they cannot match it to "cawf."

Patients cannot select functor words from multiple choice to an orally presented model; that is, given a list of written words such as of, with, by, and from, they point randomly when asked to select one of these words.

Patients are essentially at chance levels in selecting from choice a noun to match one from a list of semantically related nouns, such as choosing tiger from a list containing lion, wolf, leopard, and tiger.

Note that the last of these is a characteristic that has been described for many patients with aphasic alexia. The difference in patients with deep dyslexia is only a quantitative difference and not a qualitative one. That is, patients with aphasic alexia often have sufficient grapho-phoneme association skills or sufficient word-to-phonology skills to perform at significantly better than chance levels in tasks of this type. In the case of deep dyslexia, the phonological associational capacity is so minimal as to be totally overridden by semantically activated phonological forms.

From the foregoing, it might be concluded that the way a patient with deep dyslexia treats a word is determined wholly by the structure and meaning of the individual word. Investigation of the reading of connected text shows that syntactical influences induced by the context may dictate the patient's treatment of a written word. Andreewsky and Seron (1975) used the fact that French provides instances where a grammatical functor is written and pronounced identically with a lexical term. One such instance is the word "car," which is a conjunction meaning "because" as well as a noun referring to a minibus or passenger van. They presented their deep dyslexic patient with the sentence "*Le car ralentit car le moteur chauffe*" (The van slows down because the motor overheats). The patient's oral reading was "*Car ralenti . . .moteur chauffe*" (Van slowed down . . .motor overheated). It is apparent that the patient had a sense of which instance of "car" was a noun that he could say aloud and which instance was a functor, which he could not. Adreewsky suggested a simple formalism, introduced by Bar Hillel (1964), that allows the patient to derive the morphosyntactic category of a word from positional information. The fact that word position and not word meaning assigned its morphosyntactic role to the written word was demonstrated in a complementary task. This time, Andreewsky and Seron chose the word "mer" (ocean) which is short enough to masquerade as a functor, but which has only one meaning. They created another test sentence similar in structure to the first, but with the word "mer" in the position of the conjunction (Le train ralentit mer le moteur chauffe). This time, the patient read "train ralenti . . .moteur chauffe." The patient's implicit syntactic analysis had assigned the role of functor to the common noun "mer," making it impossible for him to utter in this context.

A RIGHT HEMISPHERE PHENOMENON?

A suggested mechanism for the semantic paralexias produced by patients with deep dyslexia is that they represent the work of the right hemisphere (Coltheart, 1980; Saffran *et al.*, 1980). According to this conjecture, the normally dominant left hemisphere routes to phonology, via either whole-word processing or grapho-phonemic conversion, are disabled, but the capacity of the right hemisphere to extract semantic information from the written word may still be functional. Such semantic activation, then, results in the attempt to name the activated concept; but semantic activity mediated by the right hemisphere has been shown to be sensitive to parameters that are similar to those seen in deep dyslexia. For example, studies of split brain patients have shown them to be able to identify concrete object names presented to the left visual field (i.e., to the right hemisphere), but to be unable to deal with verbs. Zaidel and Peters (1981) have shown that the isolated right hemisphere of these patients is unable to appreciate phonological similarities between words. We have noted earlier the studies by Landis *et al.*, (1982, 1983) that indicate that right hemisphere reading is facilitated by word concreteness and emotionality.

While all of these considerations favor the plausibility that direct semantic activation by the written word accounts for the successes of deep dyslexics, they do not directly explain the failures—that is, the reason for semantically based errors. Here it is necessary to postulate that the semantic activation produced by the whole word is not always precise; it carries the sense of the word stem, but not the sense of the inflectional or derivational affixes. The latter, like free grammatical morphemes, have little semantic weight and tend to be ignored. It is also possible that if the semantics of the written word arise originally in the right hemisphere, they are received in degraded form by the left hemisphere, where the oral response is implemented. The patient then assigns the best label he can to the more-or-less imperfectly experienced concept and, having done so, he has no way of being sure whether his response is accurate or not. In this way the mechanism for the semantic paralexias of the deep dyslexic is closely analogous to that suggested in Chapter 8 for the deep dysphasic patient. They need not be paralleled by equally severe semantic paraphasias in the task of picture naming.

ALEXIA IN A NONALPHABETIC SYSTEM—JAPANESE

The written language for Japanese consists predominantly of ideographic characters taken from Chinese. These are referred to as "kanji." Kanji constitutes the bulk of normal Japanese text, being used for all of the lexical terms: nouns, verbs, adjectives, and adverbs. Individual kanji characters or combinations of two or three characters directly represent meaning and have phonological labels that are assigned directly to the character. Because spoken Japanese is largely made up of sequences of consonant–vowel (CV) syllables, there are a great many homophones among short words and many kanji characters are homophonous with each other. They are, of course, readily distinguished in written form.

Side by side with the kanji code is a phonetic code, referred to as "kana." Kana is a syllabary consisting of 69 characters, one for each syllable of spoken Japanese. It is therefore possible to spell out in kana characters any word or sentence in Japanese. Kana is used to write foreign loan words or foreign names for which there are no kanji symbols. Kana is also used to encode inflectional morphemes in writing. Although an educated Japanese reader can understand text that is written entirely in *kana* characteristics, this is a somewhat unnatural exercise because kanji is normally used for native words. Oral reading of kana is similar to the oral reading of regularly spelled words in English—but the analogy is only partial. Kana characters denote entire CV syllables and they are assembled strictly phonetically. This contrasts with the requirement for blending sequences of individual consonants and individual vowels that face the reader of an unfamiliar, but pronounceable English letter string. Oral reading of kanji is most nearly analogous to the oral reading of English abbreviations. In reading connected text, the Japanese reader slips automatically and unconsciously between decoding logographs and phonetic symbols, much as the English reader does with a text that contains regularly spelled words, abbreviations, and unfamiliar foreign words.

Just as dyslexia causes dissociation of the ability to read various written symbols in English, the kana/kanji dichotomy is the basis for highly analogous dissociations in Japanese-speaking alexia patients. The typical observation is that the meaning-to-sound route (i.e., *kanji* reading) is more robust than the grapho-phonological route (reading words in kana form); Sasanuma and Fujimura, 1971).

PHONOLOGICAL ALEXIA

A disorder with some of the features of deep dyslexia was first described by Beauvois and Desrouesné (1979) under the term "phonological alexia." The patient with phonological alexia does not make semantic paralexias. However, he or she has extreme difficulty in applying graphophonemic correspondence to the reading of pseudowords. Difficulty in reading grammatical functors is sometimes present, but is not so marked as in deep dyslexia. Glosser and Friedman (1990) have argued that phonological dyslexia is on a continuum with deep dyslexia because patients may progress in recovery from the pattern of deep dyslexia to that of phonological dyslexia as semantic paralexias disappear from their oral reading.

As we have seen, the deficit in accessing phonology from print can be demonstrated through the failure of patients with deep (or phonogical) dyslexia to select written words that match a particular phonological model. However, the inability to read words aloud correctly does not constitute evidence that the patient does not fully or partially understand the word. Such comprehension, in fact has been demonstrated for several categories of grammatical functors by Morton and Patterson (1980a,b). These authors probed the comprehension of written functors on the part of one patient who had a severe deep dyslexia and was agrammatic as well. They examined their patient's comprehension of the functors that he could not correctly read aloud. He achieved nearly perfect scores in discriminating the number (e.g., "he" versus "they") and gender (e.g., "him" versus "her") of personal pronouns, but was barely above chance in discriminating first from second from third person forms of pronouns. He was usually accurate in his understanding of the dimension of the relationship denoted by a preposition (e.g., order in time, vertical order, linear order), but he made many errors of reversal in the direction of the relationship. For example, given the written command to "put the cup on the saucer," he put the saucer on the cup. The authors concluded that when a functor included both semantic and syntactic features, their patients appreciated the semantic component better than the syntactic one. Functors that were fully or partly understood were not read aloud any better than those that could not be interpreted at all. Thus access to phonological realization involves a different process from access to meaning—in functors, as in lexical items.

SURFACE DYSLEXIA

A syndrome of disordered reading and spelling that appears to be almost the reverse of deep dyslexia was described in 1973 by Marshall and Newcombe. Their patients appeared to gain some meaning from print, but exclusively by applying grapheme-to-phoneme rules and interpreting the phonology that they achieved in this way to guess the meaning of the word. This strategy often worked well for regular words, but did not work at all for irregular words because they regularized the latter in their oral reading to produce either a nonword or a guess at a somewhat similarly written but totally wrong word. The term "surface dyslexia" was coined because the patients lacked any access either to meaning or to phonology on a whole-word basis. Strange misapplications of grapheme-to-phoneme correspondence might arise because the patients did not segment a letter string at syllable boundaries. For example, Marshall and Newcombe's patient did not recognize a silent final e as part of the preceding syllable and was likely to read the word "home" as "hommee." An interesting illustration of the patient's strategy in achieving correct (or incorrect) word meaning was given by the authors. When attempting to read the word "listen," he read the syllables lis and ten and put them together as the name of the boxer (Sonny) Liston, who was well known at the time.

The publication of additional cases of surface dyslexia has made it apparent that the details of symptomatology are sufficiently varied so that one cannot speak of the loss of one pathway and the preservation of another as representing a standard account of surface dyslexia. Among the patients who might be placed in this category, there are some with a relative, but not absolute degradation in accessing whole-word phonology, such as the one described by Shallice, Warrington, and McCarthy (1983). This patient was relatively successful in reading irregular words that shared an irregularity with a large family of similarly irregular words (e.g., head, bread, and spread), but could not pronounce one that was a unique instance of a particular irregularity (e.g., bowl). The common feature that defines these patients is their markedly reduced ability to attach semantics directly to the printed word, their relatively reduced capacity to access whole-word phonology, and their overreliance on relatively well-preserved grapheme–phoneme correspondence for subword length letter groups.

SUMMARY AND INTERPRETATION

From the review just completed it should be apparent that normal human speakers are equipped to acquire a variety of techniques for encoding the sound units of speech and the meaning of concepts in the form of written characters, and correspondingly equipped to decode these characters into strings of sounds and meaningful concepts. Within the scope of this cognitive–linguistic endowment, various cultures have developed markedly different writing systems that call on different cognitive processes.

Logographic systems, like Chinese (and Japanese kanji), encode meaning directly, and hence call for a recognition vocabulary of thousands of different characters. Speakers of alphabetically based writing systems have the greatest flexibility in what can be represented. Individual phonemes of the language may map onto individual letters and letters may be assembled into strings that have a strictly rule-governed phonological realization, whether or not they correspond to words of the language. Also, within alphabetic systems, phonetics need not be strictly observed: strings of letters of word length or subword length may be associated to phonological strings that need not correspond to the "regular" rules of one-to-one mapping. As in the first type of encoding, word meaning need not play a role in the decoding of such letter strings into phonological form.

However, the fact that alphabetic script can be decoded phoneme by phoneme, or into larger sublexical or lexical-sized phonological units, does not mean that it can also be decoded directly into meaning via the same process that Chinese logographs are read. Indeed, it appears most likely that with practice and maturation, normal English readers decode text by calling on all of these mechanisms, slipping back and forth among them unconsciously, as needed, for the most efficient execution of the particular reading task.

Cognitive models of the reading process have created labeled constructs for each of these components, each label being a term that best describes the operation that it is presumed to govern. Such models usually include a construct for stored word knowledge (lexicon). The one proposed by Morton (1979a,b) proposes that stores of word knowledge (called logogens) exist separately for each modality of input and output—for example, a visual input logogen, separate phonological and graphic output logogens, and so on. An example of such a model (from Morton and Patterson, 1980b, p.115) is reproduced as Fig. 9.1. In this flow chart, dotted ovals indicate functional "lesions" to the system that could result in the deficits of deep dyslexia. Models of this type are internally consistent and have been progressively modified by their authors to accommodate new clinical observations. The labeled constructs, however, remain at the black box level, being specified no further than required for the internal logic of the model; they often refer to complex processes whose unity cannot be assumed (e.g., semantic system).

It is well to stand back from the constructs that one finds in flow charts of this type to recognize that the human cognitive apparatus is capable of many more and many more subtle ways of perceptually analyzing the visual input and generating associations than these labeled boxes convey. For example, we have noted that a one-to-one grapheme to phoneme conversion channel is relevant only for writing systems that attempt to represent single phonemes by single letters. The alternative (nonsemantic) route to word phonology that is recognized by these models is the whole word (lexical) route.

However, the distinction between these two routes is blurred when one considers the evidence (cited previously) of Glushko (1979) and Henderson (1982) that phonology is assigned to letters and letter groups by analogy with the phonology of other known words in which the letters appear. Seidenberg and McClelland (1989) give a detailed account of

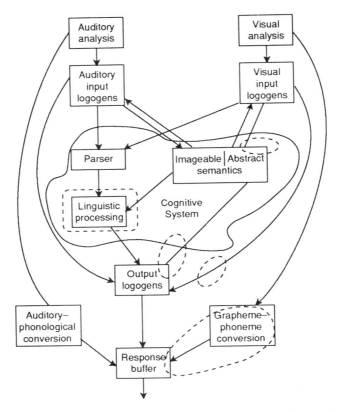

Figure 9.1. A proposed cognitive architecture for oral reading and repetition, showing sites of impairment that may be responsible for aberrant performances. From Morton and Patterson, in Coltheart, Patterson, and Marshall, *Deep Dyslexia*, p. 115, London: Routledge and Kegan Paul. Reproduced with permission.

access to word phonology by a spreading activation mechanism, close in concept to that of Glushko.

Whatever the nature of the visually perceived graphic symbol—for example, logographic, alphabetic or syllabic— all share a common pathway to the language system, beginning in the primary visual areas and visual association areas of the occipital lobes and accessing the language area of the left hemisphere through white matter connections to the left angular gyrus. Structural damage that interrupts either primary visual processing or the pathway leading to the angular gyrus may lead to a pure reading disorder, which need not affect writing or oral language. However, the operation of the principle of cerebral dominance introduces variations from case to case. Although it is generally agreed that the left hemisphere of the prototypical right-handed person is capable of all of the components of the reading process, this is not necessarily the case for the right hemisphere. Whether the individual with pure alexia is capable of recognizing letters, or of accessing some of the semantic features of words that are available for processing only in the right hemisphere, is undoubtedly a function of individual differences in the language processing potential of the right hemisphere.

We have seen that one of the controversial attributes of right hemisphere language capability is in the area of semantics. The adequacy of semantic representation of a concept is somehow linked to its picturability. At least, this dimension would account for the superior processing of concrete object names over abstract terms. It is much more difficult to reduce the superior appreciation of pronoun number and gender over pronoun person (Morton and Patterson, 1980a,b) to the dimension of picturability. It has generally been assumed that the semanticity versus the syntacticity of a word constitutes points on a continuum at the opposite poles of which we find concrete nouns and case-marking prepositions. But the semanticity of verbs may not be merely quantitatively less than that of concrete nouns, but also qualitatively different. The differences in the properties of nouns, verbs, adjectives, and functors that are expressed in the oral reading of deep dyslexics appear in the spontaneous speech of agrammatic patients, as well as in the reading comprehension that is demonstrable in the isolated right hemisphere of split brain patients.

We have placed major emphasis on the difference between the relatively uniform degradation of the cognitive components of reading in aphasic alexia in opposition to the selectivity of the cognitive-linguistic impairments of the dissociative alexias—especially deep dyslexia. It is certainly clear that in a subset of aphasic patients, previously learned associations between letter strings and phonology no longer operate, leaving them excessively dependent on associations to semantic features only. Up to now, there is little evidence of an anatomic basis for this dissociation. Although it is more often seen with agrammatic Broca's aphasia than with other forms, this is far from an exclusive relationship. Certainly Broca's aphasia need not entail deep dyslexia. It may not be farfetched to suggest that only some individuals are vulnerable to deep dyslexia (or to phonologic or surface dyslexia), and that this vulnerability is largely determined by premorbid differences in the processing of written language.

Chapter 10

Disorders of Writing

The acquisition of writing, like that of reading, is linked to the earlier knowledge of spoken language. As in the case of reading, the breakdown of writing in aphasia may coincide with and appear to be the result of a loss of oral language and thus deserve the name "aphasic agraphia," appearing in conjunction with "aphasic alexia." But the complex graphomotor skills of writing also expose it to impairments specific to this form of motor execution. On the other hand, writing may remain functional, if not normal, in cases of aphasia that primarily affect articulatory output. In still other, rare cases, writing behaves as though it provides an autonomous channel for language output, bypassing speech entirely. We first review the component input and output processes that are integrated for the act of writing and see how selective impairments in certain areas may result in observed patterns of writing impairments.

MECHANISMS IN THE ACQUISITION OF WRITING

Introduction

As we review the various mental links that form between graphomotor movements and their visual product on the page, the associations between graphic movements and letter names, oral spelling via phoneme–grapheme associations, and direct associations between concepts and letter strings, there is one principle that we must bear in mind: that is, that the human language apparatus can and does utilize every one of these links and associations in the acquisition of writing and in the execution of writing-related activity, such as oral spelling. Indeed, the features that are noted and learned by the language-using organism go well beyond those that we can list by invoking the categories available to our logical analysis. Evidence of the availability of unexpected associative fragments is constantly cropping up in the partially retrieved written product of aphasic patients. Cases in which only a single major associative pathway has been selectively impaired or selectively spared are uncommon, but such cases have been particularly instructive because of the possibility of in-depth case studies of these individuals.

Having made the strong claim that every possible associative link between all aspects of the writing experience are used in learning and in execution, we must qualify this claim. Three types of qualification are offered:

1. Some channels of association are dominant over others for the efficient performance of writing. There are individual differences in the role that a particular component (e.g., motor memory for entire words) plays for different individuals. Such a component may come to the fore as a compensatory device for one aphasic patient, but contribute little if anything to the efforts of another.

2. The second qualification—one that is made by Bub and Chertkow (1988)—is that in normal performance we deal with the longest possible organizational units, falling back on more molecular levels of written word reconstruction only to the extent that longer units are not available. For example, the normally competent writer has a considerable stock of words that will activate their letter sequences on a whole-word basis as a direct association to their phonology. In aphasic patients, such lexical-level associations may remain available for only a small set of primer level words. Most words are reconstructed by smaller units of phoneme to letter string associations, or even by mapping phonemes to individual letters or to tightly grouped letter combinations (*ch, sh, tion*, and so on). The latter type of reconstruction exposes the patient to spelling errors due to "irregularities" in English spelling. When lexical level associations are available, any spelling irregularities are simply part of the activated letter string. The most extreme form of the shrinking of organizational units (Bub and Chertkow, 1988) is in the performance of the surface dysgraphic patient who relies only on the application of sublexical sound-to-letter mapping rules to small phonological units, virtually devoid of any knowledge of whole word spelling.

3. A third qualification is that the encoding of sensory and motor representations is not in iconic form, but in a more abstract code that is not tied to a particular sensory or motor configuration. As examples, the activation of a letter string by a spoken stimulus word may lead to implementation by oral spelling, by cursive writing or by block printing, by typing, by tracing letters in the air with a finger, by foot movements, or by writing on a blackboard using movements from the shoulder. To be sure, to say that letter strings are retrieved in abstract form does not solve

the problem of what this abstract form is in terms of a cerebral operation; it is simply to emphasize that it is not the image of a particular visual memory, auditory memory, or motor memory.

Graphomotor, Visual, and Oral Associations

The process of learning to write has traditionally been segmented by educators into components that can be mastered through standard teaching procedures, adapted to the learning capability of the young child. Of these, the first component is the mastery of the graphic forms, almost always in association with their letter names (in alphabetic languages). Repetitious letter copying followed by the copying of short words assures that the representation of the letter as a visual form, its name as a phonological form, and its grapho-motor representation are tightly linked and that the same is true for the common short words that may have been taught in this way. In spite of the high degree of overlearning of graphic movements as an association to letter names, these movements are highly vulnerable to aphasia, particularly in association with anterior speech zone lesions. The impairment is greatest for the recall of cursive letter forms by patients who are forced by hemiplegia to use their nonpreferred left hand. They use block-printed capital letters, laboriously formed, even though this was never their preferred premorbid writing style. This extremely common strategy adopted by agraphic patients suggests that the block-printed letter is closest to the mental prototype of the letter form, as opposed to the cursive form. Cursive writing as a motor skill is linked to a facility of motor-graphic performance. Patients who are not hemiplegic (e.g., many Wernicke's aphasics), may produce cursive letter forms with facility, even though they may have profound impairment in recall of spelling.

During the early acquisition of letters and primer words, a child is exposed to the written forms that he or she has created, so that the processes of reading and writing are tightly interrelated.

Sublexical and Lexical Phonology and Letter-String Activation

Oral spelling plays a large role in the teaching of writing to English-speaking children because of the large number of irregularly spelled words that must be memorized. Oral spelling also plays a large part in mediating the writing of corresponding letters in the early stage of written word acquisition, but it becomes superfluous as the graphic motor sequences and the visual feedback from the page become attached to the phonology of individual sounds, syllables, and to whole word phonology. Nevertheless, the immediate link between the recall of a letter string for writing and the oral production of that string remains part of the skill of the average literate English-speaking person, from a relatively early school grade. Even in aphasic patients who have reduced writing skills, one often finds a stock of words the spelling of which can be rattled off orally as unthinkingly as they would be written by a normal writer. Often such patients can spell correctly aloud, but are unable to use their oral spelling accurately to guide their written production. Longer or less common words are reconstituted by more piecemeal retrieval of letter groups that correspond to morpheme or syllable-sized units. As in the case of reading, the word's concept may determine what letter string is activated when concepts with different spelling share the same phonological form (e.g., soul/sole; bough/bow). Obviously, if one can retrieve a letter string directly from a concept in the case of sound-alike words, this must also be a route available for a great many words that have a unique phonology.

Thus, writing shares with reading virtually every level at which correspondences between letter strings, word concepts, word phonology, and subword phonology may be evoked, although the direction of the association is reversed. As in the case of reading, although these associative links are acquired without deliberate effort by the normal literate person, they can be sufficiently autonomous from each other so that dissociative forms of agraphia appear in which a particular one of them is nonfunctional (e.g., loss of phoneme or syllable level phono-graphemic associations), or in which only one of them functions, imperfectly. However, two major components of writing are unique to that modality. One is the part played by the motor-kinesthetic representations of letters and of the highly overlearned multiletter groupings. The other is the role of oral spelling as either an independent form of writing or as a mediator of written spelling.

We referred earlier to the use of features other than those that we have cited in the preceding analysis. One that frequently appears is the recall of various visual characteristics of a word—its contour of tall and short letters, or the position in the whole word of particular letters that are salient for the patient. Patients with agraphia not uncommonly place the first and last letters in their positions and attempt to fill in the blanks. Even metaknowledge about word spelling enters into the retrieval of whole word letter strings when subjects are aware of the presence of a double letter but attach the doubling to the wrong letter. It is undoubtedly the case that visual configurational features are of low influence in their contribution to the retrieval of graphic word forms, with rare exceptions. Even in cases that have been cited because of the patient's reliance on visual features of the written word (e.g., Roeltgen and Heilman, 1984; Baxter and Warrington, 1987), the visual features recalled are fragmentary and rarely result in correctly retrieved spelling. The structure of an alphabetic language would seem logically to place a premium on channels related to the mapping of sound onto graphic symbols. However, it is a matter of empirical observation that the capacity to acquire a lexicon of letter strings (for production through any of multiple possible media) in direct association to whole word phonology (or in association to word concepts) is part of the human language learning endowment. This fortunate gift probably makes writing much faster and error free than if it depended entirely on sound-to-grapheme mapping. Undoubtedly, nonalphabetic languages place a much higher premium on visual configurational features and much less on phono-graphemic mapping.

Graphemic Buffer

Any model of production of written or oral language must provide for a mechanism that holds in readiness for motor implementation the motor sequence for the end of a word while the beginning of the word is being produced. In a number of reported cases (e.g., Caramazza *et al.,* 1986), it appears that the only way to account for the spelling errors that are observed is to postulate inadequate short-term storage capacity within the graphemic buffer.

Writing at the Sentence Level

The subjective experience of writing connected text is one of transcoding "inner speech" word for word into graphic form. To the extent that such transcoding actually occurs, we may consider writing to be parasitic on speech. When aphasic patients have adequate command of motor-graphic and whole-word writing skills, the most usual observation is that their written output mirrors their spoken output in terms of access to vocabulary, sentence structure, and error types. However, there are many instances that demonstrate autonomy of written from spoken language. In these cases, the patients produce written text that does not resemble either their speech output or the sentences that have been dictated to them. Patients who typically produce grammatically organized speech may write in telegraphic form, omitting grammatical morphemes; patients who speak agrammatically may produce writing that is much more syntactically organized than their speech. Examples of varieties of dysgraphic performance will be presented.

CLINICAL FORMS OF AGRAPHIA

Aphasic Agraphia

We apply this term to the disorders of writing seen in the great majority of patients with aphasia. We refer to writing disorders that touch on virtually every associative channel, without notable impairments in one particular aspect (e.g., phono-graphemic matching) as opposed to another. Within the scope of this term, there is room for considerable variation because the writing of many patients embodies features of their oral language, and tends to be commensurate with the severity of their speech output disorder. For example, many patients with the fluent paraphasic speech of Wernicke's aphasics produce a fluent paragraphic jargon that has a similar linguistic structure to their speech. The converse is true for many patients with agrammatic speech output.

Agraphia in Severe Mixed Aphasia

At this level of impairment, the recall of letter shapes may be defective, although the patient has adequate motor control for copying and may be able to produce a few highly overlearned motor-graphic sequences such as his or her name. Patients who are free of hemiplegia may attempt cursive writing, but produce little that is intelligible beyond their name. Block printing is the usual style for patients using their nonpreferred hand. They can commonly write the beginning of the alphabet, breaking down in both the recall of letter identities and the letter forms after the opening sequence. Whole word recall from dictation is limited to no more than a few primer level words. Dictation of other simple object names rarely reveals any useful control of phono-graphemic correspondence as, for example, by using the correct first letter in attempting to retrieve the written word. Patients at this level cannot usually produce single letters that are requested by name, nor can they produce grammatical functors such as "and" or "the."

Agraphia in Nonfluent Aphasia with Moderate or Mild Comprehension Impairment

As compared to the patients just described, the performance of patients in this group reflects some recovery of function along virtually every channel of motor and linguistic association contributing to writing: graphomotor memory for letter forms and for name and address, recall of some whole-word letter strings, and utilization of phono-graphemic associations of subword segments. These aspects of recovery are reflected in the ability to write common irregularly spelled words from dictation, and to initiate the spelling of less familiar words with correctly chosen first letters. Many patients of this type have considerable success in conveying information by writing words that they cannot retrieve for oral production. Even though most of these words are incompletely spelled, they reflect partial autonomy of written word retrieval from speech. The degree of proficiency in recovery of written word retrieval naturally reflects the recovery of speech output. In patients who have a persistent, severe articulatory impairment, writing may far exceed speech recovery; on average, however, writing lags behind speech in functional recovery.

For patients who have recovered usable access to a written vocabulary, the chief limiting factor in functional writing is access to syntax; that is, the written counterpart of agrammatism. Agrammatic writing is to be found not only in patients with agrammatic Broca's aphasia, but occasionally in other nonfluent aphasics and, more rarely, even in fluent paraphasic patients. These patients fail to use prepositions, articles, or noun and verb inflections, and show the predilection for using nouns in preference to verbs that is observed in spoken agrammatism. When pressed to produce a written sentence, they commonly fall back on a formulaic construction often beginning with "The." For example, a patient asked to tell about the weather that he could see through the window, wrote "The morning and sun."

Some patients who write individual words successfully respond to the task of writing sentences with the production of highly confabulated strings of words that include ill chosen lexical terms, wrong inflections, and wrongly chosen functors, including forms that never appear in the patient's speech. Figure 10.1 is an example of such writing by an agrammatic patient.

Aphasic Agraphia in Fluent Aphasia

In the severe stages of Wernicke's aphasia, writing is likely to appear as unintelligible jargon, even though letters may be well formed in cursive script. Figure 10.2 illustrates such syntactically disorganized jargon produced by a fluent aphasic, although one whose speech output is far superior to his writing. At milder levels of impairment, the parallel between written and spoken output is usually more striking. For one thing, grammatical morphemes, both free and inflectional, appear in the written sentences of these patients, just as in their speech. Within-word spelling problems are not different from those of nonfluent patients. Written whole-word retrieval and phoneme to grapheme mapping have fairly constant characteristics that are not determined by the character of the speech output disorder.

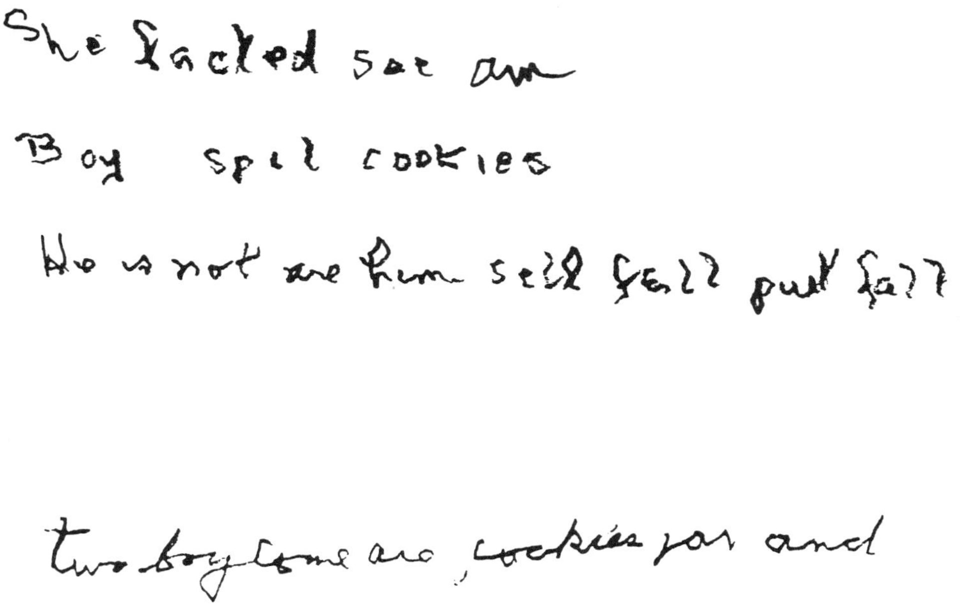

Figure 10.1.   Writing produced by two agrammatic Broca's aphasia patients.

SELECTIVE FORMS OF AGRAPHIA

Apraxic Agraphia

This term is applied to writing disorders in which the patient appears unable to direct the pencil to form graphic symbols, even when given a model to copy. It appears in association with several different syndromes. Marcie and Hécaen (1979) describe several such cases that were associated with lesions of the left parietal region. In some cases it is seen in the syndrome of alexia with agraphia, where the only disturbance of oral language is an anomia. In other instances, the apraxic agraphia is unaccompanied by reading disorder. For example, Coslett *et al.* (1986) reported a patient who developed an apraxic agraphia with little in the way of aphasic language deficit and normal praxis for nonwriting movements. He was able to spell words with anagram letters and typed 9 out of 10 words correctly. This case clearly shows that motor graphic skills can be damaged in isolation from other praxic and paper and pencil skills, as well as in isolation from the access to orthographic letter strings.

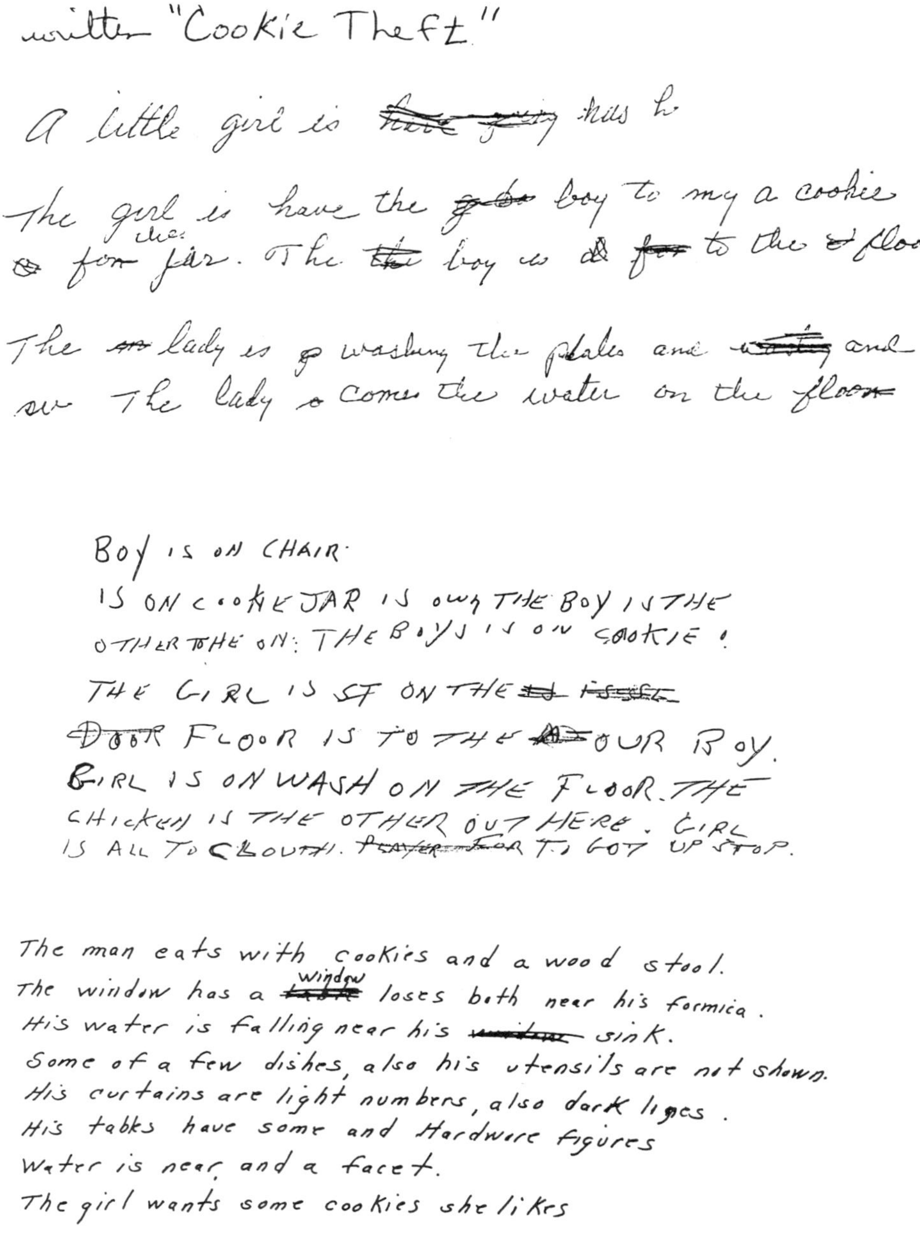

written "Cookie Theft"

A little girl is ~~not going~~ has h.

The girl is have the ~~g bo~~ boy to my a cookie
& for jar. The ~~the~~ boy is d ~~for~~ to the & floor

The ~~an~~ lady is g washing the plates and ~~wating~~ and
sw The lady o comes the water on the floor

Boy is on CHAIR.
IS ON cookie JAR IS own THE Boy IS THE
OTHER THE ON; THE Boy is on cookie !

THE GIRL IS SF ON THE ~~is~~ ~~first~~
~~Door~~ FLOOR IS TO THE ~~A~~ OUR Boy.
GIRL IS ON WASH ON THE FLOOR. THE
CHICKEN IS THE OTHER OUT HERE . GIRL
IS ALL TO CLOUTH. ~~frayer for~~ TO GOT UP STOP.

The man eats with cookies and a wood stool.
The window has a ~~late~~ window loses both near his formica.
His water is falling near his ~~water~~ sink.
Some of a few dishes, also his utensils are not shown.
His curtains are light numbers, also dark liges.
His tabks have some and Hardware figures
Water is near and a facet.
The girl wants some cookies she likes

Figure 10.2.   Samples of paragraphic writing produced by three patients with Wernicke's aphasia.

Apraxic attempts at writing are also seen as one component of severe ideomotor apraxia affecting all purposeful movements, or of an apraxia that affects not only writing but any form of paper and pencil activity such as drawing or copying designs.

Psychological accounts of these disorders have traditionally been stated in terms of a breakdown in coordination or connection between centers for spoken and written language (Kussmaul, 1884, as cited by Marcie and Hécaen, 1979).

Anatomic disconnection between the left hemisphere and the motor system of the right hemisphere can result in a unilateral apraxic agraphia affecting the left hand, but not the right, as a result of lesions of the corpus callosum. This phenomenon was first reported by Liepmann and Maas (1907). Geschwind and Kaplan's (1962) patient, who had an anatomically proven infarct of the anterior two thirds of the corpus callosum, was able to write with normal spelling with his right hand, but, as can be seen in Fig. 10.3, his attempts to write the alphabet with the left hand degenerated into formless scrawls after a few letters.

Agraphia with Alexia in Parietal Lobe Lesions

Dejerine (1891) first reported the anatomical correlates of the breakdown of written language affecting both reading and writing, but largely sparing oral language. The left angular gyrus has since been regarded as the crossroad between oral and written language (see discussion in Chapters 3 and 9). These impairments affect the most elementary associations between letter strings and semantic or phonological representations. That is, patients neither spell, recognize oral spelling, nor retrieve the graphic form of letter strings. Even their ability to retrieve the visual or motor graphic form of individual letters may be disrupted. In most cases, the ability to copy print is retained. It is important to note, however, as Marcie and Hécaen (1979) point out, that the degree of impairment of reading and writing in this syndrome do not necessarily go hand in hand. Some instances of virtually pure agraphia are associated with lesions of the left angular gyrus.

Pure Agraphia

Cases of agraphia in which there was little or no impairment of any other language function have been described by a number of authors. However, these cases have involved a number of different anatomic sites and have differed from each other in clinical details, such as the prominence of the praxic factor, the ability to write letters versus words, and

a)

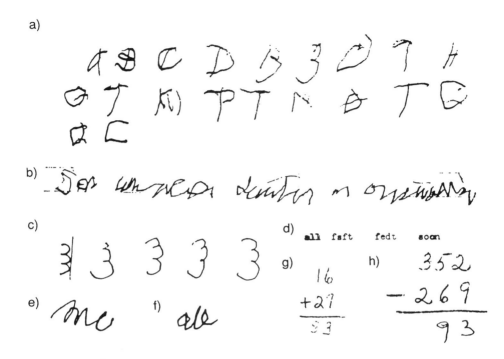

Figure 10.3. Writing with the left hand by a patient with a lesion of the corpus callosum. From Geschwind and Kaplan (1962). A human cerebral disconnection syndrome. *Neurology, 12,* 675–685. Reproduced with permission.

the preservation of oral spelling. There is currently no anatomical site where a lesion can confidently be predicted to result in pure agraphia, nor is there an anatomical schema, such as that underlying pure alexia, that would give a plausible explanation for pure agraphia. Historically, however, claims of a center for writing have been made.

Exner (1881) proposed an independent writing center in the foot of the second frontal gyrus of the left hemisphere. However, independent clinico-anatomic verification of this claim has been scant. Four cases of pure agraphia, reported by Dubois, Hécaen, and Marcie (1969) had frontal lesions, as did a case reported by Assal, Chapuis, and Zander (1970), but in none of these was localization exact enough either to support or conflict with Exner's proposal. Other cases have been found in association with parietal lobe lesions (Russell and Espir, 1961; Dubois *et al.*,

1969; Kinsbourne and Rosenfield, 1974). The specifics of clinical sympto-matology have also failed to point to the disruption of any particular component of writing in these cases. Dubois *et al.* observed that spelling was disrupted in their cases, rather than the motor aspect of letter for-mation. However, some sense of phoneme–grapheme correspondence was retained, and patients could often spell aloud better than they could write. Kinsbourne and Rosenfield's case was particularly notable for the relative preservation of oral spelling in a patient who could neither write words, nor build them from anagrams.

DISSOCIATIVE AGRAPHIAS

We have noted that agraphia in aphasic patients is commonly mani-fested in reduced access to the orthographic letter string through all of the associative channels that contribute to normal spelling. That is, at the whole-word, or lexical level, there is reduced activation of orthography both as an association to the word concept and as an association to whole word phonology. At the sublexical level, there is impairment in the ac-cess of phoneme-to-grapheme transcoding at either the syllable or the in-dividual phoneme level. Incomplete impairments in all of these channels are commonplace, as is partial compensation through a partially pre-served channel. In this section we review instances in which a single as-sociative channel is profoundly impaired, or selectively spared. These dissociative disorders are analogous to the phenomena of deep dyslexia, phonological dyslexia, and surface dyslexia, but they may appear only under conditions of written output, without implicating the parallel phe-nomenon in reading. In the sphere of writing, we also observe cases in which oral word retrieval is profoundly impaired, but orthographic re-trieval is preserved. These cases of dissociative agraphia are not com-mon, but a number of them have been studied in depth.

Phonological Dysgraphia

Patients with this disorder succeed relatively well in writing real words, but are almost totally unable to write the easiest pseudowords. Their success in writing actual words is independent of word frequency or of spelling irregularity. This disorder is conceived as being caused by the loss of capacity for sound-to-grapheme conversion, at the level of individual sounds as well as for sublexical sound clusters. Patients are probably depending primarily on the activation of word orthography by the phonology of the whole word as well as by its meaning. Well studied cases involving phonological agraphia have been reported by Shallice (1981), Bub and Kertesz (1982b), and Roeltgen and Heilman (1984). The latter authors found that their patient's spelling errors were likely to preserve the visual contour of the target word, substituting visual associations for the deficient phono-graphemic ones. Roeltgen (1985) reported that this disorder has been consistently associated with an injury to the supramarginal gyrus or the insula underlying it.

Deep Dysgraphia

Patients with deep dysgraphia make errors that indicate they are guided neither by phoneme–grapheme correspondence nor by whole word phonology. Rather, like patients with deep dyslexia, there is a direct but imperfect route between word meaning and the written word form. Many errors take the form of a word semantically related to the dictated word, but having no phonological resemblance. One of the author's patients, when asked to write "agriculture," wrote "industrial." Bub and Kertesz' (1982a) patient wrote "funny" when asked for "happy" and "smile" when asked for "laugh." In further analogy with patients with deep dyslexia, patients with deep dysgraphia are at their best in writing concrete nouns, less reliable with abstract nouns and verbs, and almost incapable of writing grammatical functors.

The borderline between phonological dysgraphia and deep dysgraphia is not sharply drawn. A case in point is that of Baxter and Warrington (1987) that is reported as one of "phonological dysgraphia," but in which success in spelling was a function of part of speech. This patient was maximally successful in writing nouns, less so for verbs and adjectives, and most impaired in writing grammatical function words. She made a number of semantically based word substitutions (memory became remember; drag became slow), and many instances in which a verb was changed derivationally to turn it into a noun (injure became injury; applaud became applause; fail became failure).

SELECTIVE PRESERVATION OF WRITTEN NAMING

A fairly common observation in patients with severe speech output disorders is that they reach for a pencil to write a word that they cannot say. Many of these instances involve patients with articulatory problems that are so severe that it is conceivable that the spoken phonology for the word was also available, but blocked at the point of motor realization. However, the same behavior is frequently seen in patients who have little or no problems with articulation, per se. In fragmentary form, it may appear through the patient tracing the first letter or two of the word on his knee or in the air, or by beginning to spell it out loud. Thus, partial retrieval of the orthographic string is very similar to partial retrieval of oral phonology by patients who are attempting to name aloud.

It is rare, however, to encounter a patient with well preserved written naming in the presence of severe anomia and fluent aphasia. Bub and Kertesz (1982b) described such a patient who succeeded in writing correctly 34 of 40 objects or drawings of objects, of which she could retrieve the spoken names for only three. In other respects, she showed the deficits of phonological agraphia, as previously described. That is, she was totally unable to apply phoneme-to-grapheme conversion to the spelling of simple nonsense words.

PART-OF-SPEECH EFFECTS

We have noted that as part of the syndromes of phonological and deep dysgraphia there is a clear gradient based on parts of speech. In this scheme, nouns have a strong advantage over other form classes, whereas grammatical functors are the most difficult. Usually, verbs and adjectives occupy a middle ground. It is notable that this gradient appears in the same sequence of difficulty in the speech production of agrammatic patients and in the word-reading comprehension of the right hemisphere of patients who have undergone section of the corpus callosum. It has commonly been assumed that this gradient has a relationship to the concreteness or picturability of the concept. In the case of patients with deep dyslexia, it has been amply demonstrated that concrete, picturable nouns have an advantage over abstract ones in the patient's oral reading. It would therefore be parsimonious to attribute the part-of-speech effect to the same principle.

In their analysis of the spelling problems of their phonological dysgraphic patient, however, Baxter and Warrington found that the part-of-speech effect totally overrode any effect of word concreteness. That is, their patient spelled abstract nouns as well as she did concrete ones, and abstract verbs as well as concrete verbs. However, verbs were at a disadvantage in comparison with nouns. This result throws into doubt the contribution of concreteness or picturability to the part-of-speech gradient in each of the previously mentioned disorders. The gradient may simply represent independently determined levels of difficulty of three psychologically distinct types of linguistic elements: nominals, verbs, and semantically empty functors.

The special status of verbs is highlighted by cases in which the writing of verbs is almost wholly suppressed in comparison with that of nouns. We have recently examined such a patient, LR, a Broca's aphasic with an almost complete incapacity for oral production, but having fairly well recovered auditory comprehension. LR belongs to the group of patients who spontaneously reach for a pencil to communicate concepts that they cannot say. He usually correctly spells words of four or five letters, but makes errors of partial retrieval on longer or less common words. This spelling pattern is not remarkable, showing some reliance on each of the associative routes to the orthographic string. What is remarkable is that it is impossible to get him to write a verb to dictation. His response is to write one or more closely associated nouns. For example, when required to write "sleep," he wrote "bed," then "pillow," then "cover." When asked to write "run," he wrote "race;" for "eat" he wrote "breakfast." This pattern does not extend to reading comprehension, he easily selected the correct verb form from a list when the word was given orally.

Caramazza and Hillis (1991) describe a patient in whom the selective dissociation of verb writing was extensively studied. The patient, SJD, developed a fluent form of aphasia following a stroke in the left fronto-temporal region. Her comprehension of both nouns and verbs was good through both the auditory and the written modalities and her oral reading and naming of both verbs and nouns was nearly error free. However, her writing of single words was marked by many semantic errors, and these were almost entirely confined to verbs (56% correct). An ingenious feature of the experimental design was the use of words that can commonly serve as either nouns or verbs, for example, "crack." To examine performance with verbs, the patient was instructed to write the word "crack" in the sentence "Don't crack the nuts in here." To examine performance with nouns, the patient was given the sentence frame "There's a crack in the mirror," and again asked to write the target word. Errors occurred almost exclusively in the verb condition. A similar pattern of errors was observed when pictures of objects and pictures of actions were presented for written naming. Like Baxter and Warrington (1987), they were able to show that abstractness versus concreteness of words had no effect on performance.

Caramazza and Hillis argue that their results indicate that modality-specific representations of lexical items are organized by grammatical category. Because the words in the output lexicon for the written modality are strings of letters, Caramazza and Hillis suggest that these are organized into sublexicons, one for nouns and one for verbs (and presumably other sublexicons for other parts of speech). Even though many verbs have almost complete phonological and semantic overlap with many nouns [e.g., jump (v)—jump (n); love (v)—love (n)], they would be accessible only from one or the other sublexicon, depending on whether the nominal or verbal meaning was intended. A subset of aphasics, like SJD, has selective difficulty in accessing the sublexicon for verbs. Caramazza and Hillis contrasted SJD with another patient, HW, who also had a selective retrieval disorder for verbs, but only in oral production and not in writing.

The concept of separate lexical lists for nouns and verbs lacks parsimony, but it cannot be rejected on that ground alone. There are, however, other considerations that make this an unattractive solution. First, because selective difficulty for verbs as opposed to nouns appears in the speech production of agrammatics, the oral reading of deep dyslexics, and the reading comprehension of the right hemisphere of split brain patients, one would be forced to postulate separate noun and verb lexicons in each of these other three modalities. Second, the errors in which a dictated verb is nominalized in the patient's writing (e.g., applaud becomes applause, and similar errors by Baxter and Warrington's patient) strongly suggest that, for the patient, a single morpheme stem may be used in either a nominal or a verbal functional role. The literature on deep dyslexia contains innumerable errors in which verbs are nominalized in oral reading.

An even stronger argument for believing that homonymous nouns and verbs often share a single lexical representation is the frequency with which nouns are verbalized in both colloquial and technical language. For example, in baseball jargon, "he flied out," and "he homered over the left-field wall"; in neurological jargon, we speak of "a lesioned area." Improvised nominalizations of verbs and verbalizations of nouns may grate on the purist's ear and never enter common usage. In many instances, such a form is accepted, but may have a restricted meaning or survive in a metaphorical sense which differs semantically from the word of origin, for example, a "claim" referring to a piece of land that is "claimed." In this case, the noun and verb are merely homophones that have separate meanings.

From this standpoint, the difference between love (n) and love (v) is the functional role that the speaker (reader or writer) imposes on a single lexical term. The author proposes that the speaker has a particular "functional attitude" in the utterance (reading or writing) of each lexical unit, whether in running speech or as an isolated word. The construct that we have just labeled as a functional attitude falls neither in the conventional notion of the lexicon, nor in the realm of syntax. Phenomenologically, the nominal functional attitude is the most facilitating for the retrieval of the phonological or the orthographic form of concepts for most aphasics.

The verbal functional attitude, however, produces modality-specific impairments in aphasics of different types; in many instances, patients appear incapable of adopting the verbal functional attitude, reverting to the
nominal one when operating in a particular modality of input or output.

How do the notions of verbal and nominal functional attitudes differ
from the concept of "part of speech"—verb versus noun? The functional
attitude is active before the retrieval of the lexical item. While the functional attitude may be construed as a component of the semantics of the
lexical item to be chosen, we propose that it is distinct from other semantic features, and whereas semantic features are aspects of the concept, the functional attitude refers to the speaker/writer's intention
concerning his or her use of the concept. The result of the functional
attitude is the output of a term that can then be given a part-of-speech
classification.

The distinction that we propose here is somewhat similar to Luria's
(1970) distinction between the nominal and the predicative use of language. Luria used the term "predication" in a broad sense to define the
basic deficiency underlying agrammatism in speech production. What
we have labeled the "verbal functional attitude" is conceptually similar
to predication, but in a much more restricted sense because it is applied
to the functional role of a single word.

The verb–noun problem has been considered in depth by Miceli *et al.*
(1984) in relation to the verb retrieval problems of agrammatic aphasics.
These authors consider the possibility that verbs are difficult for agrammatic speakers because of their implied syntactic link to other words in
a sentence. They reject this account because of the fact that verb usage is
impaired even in isolated word production. Furthermore, they cite the
existence of cases in which the verb-retrieval deficit clearly dissociates
from the hallmark of agrammatism—that is, difficulty in using syntactic
markers.

Miceli *et al.* suggest that the problem should be viewed in terms of a lexicon that is differentiated by form class. This view is identical with that expressed by Caramazza and Hillis (1991). We are critical of this approach
because it is bound by the orthodoxy that the traditional linguistic categories of phonology, semantics, lexicon, and syntax define all conceivable
language operations. We construe the behavior of patients with selective
verb production deficits as requiring us to step outside of this framework.
The behavior in question is that the function of verbs appears at times to
be nonexistent for certain aphasic speakers and that verb-demanding situations have to be met by the use of nominals. However, our proposed
"functional attitude," determining the part of speech in which a concept

is to be used, does not solve the problem of modality specificity. We cannot account for why the verbal functional attitude should fail some aphasics only in oral output and others only in graphic output.

Bates *et al.* (1991b) report that Chinese-speaking Broca's aphasics have the same selective difficulty in accessing verbs, in comparison with nouns, as do English-speaking Broca's aphasics. This disparity is not found in Chinese-speaking Wernicke's aphasics. Bates *et al.* agree with Caramazza and Hillis in rejecting a syntactic deficit explanation for the verb access problem, but for reasons that arise in the Chinese language. First is the fact that Chinese verbs carry no more inflectional morphology than do Chinese nouns. Second, Chinese Broca's aphasics performed competently in ordering the constituents of a sentence in relation to the verb, even when they could not produce the verb. Bates *et al.* see the verb access problem as lying in the lexical–conceptual sphere. They are not concerned with modality specific part-of-speech access problems.

SUMMARY

Writing is probably the language skill with the most complex network of relationships to other input and output channels. Hence, the disruption of writing (agraphia) can result from many sites of injury in the language zone of the left cerebral hemisphere. We have noted that some degree of impairment in all of the channels that mediate written output are likely to follow both anterior and posterior forms of moderate and severe aphasia, producing what can be termed "aphasic agraphia." The linguistic aspects of aphasic agraphia, that is, word retrieval, syntax, and written paraphasia, tend to mirror the level and quality of the oral language defect—but there are many exceptions to this tendency. The visual-motor aspect of writing skill is most susceptible to anterior speech zone lesions.

Although pure agraphia has been found with both frontal and parietal lobe lesions, the relative prominence of grapho-motor versus spelling components has varied from case to case. The relationship between lesion site and the detailed features of pure agraphia are not sufficiently clear to support an anatomical model of writing disorders. At the present time, a conservative interpretation is that the region of the angular gyrus of the left hemisphere is a crossroad for the auditory–visual input to graphic processes and that the motor representations for writing movements are proximal to the anterior speech zone controlling articulatory output.

Cognitive Aspects

Contrary to common assertions that orthography is based on a visual word representation, clinical observations suggest that the primary representation for the written lexicon is in the form of abstract letter sequences, implemented by graphic movements or, optionally, by oral spelling. These representations are termed "abstract" because the activated sequences can be realized graphically in many styles of writing, with either hand, foot, or arm movements, or by oral spelling or by typing. In most instances, recourse to visual memory to supplement impaired recall of letter strings results in only fragmentary retrieval. Figure 10.4 illustrates the unsuccessful effort to use visual representation in reconstructing written words.

We have approached the cognitive components through which the orthographic forms of words are acquired and re-evoked by an analysis of the learning process, beginning with the association of a graphomotor movement with letter names, primer words, and visually presented models of those letters and words. These associations are, of course, linked to the appearance of the written product. We may assume that this visual feedback becomes integrated with the motor-graphic activity, reinforcing and guiding it, but it is also indistinguishable from reading. (The phenomenon of pure alexia shows that writing is possible without the ability to read, the possibility of monitoring one's writing by reading the output may nevertheless serve to speed the process and make it more accurate.)

We have presented the process of acquiring and retrieving word orthography as engaging many concurrent associative paths, of which some are dominant over others because they contribute more quickly and efficiently to the realization of writing. We propose that the dominant mechanism in normal readers of an alphabetic language is the direct activation of an orthographic string by the meaning and/or the phonology of the target word. But these whole word (or lexical) associations are believed to make their appearance relatively late in the learning process. The basis for alphabetically based reading and writing is the possibility of phoneme by phoneme mapping of sound to letter, which is referred to as phoneme–grapheme conversion. While fine-grained phoneme-by-phoneme mapping is prominent in the early acquisition of reading and spelling, it is soon supplemented by the coarse-grained mapping of larger sublexical phonological segments (i.e., syllable-length and longer segments) to multiletter clusters. We have emphasized the role of oral spelling as an optional parallel output channel to writing, not because it plays a role in most writing situations, but because it illustrates

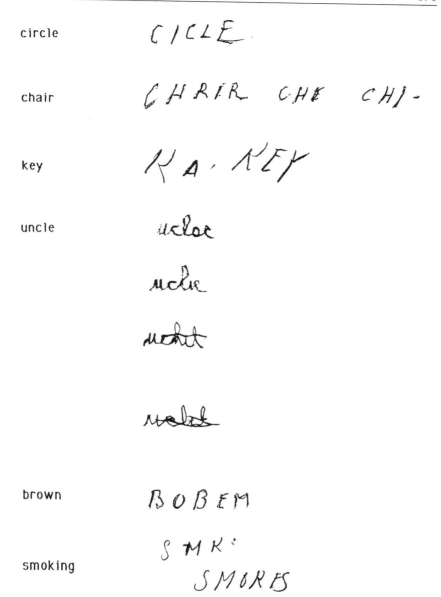

Figure 10.4. Examples of attempts at written word retrieval, guided chiefly by recall of visual features.

the fact that the written word lexicon takes the form of a letter sequence that can be implemented by many modalities of output, without going through a conscious process of conversion from one modality to another.

In addition to the foregoing major channels of association for the retrieval of the letter string, there are supplementary routes that may become dominant for short common words and may provide partial compensation, in aphasia, for the disablement of the major phonological routes. Among these are (1) graphomotor memory for highly overlearned sequences, such as one's signature and the most common grammatical functors, and (2) retrieval of visual features of the written word.

As in the case of reading, the effect of brain injury in the language zone is to produce partial or total dissociation among these various associative routes to the orthographic string. From cases of so called "deep dysgraphia," we observe that the phonological routes, from the most fine-grained phoneme-to-grapheme mapping to the coarsest whole-word phonology, can be so disabled that meaning-determined orthographic retrieval takes over and phonological relationships are violated (as in writing "slow" for "drag"). In contrast, instances of surface dysgraphia (analogous to surface dyslexia) show that fine-grained phoneme–grapheme associations may be used almost to the exclusion of other mechanisms, which appear no longer to be available to the patient.

Chapter 11

Apraxia and Aphasia

HISTORICAL INTRODUCTION

Any observer of the communicative efforts of aphasic patients cannot help noticing that most patients make little effort and have little success in circumventing their handicap in oral language by means of pantomime or gesture. When patients are directly asked to demonstrate a pretended gesture (such as beckoning someone over) or to pantomime the use of a familiar object, the result is often a vague movement that is unintelligible to someone who does not know in advance what the requested action was.

Impairment in the ability to perform purposeful movements on request was recognized as a discrete deficit by J. Hughlings Jackson in 1866 and by 1870, Steinthal (in Weisenburg and McBride, 1935) had coined the term "apraxia" for disorders of purposeful movement that could not be accounted for by muscle weakness or incoordination. In the same year, Finkelnburg (1870) used the term "asymbolia" to include any disorder that entails impaired ability to encode a concept for communicating it, whether through language or through gesture. Finkelnburg's position has been interpreted as linking aphasia and the impaired use of gesture and pantomime as aspects of a single underlying deficit.

In a series of case studies and comparisons of patient groups, Liepmann (1900, 1905, 1908) presented both an anatomic schema and a taxonomy of types of apraxia. Liepmann's work has been the center around which a great deal of subsequent investigation has revolved. Although his classification is not rigorously adhered to by contemporary writers, no alternative system of terminology has been offered.

CLINICAL FEATURES OF APRAXIA

Apraxia is a disorder in the deliberate execution of purposeful movements that cannot be accounted for by weakness or incoordination of the muscles involved, or by impairment of motivation, attention, or comprehension of verbal commands. Characteristically, apraxia becomes manifest when a patient fails to carry out a movement adequately on verbal command, although other forms of elicitation may result in identical difficulty; for example, requesting the pretended use of pictured or real objects or requesting imitation of movements demonstrated by the examiner. The same movements, however, may be carried out normally by the apraxic patient when the occasion for their use arises in a real-life context, or even when a situational context is created for the patient by the examiner. For example, the patient who cannot pretend to use a hammer may handle a real hammer unhesitatingly; the patient who cannot pretend to blow out a match, or even to imitate the movement accurately, often blows in a totally natural way when a lit match is held up before him. It is undoubtedly because of the fact that apraxic problems rarely appear in everyday life that the patient and family almost never mention the problem as a complaint.

Although the examples given so far involve representational depictions of meaningful acts (i.e., gestures and pantomimes), apraxia equally involves the performance of nonmeaningful movements carried out by imitation. These may be either static hand or limb positions or arbitrary movements that have been modeled by the examiner. The issue as to whether meaningfulness plays a role in the disorder will be elaborated.

CLASSIFICATION OF APRAXIA

Liepmann proposed a three-fold classification of apraxias based on the level of organization at which movements were disrupted.

Limb Kinetic Apraxia

Limb kinetic apraxia refers to apraxic impairment in the form of clumsiness or inability to position the hands for the execution of elementary movements, as in grasping an object or carrying out simple manipulations. Few authors continue to refer to limb kinetic apraxia, possibly because it is so difficult to distinguish an apraxic disorder of this type from a primary disorder of motor coordination.

Ideomotor Apraxia

Most usages of the term "apraxia" refer in fact to what Liepmann called "ideomotor apraxia." Here, elementary movements are adequately coordinated, but the motor plan for the intended action appears to be absent, inadequately formulated, or else poorly related to the patient's actual movement. A typical command in an examination for ideomotor apraxia is "Show me how you brush your teeth," and a typical performance of an apraxic patient is to bring his hand toward his mouth and rub his lips with his fingers or to part his lips and rub his teeth. This performance is likely to change little if the examiner provides a demonstration of a well-executed pantomime. It is common for an apraxic patient to bring his limb to approximately the right position in space for the required movement, but fail to assume the appropriate hand posture or the movement direction of the hand or arm.

Ideational Apraxia

Most authors interpret Liepmann's definition of "ideational apraxia" as involving a disorder of a complex sequential movement in which the individual elements are performed with normal facility but in a disordered sequence. Ideational apraxia is usually elicited with the manipulation of actual objects in a task such as having the patient fold a letter, place it in an envelope, seal it, and stamp it. Given the foregoing task, ideational apraxia might be manifested by the patient's applying the stamp to the letter and inserting the envelope in the fold of the letter. De Renzi (1989) reviews the history of the use of this term in the clinical literature and points out that it has commonly been applied to the inappropriate use of a single object, as in attempting to use a key to comb hair. De Renzi and Lucchelli (1988) tested a group of left brain damaged patients on a series of tasks involving two objects (e.g., opening a padlock with a key) as well as a series involving the use of a single object. Misuse of objects was as common in the single object tasks as in the dual object tasks, whereas errors of serial ordering were uncommon.

Another problem that has dogged the concept of ideational apraxia is that this form of behavior is commonly observed in demented patients suffering from disorders of attention. In these instances, the behavior may be considered confused rather than apraxic. However, there is no doubt that it has been observed in cases of focal lesions of the posterior left hemisphere in patients who were neither confused nor demented.

Bucco-Facial Apraxia

Failure to carry out movements of the face and upper respiratory apparatus may occur without limb apraxia. The type of movements affected include licking the lips, pretending to blow, cough, or swallow, and sipping through a straw. As noted elsewhere, bucco-facial apraxia is a common accompaniment of Broca's aphasia. Its clinical manifestations are analogous to those of ideomotor limb apraxia in that it is usually elicited by requesting a pretended action. Normal performance of a movement that could not be done as a pretended action can generally be elicited by providing a real object: For example, a match to be blown out; a real straw to sip through.

Callosal (Unilateral) Apraxia

This disorder, discussed in relation to the anatomy of apraxia, affects performance of the left hand in right-handed individuals who have suffered a lesion affecting fibers passing through the anterior corpus callosum.

LATERALIZATION AND RELATION TO APHASIA

The bulk of evidence indicates that apraxia is the result of left hemisphere lesions within a region that almost completely overlaps the language zone. Most patients with severe aphasia are apractic. Praxis recovers more rapidly than language however, and among milder aphasics the proportion with apraxia is smaller. Some aphasic patients are remarkably adept in using pantomime, and may do so spontaneously. A survey of the literature bearing on these relationships has some inconsistencies that may be traced to differing task and scoring criteria for considering patients to be apraxic. The inconsistencies bear particularly on whether apraxia occurs without aphasia following right hemisphere lesions.

The original observation on this issue was by Liepmann (1908), who found apraxia for the execution of gestures to be present in half the population of 41 left-brain damaged subjects and totally absent in a similar number of right-brain damaged patients. The great majority (16 out of 20) of those who were apraxic were also aphasic. The left-brain injured patients who were not aphasic were also unlikely to be apraxic. Further evidence of the association of apraxia with aphasia comes from the work of Kertesz, Ferro, and Shewan (1984). These authors found that in the acute phase, 53 of 57 severe aphasics were apraxic, and that 30 of 86 mild or moderate aphasics were also apraxic. In the chronic phase, the proportion of severely aphasic patients who are apraxic remains high, whereas the incidence of apraxia among the milder patients is somewhat lower than in the acute stage. De Renzi (1989) summarizes the findings of five published investigations of sizable series of left- and right-brain damaged patients who had been tested for praxis, chiefly through tests of imitation. The incidence of apraxia ranged from 28% to 46% in the left-brain damaged, and from 2% to 9% in the right-brain cases. A conflicting observation was reported by Haaland and Flaherty (1984), who found equal impairment in right- and left-brain injured groups in the imitation of meaningless movements, as well as meaningful intransitive gestures. In their data, it was only on transitive, pretended object manipulations that the left hemisphere damaged subjects were at a disadvantage. Whereas this report stands alone in suggesting a high degree of susceptibility to apraxic disorders in right-brain damaged subjects, it is also clear from the other studies that praxis is not quite so strongly and consistently lateralized in the left hemisphere as is language.

There have been a number of cases reported of left-handed individuals for whom the lateralization of praxis and of language appear to be dissociated, either through the presence of severe aphasia without apraxia following left hemisphere injury, or apraxia without aphasia following right brain damage (Heilman *et al.*, 1973). As De Renzi (1989) points out, however, these cases are too uncommon to support the thesis that hand preference determines the lateralization in the brain for the control of purposeful movements. In left-handers, as in right-handers, apraxia is most likely to result from an injury to the left hemisphere.

THE ANATOMIC BASIS OF APRAXIA

Several authors (Liepmann, 1900; Geschwind, 1975; Heilman, 1979) have offered explicit anatomical models for the realization of purposeful movements that are also intended to account for the occurrence of apraxia.

Liepmann's proposal was based on his analysis of two cases of unilateral apraxia associated with lesions of the corpus callosum (Liepmann, 1900; Liepmann and Maas, 1907), as well as on a large number of cases of bilateral apraxia or apraxia involving a nonhemiplegic limb, which is also presumed to affect the paralyzed side. In Liepmann's view, the immediate locus of control for simple purposeful movements is in the frontal premotor association zone of the left hemisphere. Acting by itself, however, this region is adequate only for overlearned, simple movements that do not require coordination with visual or somatosensory input. In every case, however, this region is a way station for outflow to the motor implementation system. Purposeful movements that are at all complex require polysensory input that traverses deep in parieto-frontal pathways to the motor association area. Purposeful movements of the left limbs are mediated by fibers carrying information across the corpus callosum, from the left to the right premotor association area. Damage to these fibers anywhere along their path results in unilateral apraxia affecting the left side only. This apraxia includes the inability to write with the left hand (unilateral agraphia) without entailing any other aphasic symptoms. Liepmann and Maas' case (1907), as well as Geschwind and Kaplan's case (1962), both showed these features as a result of a lesion in the corpus callosum. A further feature of Liepmann's anatomical model is that it accounts for the apraxia that is often observed in the left, non-hemiplegic limbs of patients with left hemisphere lesions; that is, that they have an underlying bilateral apraxia that can only be observed on the left because the right limbs are hemiplegic. Liepmann termed this "sympathetic apraxia."

Geshwind (1975) largely espoused Liepmann's account of the anatomy of apraxia, but added a feature that emphasized the nature of apraxia as a disconnection of pathways within the left hemisphere, in addition to allowing the unilateral left limb apraxia that results from a callosal disconnection. The salient feature in Geschwind's account of aphasia is that the comprehension of a command in Wernicke's area constitutes the input stimulus for purposeful movements. These instructions are then transferred via one of the bundles within the arcuate fasciculus to the left premotor area. Apraxia is the result of a lesion anywhere along this path that prevents this information from reaching the premotor area.

Geschwind also points out the existence of apraxia limited to commands involving the facial-upper respiratory apparatus (e.g., blowing, sniffing, coughing, or licking lips). This apraxic component is most often seen in aphasics with lesions affecting the left precentral face area, in conjunction with Broca's aphasia.

Preservation of Axial Movements

An important feature of Geschwind's model of the anatomy of apraxia is based on the clinical observation that movements involving the trunk and midline structures, including the eyes, are exempt from the apraxias involving the limbs. He demonstrated the readily replicable observation that some patients who are unable to carry out limb commands can readily execute such instructions as "turn around," "take two steps backwards," "bow," "kneel," and so on. Geschwind's argument to account for these cases is that, because midline movements involve non-pyramidal motor systems, they are not involved in the Wernicke's area -arcuate fasciculus- premotor area circuit that is the basis for purposeful limb movements and limb apraxia. He cites evidence that one point of origin of the nonpyramidal motor system is in the temporal lobe itself.

Geschwind acknowledges that there is a troublesome clinical observation involving axial movements that is not accounted for by this schema. This is the fact that occasional patients who have suffered destruction of Wernicke's area and who have profound auditory comprehension disorders have an island of spared comprehension for axial commands. These individuals cannot understand limb commands or point to objects that are named, yet they may promptly follow complex verbal commands involving trunk activity. The problem for Geschwind's model is that its account, up to this point, has required that the command be understood in a functioning Wernicke's area. The preservation of axial movements to verbal command in the presence of Wernicke's aphasia raises the question as to whether the right hemisphere may somehow be capable of processing these commands.

Recognizing that not all apraxic behavior is in response to a verbal command, Geschwind invokes the principle, already suggested by Liepmann, that the left hemisphere is dominant for the learning of motor movements, and that this dominance is associated with hand preference. He does not suggest any locus in the hemisphere as the site most responsible for this motor control.

Although Geschwind's model unifies the concept of interhemispheric disconnection with that of intrahemispheric disconnection, it leaves a number of troublesome questions. For one, he makes no effort to deal with how (or whether) an auditory command is converted in the premotor area into a series of organized goal-directed movements. In his account, it is sufficient to designate a pathway, which, if damaged, results in defective performance. Having introduced the notion of disconnection of an auditorily perceived command from the motor system, he then sets this mechanism aside in order to account for apraxic responses to nonauditory stimuli, citing the principle of left-hemisphere cerebral dominance for motor learning. If this principle suffices to account for apraxic responses to imitation, or to visual confrontation with an object to be pantomimed, why does it not also account for apraxic responses to auditory commands?

It is difficult to conceive of a theory of praxis that does not address the question of how plans for purposeful movements are represented in the brain and activated for motor realization. Such a theory would have to deal with the fact that pantomimed movements involving object manipulation are often only approximations of the veridical activity. As such, they are created on the spot by the subject to represent the idea of a movement. Verbal instructions to elicit a gesture or pantomime do not necessarily use a standard label for the movement. For example, to elicit the gesture for "hitchhiking," one can also say "Show me how you would thumb a ride" or "Show me how you would signal for a lift at the roadside." After the subject makes his response, one can ask "Show me that one again." Obviously, there is no storehouse of movements labeled by name. It is hard to escape from the conclusion that intervening between the stimulus (whether in the form of a verbal request or otherwise) and the response is some form of conceptualization of the goal to be achieved by the gesture or pantomime to be performed, which can be conceived of as a script.

Heilman (1979) offers an alternative anatomical model that differs from those of Geschwind and Liepmann in postulating a center for visual-kinesthetic memories in the left parietal lobe—a center that would be responsible for planning the sequence of movements that are involved in most pantomimes. Verbal commands given by an examiner would, as in Geschwind's model, first be processed linguistically in Wernicke's area, then converted into a motor plan in the parietal lobe. The pathway for execution of purposeful movements would then lead from the parietal lobe to the frontal motor association pathway. Apraxia would result either from injury to the left parietal lobe, damaging the center for visual-kinesthetic engrams, or else from injury to the pathways leading to the frontal motor association area. Liepmann's proposed mechanism for unilateral apraxia of the nondominant limbs is accepted by both Heilman and Geschwind.

Heilman's suggestion that a center for the representation of visual kinesthetic memories plays a role in praxis leads to the expectation of different symptoms resulting from injury to this center in the parietal lobe, as compared to the result of injury in the pathway to the frontal motor areas or to the frontal area itself. This means that damage to the memory store for movements might impair the recognition of movements, as well as their performance. Injury to any portion of the system that lies anterior to the parietal lobe should spare the ability to recognize movements, but produce an apraxia for their execution. In order to test this hypothesis, Heilman, Rothi, and Valenstein (1982) compared the ability to discriminate between correctly and incorrectly performed pantomimes on the part of apraxic patients with lesions involving the left parietal lobe and those whose lesions spared this region. They reported that patients with parietal lobe involvement were, in fact, significantly more impaired in the judgment of pantomimes than the other subjects. Additional data supporting the concept of a parietal locus for visual-kinesthetic motor engrams has yet to be reported.

Parietal versus Frontal Source of Apraxic Symptoms

Taking literally any of the anatomical models cited (e.g., those of Liepmann, Geschwind, or Heilman), there is no basis for expecting differences in the severity or symptomatology of apraxias arising from lesions anywhere in the pathway from the parietal lobe to the frontal motor association zone. The bulk of studies of lesion location, in relation to apraxia, indicates that parietal lobe lesions are more damaging than those in the anterior areas. For example, Kolb and Milner (1981) compared patients with unilateral tissue ablations from frontal, temporal, or parietal regions in either hemisphere in carrying out complex serial movements. The most severe impairments followed left parietal lobe damage, with milder impairments following frontal lobe removals. De Renzi *et al.* (1983) as well as Kertesz *et al.* (1984) also reported that more severe apraxic impairments were associated with parietal than with frontal lobe lesions in stroke patients. Of the recent studies on the relationship of lesion locus to apraxia, only that of Basso, Luzzatti, and Spinnler (1980) reported no differences in the incidence of aphasia as a function of the anterior–posterior location of left hemisphere lesions.

THE RELATIONSHIP BETWEEN LANGUAGE AND PRAXIS

Two principled opposing views have emerged among investigators who have considered the basis for the relationship between aphasia and apraxia. At the heart of the controversy is the question of whether there is a distinction between apraxia for the communication of meaningful messages, as in pantomime and gesture, and apraxia for the execution of nonmeaningful movements by imitation. Closely related to this issue is whether the ability to interpret pantomime and gesture is related to the ability to perform them, and to the presence and severity of aphasia.

The notion that the execution of pantomime is a form of symbolic behavior closely related to language dates to Finkelnburg (1870) and has been restated by a number of investigators, most recently Duffy and Duffy (1981). In this view, impaired pantomime and aphasia are parallel manifestations of "asymbolia." Duffy and Duffy, in particular, press the point that the impairment of symbol use that results in the loss of pantomimic expression also results in the loss of the ability to interpret communicative gestures.

The more widespread classical view, dating to Liepmann's writing (1900), holds that apraxia is a disorder of movement planning that is equally manifest in nonmeaningful gestures and in communicative ones. The many authors who have studied the phenomenon from this standpoint have given no consideration to the interpretation of pantomime and gesture, which would appear irrelevant from their perspective.

One of the first studies to address explicitly the relation between pantomime and language disorder was that of Goodglass and Kaplan (1963). They examined 20 aphasic patients (predominantly nonfluent, but excluding global aphasics) and a matched group of 19 nonaphasic brain injured patients. Their tests of pantomime consisted of natural expressive gestures (e.g., holding one's nose to indicate a bad smell) and conventional gestures (e.g., saluting), both elicited by verbal command. Simple pantomimes of object manipulation were elicited by presenting a picture of the object to be demonstrated. Subjects were than tested for their ability to imitate the same set of gestures and pantomimes after they were modeled by the examiner. Severity of aphasia was rated on measures derived from the Boston Diagnostic Aphasia Examination. Goodglass and Kaplan found that the correlation of pantomime and gesture scores with severity of aphasia was low and insignificant. Further, performance on imitation showed little improvement over performance without a model. On the basis of these findings, Goodglass and Kaplan concluded that the ability to execute meaningful gesture or pantomime was not related to the severity of aphasia, but was rather a manifestation of a disorder of purposeful movement.

A more ambiguous result was obtained in a study by Dee, Benton, and Van Allen (1970), who divided their subject population into nonaphasic, mildly aphasic, moderately aphasic, and severely aphasic patients, using the Token Test (De Renzi and Vignolo, 1962) as the basis for classification. They, too, used tests of verbally elicited gestures, pantomime of object use, and imitation. They found that the severely aphasic patients scored more poorly on the performance of gestures and pantomimes on request than did the mild and moderate aphasics. Performance on request was paralleled by performance to imitation. These results were seen as indicating a link between aphasia and apraxia, but not sufficient to define the pantomimic disorder as simply one of symbolization.

Several investigators (De Renzi et al., 1980; Lehmkuhl et al., 1983) compared left brain damaged patients' execution of meaningful and nonmeaningful gestures and found them to be equally affected. Kimura (1982) similarly takes the strong position that the presence or absence of communicative intent is irrelevant to the characterization of apraxia.

Kimura develops the thesis, in a series of studies done with various collaborators (Kimura and Archibald, 1974; Mateer, 1976; Kimura, 1982), that praxis, the execution of serial motor movements, and cerebral dominance for language are intimately related. The basic skill in question is the performance of any movement that goes beyond assuming a static posture to involve sequential action. Kimura (1976, 1979) argued that the lateralization of language itself is due to the fact that speech entails serial motor activity, for which the left hemisphere is dominant. Kimura proposes that the role of the left hemisphere in symbol use is totally secondary to the dominance of that hemisphere for speech, which, in turn, is an expression of left hemisphere control for serial movements. Kimura and Archibald's (1974) study found that left-brain damaged subjects and right-brain damaged subjects did not differ in their ability to copy simple finger flexion or to imitate static hand positions that were demonstrated. Left-brain damaged aphasic patients were more impaired than the right brain damaged subjects in carrying out serial hand movements and equally impaired in performing the pantomimes and gestures of a traditional apraxia examination.

Contrasting with the foregoing view is the position that originated with Finkelnburg's (1870) paper—namely, that the impairment of pantomime and gestural use is due to a deficiency in symbolic capacity that extends to and includes spoken language. Pickett (1972) saw the significance of including a test of the comprehension of gestures along with measures of the severity of aphasia and of the ability to perform pantomimes on request and by imitation. There were significant correlations between all of the measures of pantomime production and of pantomime comprehension with severity of aphasia, as measured by the Porch Index of Communicative Ability (PICA; Porch, 1971). Pickett concluded that communicative competence was a common factor in all of the measures.

Duffy and Duffy (1981) attempted to distinguish between communicative movements and nonmeaningful movements in drawing a distinction between apraxia as a motor disorder and impaired pantomime use as an expression of asymbolia. The authors' measure of apraxia was a movement imitation test (the Manual Apraxia Test) comprising the imitation of both meaningful and nonmeaningful movements. Their measure of pantomime production was a subtest for the representation of an object concept by demonstration of its use. The measure of pantomime comprehension was a series of pantomimes to be matched with a multiple choice picture array that included the target. The PICA served as the measure of aphasia severity and Ravens' Matrices were administered as a measure of postmorbid cognitive functioning. Duffy and Duffy, like

Pickett, found that pantomime production and pantomime comprehension were correlated with each other and that both were strongly correlated with the severity of aphasia. General cognitive impairment as reflected in Ravens' Matrices was ruled out as a factor. Performance on the Manual Apraxia Test of movement imitation was not related to severity of aphasia and it is considered by authors to serve as a measure of apraxia, uncontaminated by any communicative intent.

Duffy and Duffy's position has the merit of challenging the more widely held view that the communicative content of movements does not enter into the definition of praxis. Their suggestion that meaningful gestures have both a conceptual and a motor aspect, whereas imitation of nonmeaningful movements has little or no conceptual content, has the appeal of plausibility. However, a weakness in their results is that their pantomime test was said to show no relationship to motor praxis but was exclusively related to the severity of aphasia.

Few investigators have concerned themselves specifically with the ability to recognize pantomimed actions. Varney (1978) examined the relationship between pantomime recognition and various components of aphasia, as well as performance IQ, in patients with aphasia. He reported that reading comprehension alone exhibited a significant correlation with pantomime recognition. Only one study, by Seron et al. (1979), reported a similar finding.

The issue posed by Duffy and Duffy was reexamined by Wang and Goodglass (1992). Their tests of pantomime production used pictures to elicit pantomimes of object use nonverbally and oral requests to elicit intransitive gestures. Imitation of gestures was tested for both nonmeaningful and meaningful gestures separately by having the subjects copy from a videotaped demonstration. Comprehension of gestures was measured with a Pantomime Recognition Test. In this test, 20 short videotaped pantomimes involving the use of an object are played for the subject who is asked to select a picture of the correct object from a multiple choice of four objects. The distractors included one that was semantically related, one structurally related, and one unrelated to the target. Language impairment was measured through the subjects' scores on the Boston Naming Test (Kaplan, Goodglass, and Weintraub, 1983), on the composite auditory comprehension subtests of the Boston Diagnostic Aphasia Examination (BDAE; Goodglass and Kaplan, 1963), and on the Sentence Reading subtest of the BDAE. The subjects were 30 aphasic patients from the Aphasia/Neurobehavioral Unit of Boston VA Medical Center and represented a range of types and severity of aphasia.

Data were analyzed by intercorrelations, multiple regression analysis, and factor analysis. All of these approaches concurred in revealing a strong intercorrelation linking all of the movement production subtests and the *pantomime recognition subtest* with each other. The auditory comprehension measure from the BDAE was significantly related with the production tests of pantomime and gesture as well as with the pantomime recognition subtest. It was not related with the imitation of nonmeaningful gestures. Whereas auditory comprehension accounted for a significant portion of the variance of both the pantomime production task and the pantomime recognition task, the relationship between all the tests of movement production and recognition was much stronger than their relationship to auditory comprehension. Of the two remaining language tasks, the naming measure had weak relationships with intransitive pantomime production and with pantomime recognition. Reading was unrelated to any of the movement measures. There was, however, a strong common factor linking the three language measures with each other. The Wechsler Adult Intelligence Scale (WAIS) performance IQ scores were not a significant determinant of any of the movement or pantomime comprehension measures.

Wang and Goodglass' results provide some justification for Duffy and Duffy's assertion that there is a common factor linking communicative gestures with language capacity, and that this factor does not extend to nonmeaningful movement imitations. There are, however, two important qualifications. The first one is that the relation between communicative gesture and language is minor in comparison with the relationship among all of the gesture-related tasks, both expressive and receptive. The second qualification is that it is only auditory comprehension—and not a general language factor—that is associated with pantomime production and comprehension.

Special note deserves to be made of the strong correlation between the pantomime recognition and the pantomime production tasks. This lends some credence to the notion, suggested by Heilman, Rothi, and Valenstein (1982) that the receptive and expressive aspects of purposeful movement are governed by a common set of representations. The author would avoid the implication of the term "engrams" as used by Heilman *et al.* because this can be taken to refer to a set of memories of previously learned movements. The idea that pantomimes are evocations of items from a store of memories of movements does not stand up to scrutiny. In particular, the ability to encode, briefly store, and reproduce newly demonstrated meaningless movements would appear incompatible with the reliance on a store of movement memories. A more plausible notion, in the author's view, is that the ability to perceive and encode limb movements in either immediate or long-term memory shares a mechanism with the planning of limb movements for production.

SUMMARY

Apraxia, a disorder in the organization and execution of purposeful movements, was recognized as a discrete functional impairment only in the mid-nineteenth century. One reason for its late recognition is that it usually appears only when gestures are to be performed on request, but it does not usually handicap patients in the context of daily life. By definition, apraxia is a disorder in the execution of movements elicited by specific request, which cannot be accounted for by impairment of strength or motor coordination, or by failure to comprehend, to attend to, or to attempt to carry out the requested action.

The most common type of apraxia (following Liepmann's taxonomy) is ideomotor limb apraxia which renders the patient incapable of clearly executing such conventional gestures as waving goodbye, saluting, or hitchhiking, or to pantomime the use of common objects. Offering a model for imitation usually provides slight facilitation of the movement. Bucco-facial apraxia, specific to movements of the oral and upper respiratory apparatus (as in sniffing, coughing, and blowing) may appear, with or without limb apraxia, in patients with aphasia involving lesions of the anterior speech zone.

A second form of apraxia, referred to by Liepmann's term "ideational apraxia" involves the inappropriate use of real objects. There is some disagreement as to whether this term refers only to the interchange of elements in a series of object manipulations (e.g., placing a match in one's mouth, striking a cigarette on the matchbox, and attempting to light the match with the cigarette) or whether it includes misuse of individual objects, as in demonstrating the use of a key by trying to comb one's hair with it. Similar behavior is observed in patients who are confused, but the term "apraxia" is probably inappropriate for confused patients.

Apraxia is most commonly observed with left hemisphere lesions in the presence of aphasia. The incidence of apraxia in cases of very severe aphasia has been reported to be as great as 90% and in moderately severe aphasia, as much as 35%. Impairment in the performance of communicative movements is uncommon after right brain injury, although one study reports that right brain injured patients are equally impaired with left brain injured in their ability to *imitate* movements.

The basis for the cerebral lateralization of purposeful movement has had various explanations. One of these is that it is strongly linked to the laterality of the preferred hand. If this were the case, one would expect many instances in which aphasia and apraxia are dissociated in left-handed patients with a unilateral lesion. Although such cases have been described, they are very rare and most left-handers who develop aphasia and/or apraxia have had unilateral left hemisphere lesions.

On the basis of current evidence, the most conservative interpretation of the laterality of purposeful movement is that, like language, it is strongly left hemisphere dominant in the great majority of people so that the lateralization of language and of praxis usually coincide. As in the case of language, the lateralization of purposeful movement is subject to variation in the population, with bilateral control or complete right hemisphere control in some individuals. There is some indication that non-right-handers are more likely to be deviant in their lateralization for movement. However, there is no basis for considering a direct causal link between the lateralization of hand preference, language, and movement.

Clinico-pathological data support an anatomical model in which the major crossroad for praxis in either limb is the premotor area of the dominant hemisphere. Information for the control of movements of the non-dominant limbs is conveyed from this area to its homologue in the other hemisphere through fibers traversing the corpus callosum. While apraxia may be produced from injury to the dominant premotor area, most reports find that apraxia occurs most consistently and in most severe form from lesions involving the dominant parietal lobe and deep-lying fibers in the fronto-parietal subcortex that can be conceived as bringing poly-sensory information to bear on the premotor area. In some accounts (e.g., Heilman *et al.*, 1982), the parietal lobe is the center for the formulation and storage of movement plans.

Apraxia is found to affect both meaningful communicative gesture and pantomime, and the imitation of arbitrary, nonmeaningful movements. The fact of the correlation of these two types of performance has led to the dominant position that the meaningfulness of a gesture is irrelevant to the definition of apraxia. This position has been challenged by investigators who regard the content of meaningful gesture (e.g., pantomime) to involve a symbolic component that is absent in the imitation of non-meaningful movements.

A somewhat different view has recently been proposed for the relationship between the production of communicative gesture and pantomime, the ability to comprehend pantomimed movements, the ability to imitate nonmeaningful movements, and the severity of aphasia. According to results obtained by Wang and Goodglass (1992), there is a strong common factor linking the production and the comprehension of meaningful movements with the imitation of nonmeaningful movements. Furthermore, there is a significant correlation between the impairment of auditory comprehension and the production and comprehension

of meaningful gestures. The imitation of nonmeaningful gestures is unrelated to any language component. These findings provide some support for the argument that both the production and comprehension of
meaningful gestures have a symbolic component that is absent from
nonmeaningful movements. They also are consistent with Heilman *et al.*
in clustering all purposeful movement, along with gesture comprehension, under a single factor.

Chapter **12**

Classification of Aphasia

At no time has there been complete consensus on how the various manifestations of aphasia should be classified. Differences in the approach to classification often imply deep differences in underlying assumptions about the basis for the various symptoms. As we saw in Chapter 2 (History), the major opposition in the twentieth century has been between those who favor an anatomically based account of the symptomatology (e.g., Geschwind and Luria) and those who propose a typology in psychological or linguistic terms (e.g., Head and Wepman).

In this chapter, we will begin by reviewing the syndrome typology espoused by Geschwind and his associates in the Boston school of aphasiology. Because this typology is an updating of that of Wernicke, as it was passed on among European scholars from the latter part of the nineteenth century, it has become dominant in the European and American literature. We will discuss the advantages and limitations of the syndrome approach and alternative approaches to classification.

This section pulls together the information on classification of aphasia that has already appeared in scattered form in connection with the deficits that primarily characterize each of the syndromes, as covered in Chapters 4 through 10.

BROCA'S APHASIA

Other terms: Motor aphasia; efferent motor aphasia (Luria); verbal aphasia (Head).

Behavioral features: Dominated by reduction or suppression of speech output with relative sparing of auditory comprehension. Speech production is effortful, usually limited to word groupings of one to three words produced with labored articulation. Quality of articulation varies as a function of the familiarity of the words in the message. That is, these patients often have a subset of well practiced words that they produce with perfectly normal articulation. Articulation may also be facile in the utterance of conversational stereotypes (e.g., "I can't say it"), but distorted during attempts at more difficult or uncommon words. Severity of output impairment may range from virtually complete inability to articulate words to mild awkwardness of articulation.

Agrammatism (see Chapter 6) is a common but not universal feature of Broca's aphasia. Vocabulary access in speech production is limited— often patients perform well on picture naming, but have more difficulty evoking needed vocabulary in free speech. Auditory comprehension at the one-word level is usually close to normal, but impairment in the processing of sentences can usually be demonstrated.

Reading for comprehension is usually functional, but patients rarely read for recreation because of the slowness and the effort required. Some degree of phonological dyslexia or deep dyslexia (see Chapter 9) is commonly found in patients with Broca's aphasia who are agrammatic. However, deep dyslexia may be present without agrammatism, as DeBleser and Bayer (1990) have shown. Writing may vary widely in Broca's aphasia; some individuals write considerably more than they can say, but for most patients of this type, writing is affected to a similar degree as their speech output.

Anatomy: A lasting Broca's aphasia involves a lesion encompassing the cortical Broca's area (*pars opercularis* and *pars triangularis* of the left frontal lobe), often extending posteriorly to include the lower portion of the motor strip. The lesion must extend in depth to the periventricular white matter, because a purely cortical or shallow lesion produces only a transient disorder.

WERNICKE'S APHASIA

Other terms: Sensory aphasia; temporo-acoustic and acoustic-mnestic aphasia (Luria); syntactic aphasia (Head).

Behavioral features: Speech output is facile in articulation and sentence structure, tending to be filled with ill chosen words and poorly formed sentences (semantic paraphasia and paragrammatism). In severe cases, speech output consists only of neologistic jargon. Auditory comprehension is defective even for the comprehension of common object names— it is even more defective for the comprehension of sentences. Word finding is severely restricted so that free conversation is often circumlocutory and empty. Patients' rate of speech is sometimes excessively rapid and they may be unaware of their many speech output errors. Early in the illness, patients who exhibit this pattern may incorporate words and phrases that are far afield from the presumed topic of conversation. Their output may consist largely of neologisms embedded in pseudo-grammatical sentences, with grammatical words, and noun and verb inflections, providing a semblance of syntactic structure. This is referred to as "jargon aphasia," observed in very severe forms of Wernicke's aphasia.

Reading and writing are affected to varying degrees depending on the boundaries of the lesion. Complete agraphia is often seen in Wernicke's aphasia; when writing is possible, the written output often resembles the patient's speech in the character of errors and the rambling, paraphasic style.

Anatomic correlates: Wernicke's aphasia is the result of a lesion that includes the entire posterior portion of the first temporal gyrus, known as Wernicke's area. Lesions that extend posteriorly to include the region of the angular gyrus are likely to produce severe reading and writing disorder.

CONDUCTION APHASIA

Other terms: Afferent motor aphasia (Luria); central aphasia (Goldstein).

Behavioral features: The general level of articulation, rate of speech, and use of grammatical elements is fluent, but speech output is usually disrupted by characteristic errors. Prominent among these is the occurrence of phonemic paraphasias—the patients sporadically become tangled in the production of a word, transposing the order of sounds, substituting or inserting extraneous phonemes, and making repeated stabs at correcting themselves. This difficulty may appear as stutterlike blocking, when the patient interrupts himself at the beginning of a word. Anomia is frequently a prominent component of the disorder and instances of phonemic entanglement are sometimes confined to the production of nouns or other key words, whereas grammatical words are produced fluently. In some instances, patients with conduction aphasia have a speech pattern that borders on that of Wernicke's aphasics, producing syntactically disordered constructions and making repeated starts to repair syntax.

Repetition of words or sentences modeled by the examiner is remarkably poor. Occasionally, repetition difficulty extends to easy one-syllable words; more commonly, failures occur only on polysyllabic words and on sentences. A defining characteristic of this disorder is the relative preservation of auditory comprehension. Whereas comprehension may not be totally intact, it is superior to the capacity to repeat; that is, conduction aphasics differ critically from Wernicke's aphasics in that conduction aphasics have paraphasia with good auditory comprehension, and Wernicke's aphasics have paraphasia with impaired comprehension. However, the paraphasia of conduction aphasics is primarily in the domain of phonological disorganization—and occasionally of syntactic disorganization. They never produce a continuous flow of disorganized or neologistic speech. Furthermore, unlike patients with Wernicke's aphasia, they are characteristically aware of their errors and make immediate self-corrective efforts. (See discussion of repetition disorders in Chapter 8.)

Reading comprehension is well preserved and on par with auditory comprehension, but oral reading may suffer from the same problems with phonological sequencing as free speech and repetition. Writing is rarely selectively impaired, and tends to parallel speech output. Spelling difficulties have been highlighted by a number of authors.

Anatomical features: The anatomy of conduction aphasia has been discussed both in Chapter 3 and, in the context of repetition disorders, in Chapter 8. To summarize, a large proportion of conduction aphasics have a lesion in the supramarginal gyrus, compatible with the anatomical account of Geschwind. However, lesions elsewhere along the border of the Sylvian fissure are sometimes the cause. Lesion extent in conduction aphasia is more restricted than in either Broca's or Wernicke's aphasia. Indeed, a patient with an extensive lesion of the posterior Sylvian zone almost inevitably has the features of Wernicke's aphasia.

TRANSCORTICAL MOTOR APHASIA

Other terms: Frontal dynamic aphasia (Luria).

Behavioral features: The dominant feature in this disorder is the preservation of a near normal span for repetition, along with the severe inhibition of spontaneous speech. Patients are characteristically unable to respond to questions that involve any type of sentence formulation. They may attempt to initiate a response with an introductory formula, such as "Well, I . . . ," and find themselves unable to progress beyond that point. Yet they perform flawlessly when instructed to repeat sentences. There is a wide range of variability with respect to word retrieval among transcortical motor aphasics. Some of these patients have excellent picture naming skills. These patients can usually provide one-word factual answers to any questions that can be answered in this way, yet they find themselves totally blocked by questions that involve organizing an answer. In other cases, severe anomia stalks the patient whenever word retrieval is demanded, whether in face to face conversation or in confrontation naming. Auditory comprehension is relatively unaffected.

Not only do these patients repeat with perfect facility, but they may occasionally have a breakthrough of a well-formed sentence of normal length in the course of conversation. Because of these occasions, it is very difficult to assign this disorder to either the fluent or nonfluent category. Other characteristics of transcortical motor aphasia are the unusual degree of preservation of memorized verbal material (e.g., the Lord's Prayer) and the sensitivity of these patients to facilitation of word retrieval when provided with the first sounds of the desired word.

Anatomical features: Lesions that result in transcortical motor aphasia are usually smaller than those associated with Broca's or Wernicke's aphasia. They impinge on a subcortical site in the anterior frontal zone that probably forms part of a circuit linking the motor speech area with the supplementary motor area and limbic structures that are essential for the initiation of speech. Lesions may extend to the cortical surface, including part of Broca's area, but it is not established whether cortical involvement affects the symptom picture.

TRANSCORTICAL SENSORY APHASIA

Behavioral features: In global terms, transcortical sensory aphasics can be described as fluent and paraphasic, having impaired comprehension but remarkably well-preserved repetition. Except for the feature of preserved repetition, the profile of disabilities of these patients very much resembles that of Wernicke's aphasia. Yet in detail, there are differences from Wernicke's aphasia. Continuous runs of mixed phonemic paraphasia and paragrammatism are uncommon in transcortical sensory aphasia, where errors generally take the form of semantic word substitutions. Perseverative intrusions of previously used words and perseveration of content are common. Auditory comprehension is impaired and patients are generally unaware of their language difficulties. Testing with confrontation naming usually reveals severe anomia. Patients are also commonly alexic and agraphic.

The sparing of repetition in these severely affected patients is striking—not only do they repeat fairly long sentences accurately, but they tend to incorporate the words of their interlocutor in framing a response to questions. Although this behavior suggests a tendency to echo, they do not echo automatically or where it would be socially inappropriate, for example, when they are not being addressed. The phenomenon of repeating without understanding (alienation of word meaning) is sometimes a feature of transcortical sensory aphasia and has been discussed in Chapter 5 (Disorders of Word Retrieval).

Anatomic features: Transcortical sensory aphasia is commonly produced by deep-going lesions in a zone inferior to the angular gyrus and between the posterior end of the Sylvian fissure and the temporo-occipital junction.

ANOMIC APHASIA

Other terms: Nominal aphasia (Head); semantic aphasia (Wepman).

Behavioral features: The defining feature of anomic aphasia is that speech output is fluent with respect to rate, syntactic form, and articulation, but that within this fluent delivery there is notable word finding failure (i.e., *anomia*), affecting primarily nouns, but also other words of high informational content, including verbs, adverbs, and so on. Speech is commonly filled with vague, circumlocutory substitutions for the intended concepts and these substitutions serve as placeholders to maintain the grammatical structure.

Of all the aphasic subtypes, *anomic aphasia* is the one that appears as a result of diverse causes and as a result of lesion sites that are remote from each other. It may be more accurate to consider this term as applying to three different syndromes, as well as to residual aphasia in which reduced vocabulary access is the primary persistent symptom. The associated behavioral features may be subtle, but serve to distinguish the forms that are associated with various lesion sites.

Anomic Aphasia of the Angular Gyrus Region

This is the form of anomia that best corresponds to Luria's "acoustic-mnestic aphasia." Patients with this disorder may show sporadic instances of "alienation of word meaning," in which, when they fail to retrieve a word, they do not recognize it when it is offered by the examiner. Because this form of anomia involves a lesion that is close to the site for alexia and agraphia, it may be accompanied by reading and spelling disturbances. It is also related, by location, to transcortical sensory aphasia and may represent a much reduced form of the latter.

Frontal Anomia

An almost pure anomic picture is sometimes seen in patients with small subcortical frontal lesions in the zone that is usually associated with transcortical motor aphasia. The one distinguishing feature of this anomic pattern is that the patients are sometimes remarkably sensitive to facilitation by hearing the opening sounds of the word. Alexander (personal communication) found them particularly susceptible to being misled by a false opening cue to give false completions.

Anomia of the Inferior Temporal Gyrus

Lesions of the left inferior temporal gyrus may result in anomia of the purest type. These patients may have severe word retrieval problems, with fluent, grammatical speech and normal or near-normal use of written language. They do not have the minimal signs of semantic dissociation that have been noted in association with the angular gyrus form of anomia.

Anomia as an Expression of Residual Aphasia

Some degree of reduced word finding is usually present in patients who have recovered near normal functional use of language after having passed through a period of aphasia of any of the foregoing types. Their test profiles at this point may indicate reduced naming ability as the only significant deficit. Objective classification based purely on the test profile may result in their being labeled as anomic aphasics. This label has little significance from the point of view of syndrome analysis.

PURE MODALITY-SPECIFIC APHASIAS

The following syndromes are repeated only for the sake of making this a comprehensive listing. They are dealt with in detail in the chapters indicated.

Pure word-deafness. This is the loss of the ability to interpret the sounds of speech in terms of their familiar linguistic value. It usually entails no impairment of auditory acuity. In its pure form, there is no impairment of oral production, reading, or writing. Most instances are produced by bilateral temporal lobe lesions, but pure word-deafness can be the result of a unilateral left temporal lesion. (See Chapter 7.)

Subcortical motor aphasia (aphemia). This is a disorder affecting only the articulation of speech, without impairing any other motor function involving the articulatory mechanism. Other aspects of language (word retrieval, syntax, auditory comprehension, reading, and writing) are unaffected. It is produced by a deep-going lesion involving the lower portion of the motor strip. (See Chapter 4.)

Pure word-blindness. Other terms for this are "letter-by-letter reading"; alexia without agraphia; and pure alexia. (See Chapter 9.) It is the loss of reading ability that may occur without any effect on other language functions. In some forms, the ability to recognize letters is preserved and written words may be reconstructed by silent spelling (hence "letter-by-letter reading"). Most instances are produced by a combination of injury to the left visual cortex and the posterior corpus callosum. In every case, there is evidence that the left posterior language area has been anatomically disconnected from visual input.

SHORTCOMINGS OF THE SYNDROME APPROACH

As long as the syndrome labels are used to provide a shorthand summary of the most prominent features of a patient's language disorder, these terms serve a useful function in communicating between clinicians. Further, depending on the clinician's experience with localization in aphasia, the syndrome label carries presumptions about lesion site and, possibly, the most likely organic etiology. To the extent that individuals who carry the same syndrome label vary with respect to a particular feature, the presence or absence of this feature may be referred to, adding precision at little extra cost in words to the listener's perception of the patient's behavior. For example, one may speak of a patient with Wernicke's aphasia, but who is without press of speech; or a patient with conduction aphasia who has an extraordinary amount of phonemic paraphasia and flawless auditory comprehension.

The syndrome label carries an additional load of implications to one who has been indoctrinated with the classical anatomo-functional model of language based on centers and connecting pathways. To such an individual, the syndrome label carries more than the expectation that the lesion has an increased likelihood of lying in a particular zone. It means that a particular anatomo-functional change has taken place that must be the result of one of a small number of anatomic possibilities.

The recent growth of neurolinguistic research has seen many instances in which syndrome classifications have been used as though they specified a fixed pattern of linguistic behaviors. For example, a group of Broca's aphasics may be pitted against a group of Wernicke's aphasics with respect to some experimental language task. The critical behavioral feature(s) leading to the choice of subject groups may not be specified. It may be agrammatism versus paragrammatism, or fluency of speech output versus nonfluency, or impaired auditory comprehension versus good comprehension. But individuals in each syndrome group may differ from each other in the severity and even in the presence of one or more features. This inconstancy is particularly true in regard to agrammatism, which is not always present in Broca's aphasics.

The most recent concerted opposition to classification by syndromes came from cognitive psychologists (Schwartz, 1984; Caramazza, 1984) who were chagrined to realize that classification by syndrome did not, nor was it designed to, specify a fixed neurolinguistic deficit. In some cases the reaction was to denounce syndrome classification as a meaningless exercise; however, calmer analysis determined several types of difficulty.

Mixing of features from unrelated domains. For any syndrome, the defining characteristics may come from different domains: for example, reference to the sensory or motor channels that are affected; reference to the linguistic character of speech errors (agrammatism, paraphasia, anomia); or reference to phenomenological impression of fluency or nonfluency. Often, the presumption is that the lesion site will fit the prototypical pattern.

Inconstancy and lack of precision (polytypicality) in feature specification. The syndromes are defined as a configuration of features, hardly any one of which is central to the classification. For example, a patient may be classified as a Broca's aphasic even if his articulation is normal, provided that he is agrammatic and has good comprehension. Another Broca's patient may have no more than one-word utterances and have profoundly impaired articulation with fairly good, but reduced auditory comprehension. One examiner may score agrammatism as present if speech is limited to single words, another may score it as present if an occasional article is omitted from otherwise well formed sentences, and yet another may insist that agrammatism can be diagnosed only when multiword utterances are attempted.

The use of subjective standards for judging the presence or absence of symptoms that vary on a continuum makes for great difficulties in documenting agreement between clinicians, except in a handful of classical, prototypical cases.

Inconstancy of anatomical criteria. Although the assignment of a syndrome label to a case of aphasia is generally determined by a match between the observed speech and language symptomatology and the accepted criteria for a particular syndrome, the link between the major syndromes and their supposed neural basis is somewhat ambiguous. Should a case that fits the speech symptomatology of Wernicke's aphasia be called by that name if the lesion does not implicate the temporal lobe? There is sufficient variability in lesion sites that produce clinically similar symptom pictures so that the standard "accepted" lesion corresponding to a syndrome has only a probabilistic, rather than a fixed, relationship to the given pattern of language disturbances. Caplan (1987) has advanced a view very similar to this.

SYNDROMES AS MODAL TENDENCIES SHAPED BY ANATOMO-FUNCTIONAL CONSTRAINTS

The nineteenth century view, fostered by the center-and-connection models of the "diagram makers," was that there was an invariant relationship between the destruction of a center or connecting pathway and a complex of resulting deficits and spared abilities. In this view, each syndrome was a disease entity that pointed to its source, just as a medical disease entity might point to a causative microorganism. This view has persisted to some extent, in spite of the decades of experience with the fuzzy boundaries between the syndromes and the variability of anatomic lesion sites. The author proposes an alternative view: one that views the familiar syndromes of aphasia as the result of modal tendencies for the functional organization of language in adult human brains. The assumption behind this position is that given the constraints of the relatively hard-wired anatomy of the primary motor and primary sensory circuits involved in speech and language, each maturing brain finds its own specific, most efficient neural organization for carrying out the operations of language production and comprehension. The specifics of the cerebral organization of a particular language operation may be presumed to depend on individual differences in the ease of acquisition of elementary components of language processes (e.g., auditory versus kinesthetic influences in guiding articulatory movements; development of semantic associations versus the development of phonological associations to letter strings). While the final product in performance may be indistinguishable between two normal language users, the underlying cerebral organization in such individuals may be based on different neural organizational strategies that most efficiently exploit the individual talents of the speaker–reader.

Once the anatomic allocation of functions is crystallized in the adult brain, it determines the pattern of deficits and the available compensatory devices likely to appear as the result of a particular lesion. Within the individual variability that the author proposes, there are common or modal self-organizing tendencies toward which many brains gravitate.

For example, to take a common syndrome, Wernicke's aphasia, following a lesion that includes most or all of the posterior portion of the left superior temporal gyrus, there is a complex of symptoms that are common but not universal. The most invariant component is the impairment of auditory language comprehension, this being closest to the primary sensory function of the temporal lobe. Even this impairment may vary widely from patient to patient—in some cases amounting to near total inability to extract meaning from individual words or from simple sentences; more often, easy words are understood and bits of conversation are at least tangentially understood, as can be judged by patients' tangential responses to the content of the examiner's remarks. In rare instances, complete destruction of Wernicke's area has little effect on auditory comprehension. The secondary features of Wernicke's aphasia are subject to much wider variation from individual to individual. Paraphasia may be so extreme in some individuals as to amount to a complete neologistic jargon, not only in conversational exchanges but also in single word repetition and attempts at single word naming. More often, however, the paraphasia of Wernicke's aphasics allows some comprehensible connected speech to be produced as well as allowing varying degrees of success in repetition and naming tasks. Overrapid, uninterruptible speech is characteristic for some patients, but by no means all. Some patients with all the other prototypical features of Wernicke's aphasia speak in a cautious, groping fashion, while making just as little sense as those who speak at a normal or hyperfluent rate. The degree of anomia also varies from moderate to complete among patients who share sufficiently in the features of the syndrome to be judged by most clinicians as having Wernicke's aphasia.

All of the foregoing variability is observed in patients who share sufficiently in the family resemblance of symptoms to earn the designation of "Wernicke's aphasics," and this variability has been accepted, for the most part, without comment by clinicians using the standard designations. Also passed over without comment are the patients who in spite of having the requisite lesion have such an attenuated form of the symptom cluster that they are assigned to a different syndrome (e.g., anomic aphasia or conduction aphasia) or are described as having a mix of several types of fluent aphasia.

Can it be that sufficiently careful analysis of fine variations in lesion distribution will eventually be found to correlate with the presence or degree of severity of each of the secondary symptoms associated with Wernicke's aphasia—that is, paragrammatism, literal and verbal paraphasia, neologistic speech, anomia, and hyperfluency? At the risk of appearing to take a pessimistic or hopeless outlook on the possibility of establishing structural correlates for all of these features of aphasia, the author argues that we can hope at best for a probabilistic relationship between symptom and lesion site. For a more precise prediction of symptoms, one would need to have access to the specifics of individual brain organizations, which are not accessible with present-day technology.

The example of Wernicke's aphasia and its associated symptoms can be extended to virtually every symptom of language dysfunction. One corollary of the position just outlined is that one can predict a lesion from an observed syndrome much more successfully than one can predict a syndrome from a known lesion. The reason for this is that the clinical presentation of a familiar syndrome is an indicator that the patient in question has a brain that has followed a commonly observed pattern of organization for the language processes involved in that syndrome. The association with the lesion site characteristic for that syndrome is therefore highly predictable. On the other hand, when only the lesion site is known, there is no way of knowing whether this particular patient has the brain organization that will cause a particular syndrome to appear in its prototypical form.

These observations apply particularly to symptoms that are rare or that have been associated with many different lesion sites. Deep dyslexia (Chapter 9) has been reported most frequently in association with agrammatic Broca's aphasia, but it has a far from exclusive relation to this disorder and is sometimes observed in fluent forms of aphasia (Coltheart, 1980). The explanation that emerges from this position is that the appearance of deep dyslexia depends on whether the cerebral organization of a patient's reading processes is one that will, on injury, display this particular pattern of deficits—that is, a disproportionately severe impairment of phonological activation by familiar lexical or sublexical letter strings while preserving semantic activation by familiar lexical letter strings. The potential for developing deep dyslexia is therefore present in some, but not all individuals. Those who do not have the predilection for this pattern of reading disorder are more likely to have a mixed aphasic alexia (Chapter 9) from the lesion which, in other patients, might produce deep dyslexia. The relation between premorbid capacities and symptom selectivity in aphasia is discussed further in the next chapter on the relation between aphasia and models of normal language.

The notion of individual variability in brain organization is more than an arbitrary *post hoc* rationalization for the inconsistencies in lesion–syndrome relationships, but can be traced to well known developmental observations. Aphasia in preadolescent children rarely takes the form of the well defined syndromes of adult aphasia. Regardless of lesion site, the disorder appears as a generalized diminution of speech, restriction of vocabulary, and reduced auditory comprehension. Fluent aphasias are rare in young children, as are severe, selective impairments of word comprehension or articulation. We can therefore infer that the representation of language in the brain is less focally organized in young children than in adults. The relation between age at the time of an aphasia-producing brain injury and the appearance of adult forms of aphasia syndromes has not been mapped out, probably because aphasia in the middle years of childhood and adolescence is too uncommon to have been studied systematically. Nevertheless, it must be the case that in the years leading to adulthood there is a transition from widely distributed, overlapping networks subserving articulation, auditory comprehension, syntax, and word finding, to anatomically more compactly organized neural systems for each of these (and other) specialized aspects of language.[1]

It must be acknowledged that the appeal to premorbid individual differences in elementary components of language leading to individual differences in cerebral organization currently lacks any direct evidence for its existence. Support for or rejection of this view could be obtained by administering to a population of normal individuals a battery of tests of elementary skills presumed to underlie language operations. The goal would be to see whether scores on such a battery fall into different modal patterns.

ALTERNATIVE APPROACHES TO DIAGNOSIS

Given the shortcomings of the syndrome-based taxonomy of aphasias, are there alternatives that would serve us better? Two approaches may be considered: one clinical, based on surface symptomatology; the other cognitive, based on the inferred integrity or deficit in the operation of postulated components of the cognitive architecture underlying the performances that are tested.

A Clinical Nonsyndromic Approach

The author proposes an approach for generating a brief, maximally communicative description of aphasic patterns that takes into account the

---

[1] There is evidence to support the idea that the representation of knowledge that is highly overlearned is vulnerable in a more restricted zone in the brain than is knowledge that is less well practiced. Ojemann and Whitaker (1978) found that word finding in the first language of a bilingual speaker could be disrupted by cortical stimulation in relatively few points, in comparison with the wider distribution of points that disrupted word finding in the second, less well practiced language.

characteristic clusters of symptoms that are common to most of the competing taxonomic schemes that are in the literature. It is shown in Fig. 12.1(a)–(e) as a decision tree that uses the most salient and diagnostically significant distinctions between patients for the first two or three steps in classification. Beyond that point, the clinician assigns severity ratings to a number of specified additional features that are vital to case description but not decisive for classification. The clinician who is trained in a particular taxonomic scheme will be able to identify both prototypical instances and borderline fits with a named syndrome. However, this approach does not require the clinician to force a borderline case or one with mixed features into a syndrome label. The proposed scheme uses technical terminology (e.g., fluent, nonfluent, and paragrammatism) that presupposes familiarity with these terms and the symptoms that they represent. It is not offered as a formula for clinically naive users.

Cognitive Analysis

It has been proposed (Caplan, 1992) that the examination and characterization of any case of aphasia may, in principle, be based on the analysis of the cognitive elements that are believed to underlie the normal execution of language processes. The "functional architecture" for any type of linguistic processing is an arrangement of processing modules

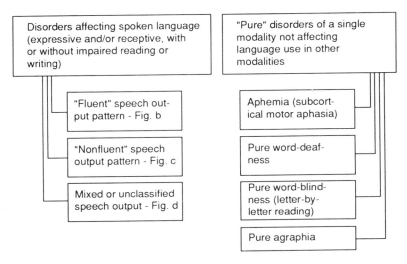

Figure 12.1a. Classification decision tree to guide a concise case description of aphasia.

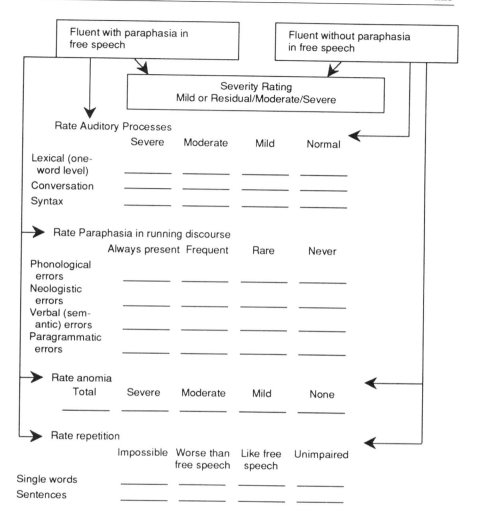

Figure 12.1b. Expansion of decision tree for fluent aphasia.

that is presumed to be common to all language users. It is an axiom of the cognitive approach to neurolinguistics that the deficits observed in aphasia are translatable into impairments in the function of specific modules of normal functional architecture. This feature is referred to as "transparency" (Caramazza, 1984). (A criticism of the transparency concept follows.) Although no one would claim that such architectures have

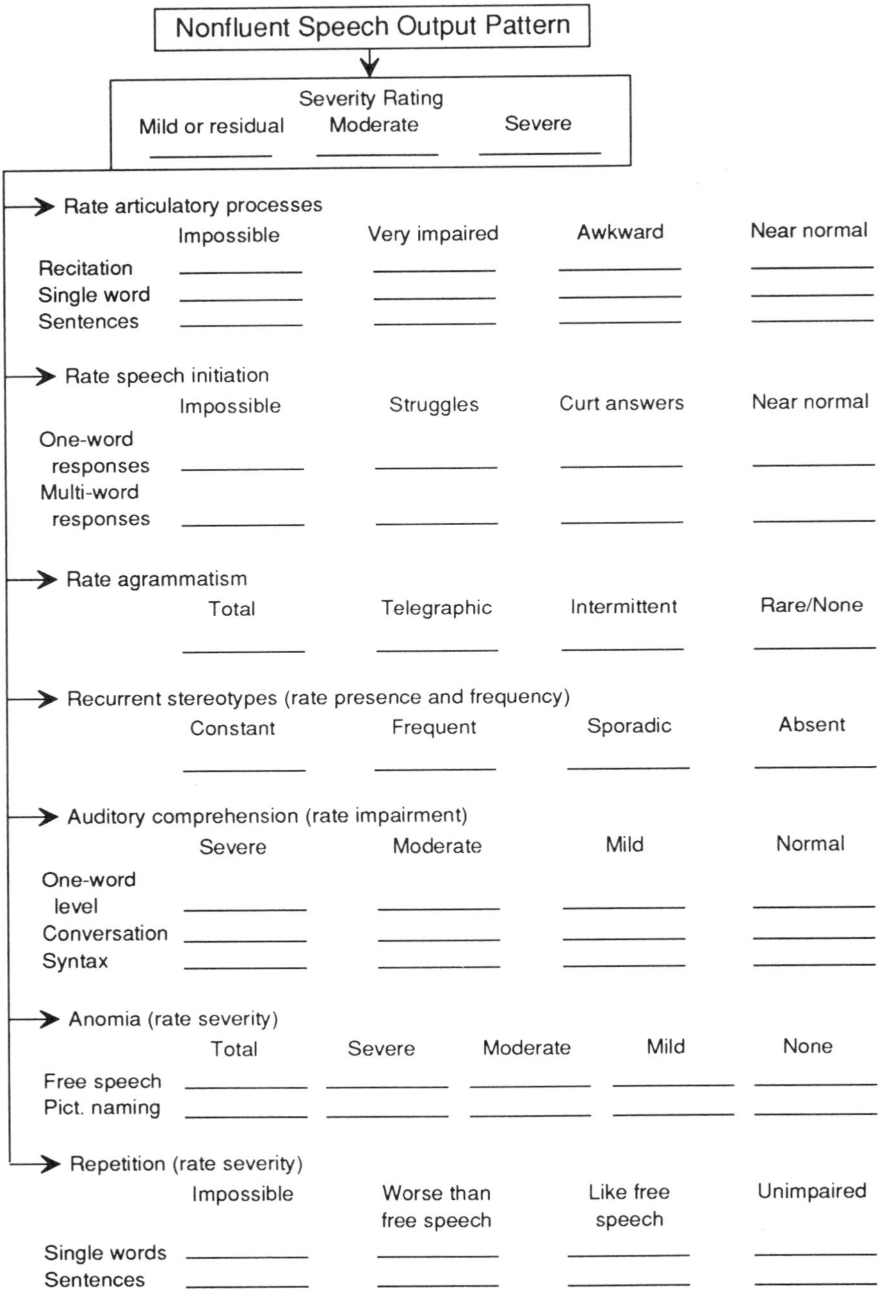

Nonfluent Speech Output Pattern

	Severity Rating	
Mild or residual	Moderate	Severe
_____	_____	_____

Rate articulatory processes

	Impossible	Very impaired	Awkward	Near normal
Recitation	_____	_____	_____	_____
Single word	_____	_____	_____	_____
Sentences	_____	_____	_____	_____

Rate speech initiation

	Impossible	Struggles	Curt answers	Near normal
One-word responses	_____	_____	_____	_____
Multi-word responses	_____	_____	_____	_____

Rate agrammatism

Total	Telegraphic	Intermittent	Rare/None
_____	_____	_____	_____

Recurrent stereotypes (rate presence and frequency)

Constant	Frequent	Sporadic	Absent
_____	_____	_____	_____

Auditory comprehension (rate impairment)

	Severe	Moderate	Mild	Normal
One-word level	_____	_____	_____	_____
Conversation	_____	_____	_____	_____
Syntax	_____	_____	_____	_____

Anomia (rate severity)

	Total	Severe	Moderate	Mild	None
Free speech	_____	_____	_____	_____	_____
Pict. naming	_____	_____	_____	_____	_____

Repetition (rate severity)

	Impossible	Worse than free speech	Like free speech	Unimpaired
Single words	_____	_____	_____	_____
Sentences	_____	_____	_____	_____

Figure 12.1c. Expansion of decision tree for nonfluent aphasia.

Indeterminate Fluency Pattern

↓

	Severity Rating	
Mild or residual	Moderate	Severe
_____	_____	_____

→ Rate articulatory processes

	Impossible	Very impaired	Awkward	Near normal
Recitation	_____	_____	_____	_____
Single word	_____	_____	_____	_____
Sentences	_____	_____	_____	_____

→ Rate speech initiation

	Impossible	Struggles	Curt answers	Near normal
One-word responses	_____	_____	_____	_____
Multi-word responses	_____	_____	_____	_____

→ Rate agrammatism

Total	Telegraphic	Intermittent	Rare/None
_____	_____	_____	_____

→ Recurrent stereotypes (rate presence and frequency)

Constant	Frequent	Sporadic	Absent
_____	_____	_____	_____

→ Auditory comprehension (rate impairment)

	Severe	Moderate	Mild	Normal
One-word level	_____	_____	_____	_____
Conversation	_____	_____	_____	_____
Syntax	_____	_____	_____	_____

→ Anomia (rate severity)

	Total	Severe	Moderate	Mild	None
Free speech	_____	_____	_____	_____	_____
Pict. naming	_____	_____	_____	_____	_____

→ Repetition (rate severity)

	Impossible	Worse than free speech	Like free speech	Unimpaired
Single words	_____	_____	_____	_____
Sentences	_____	_____	_____	_____

Figure 12.1d. Expansion of decision tree for mixed fluency types.

Written Language

Reading		Total failure	Unreliable	Good to normal
Basic skills				
Matching letters across fonts		___	___	___
Named letter identification		___	___	___
Word–picture matching		___	___	___

Text comprehension level	None	Single words	Elementary	Functional
	___	___	___	___

Presence of Dissociative Errors

a. In oral reading	Frequent	Occasional	None
Semantic paralexia	___	___	___
Omission/misreading of functors	___	___	___
Slavish misapplications of phonic rules	___	___	___
b. Matching to spoken sample			
Selective difficulty with functors	___	___	___
Inability to match nonsense words to spoken model	___	___	___

Writing	None	Copy only	Poorly formed	Good
Basic graphomotor skill	None	Copy only	Poorly formed	Good
Letters	___	___	___	___
Signature	___	___	___	___
Words	___	___	___	___
Functional writing	Pre-primer	Elementary	Limited	Near normal
Dictated words	___	___	___	___
Dictated sentences	___	___	___	___
Spontaneous sentences	___	___	___	___
Dissociative errors		Frequent	Occasional	None
Semantic paragraphia		___	___	___
Part-of-speech/category errors		___	___	___

Figure 12.1e.   Written language.

been worked out in their ultimate detail for all modalities of language, these models have been applied with some success in the interpretation of some of the most baffling dissociations in aphasia, notably those involving object naming, word reading, and spelling such as, for example, in deep dyslexia.

However, if one takes as an example the applications made so far of cognitive models to cases of aphasia, one finds that they have been used with patients who have rare selective dissociations. These patients generally have several preserved channels of language through which they can be examined. Moreover, because each such patient is the target of study of a single interesting problem, an extensive array of probe tests can be deployed to explore the theoretical underpinnings of that deficit.

For example, Caramazza and Miceli (1990) cite the performance of a patient (KE) whose semantic naming errors apparently had their origin in the "lexical–semantic system," and two contrasting patients (RGB and HW), whose semantic errors were limited to oral production tasks and therefore were attributed to a malfunction of the "phonological output lexicon." These interesting observations and conclusions were possible because all three of these patients had many input and response modalities available. For example, patient KE was able to give responses by object naming, oral reading, written naming, and writing to dictation. Thus, in response to the word "arm," tested by each of these means, he produced four different body parts. Three other words, tested in the same four modalities, elicited nine different category-related responses. Patients RGB and HW not only had these response modalities available, but had enough facility in speech to give clear and accurate (though circumlocutory) definitions of words that they had just misread semantically.

The clinician faced with the task of examining, interpreting, and classifying the disorder of the vast majority of aphasic patients rarely has the luxury of having input and output modalities available that match his armamentarium of cognitive probe tests. This is particularly likely to be true in the case of a fixed test battery designed to test the integrity of components of a postulated functional architecture. For example, given a patient with a moderately severe nonfluent aphasia with impaired auditory comprehension, a small naming vocabulary, minimal single-word reading comprehension, and agraphia, one would have questions as to the cognitive components underlying the patient's anomia, his alexia, and his impaired production and comprehension of syntax. A probe of his lexical semantic functions using auditorily presented questions about concepts (e.g., Do potatoes grow on trees? Are onions used in cooking?) would collide with his auditory input difficulty and be uninterpretable. A limited subset (i.e., those that require only a pointing response) of the tasks used to investigate the phonological routes available in word reading could be given.

Functional architectures have been well studied only at the one-word level. The functional analysis of syntax comprehension and syntax production in speech or writing has not progressed to the point that there is any agreement on an underlying functional architecture. At best, specific syntactic operations have been identified that pose particular difficulties to certain patients, such as interpreting semantically reversible relationships that are marked only by word order or by a grammatical morpheme, or by a combination of the two (see Chapter 6). Some writers have tried to paper over the gap in understanding of these complex processes by introducing the term "parser" to represent a cognitive component that interprets the syntax of sentences.

In sum, the analysis of lesions in the functional architecture of language has not achieved the state of development where it can serve as a basis for classifying the range of disorders that are seen clinically. It can provide a satisfying sense of understanding of a number of isolated aspects of aphasia—particularly difficulties at the word level. In this sense, these analyses provide a series of magnified views through tunnels. In occasional cases with highly restricted deficits, this tunnel view is able to encompass the major symptoms disabling the patient and even suggest a therapeutic approach. In most cases, probing for the cognitive components underlying language deficits is best carried out after the performance deficits have been mapped out and the areas in which further cognitive analysis is worthwhile have been determined.

From the point of view of the modal interpretation of syndromes just described, the basic axiom of transparency between deficit symptoms in aphasia and universally valid cognitive architectures is a very fragile one. Cognitive architectures based on evidence from a restricted set of patients with a particular dissociation in language function may be valid only for individuals whose cerebral language organization is such that the given symptom will appear—a point that was alluded to earlier. We must remember that if the classical anatomic associationist syndromes are based on unstable groupings of symptoms, they at least have some foundation in cerebral localization. The selective disorders that have been the prime focus of analyses of cognitive architecture do not have that sort of claim on being universally characteristic of human language breakdown. From the point of view outlined, they are, in some cases, the result of unique configurations of language organization; in other cases, they are the result of one of several alternative modal subtypes of language organization.

The case studies that take the approach of seeking definable cognitive processing components represent an elegant technique for approaching individual cases. One takes the opportunity to do such analyses with the risk that a particular case may prove to be one of a kind. The other caution is that there is the temptation to reify the components under whatever label we assign to them, forgetting that they are only temporary way stations in the analyses of language processes.

In summary, the traditional anatomic–associationist taxonomy of aphasia and the reasons that have caused many aphasiologists to bridle at its inconsistencies and shortcomings have been reviewed. The author has suggested a less rigid approach to the brief and communicative characterization of aphasia that recognizes the pragmatic validity of the symptom clusters that were respected by many of the earlier, competing systems of terminology. The author has also proposed, using the expression "syndromes as modal patterns of language breakdown," that the variability in the expression of the syndromes is a result of variability in the way different brains organize the higher processes of language around the fixed constraints of the anatomy of the primary motor and sensory systems and the fiber connections between association zones. Finally, the approach of cognitive functional architecture has been considered as a possible solution to the problem of classification, concluding that it has not yet evolved to the point of offering an alternative. Echoing Luria (1970), the author emphasizes that while aphasia includes linguistically classifiable phenomena, it is much more than a purely linguistic deficit. It includes dimensions that are not conceived of in either linguistic theory or cognitive theory. These dimensions (e.g., fluency/nonfluency; quality of articulation; characteristic compensatory strategies or "positive symptoms") must be represented in a taxonomy if classification is to succeed.

Chapter 13

Relation of Aphasia to Normal Language: Fact and Conjecture

INTRODUCTION

In the preceding chapter, we attempted to show how the shortcomings of the traditional anatomic center-and-connection interpretation of aphasic syndromes might be reduced by introducing the concept of self-organizing neural networks that mediate the acquisition and use of language. In our proposal, the anatomical basis of language is constrained by the hard-wired primary sensory input and motor output systems and by certain essential connecting fiber tracts. The constancy of this anatomy in human brains is responsible for the high predictability of lesion sites in the case of selective impairments that bear primarily on a particular sensory or motor modality. In our conception, the freedom of the individual brain to recruit computational space on demand as it acquires language competence allows for considerable individual variation in how the resources of the association areas are used to deal with *psycholinguistically* defined (as opposed to *modality* defined) operations.

This discussion will be slanted toward an interactive, spreading activation interpretation of language activity at the neural level. However, basic visual, auditory, and vocal processes have a built-in autonomy that imposes limits on interactive influences. The boundaries of subsystems within which spreading activation works freely are constrained by anatomical contiguity, by available hard-wired pathways between anatomically remote zones that form parts of a processing subsystem, and by the functional demands of particular language operations. It would clearly be incorrect to think that all of language is mediated by a single undifferentiated interactive network.

This chapter deals with subsystems of language as they are defined either by the dominant intake or output modality, or by conventional linguistically labeled domains, such as lexical processing, syntactic processing, and so on. In some areas, we will find processes that have been well studied in normals but which are relatively unaffected in aphasia, others in which there are enlightening correspondences between aphasic phenomena and analyses of normal function, and still others in which aphasic symptoms correspond to none of the preconceptions from normal language and which force the introduction of new concepts into our notions of normal language processing.

ACOUSTIC SIGNAL TO AUDITORY LANGUAGE COMPREHENSION

Research on speech perception carried out at Haskins Laboratory (Liberman *et al.*, 1967) suggests that speech engages a mode of auditory processing that is distinct from that involved in distinguishing non-speech sounds and noises. This is referred to as the "phonetic mode," as distinguished from the "acoustic mode." Thanks to the phonetic processing of speech sounds, the train of actual acoustic signals is submitted to coding processes that cause some consonant sounds to acquire their perceptual identity from acoustic information that, in real time, comes after the articulatory gesture for the consonant itself. For example, stop consonants, such as *p, t,* or *k,* may each have different acoustic features before different vowels. It is not until the vowel is under way that the consonant is identified perceptually. One such distinguishing acoustic feature is the length of the interval of silence (20 msec versus 60 msec) between the release of the closure for a stop consonant and the beginning of the voicing of the vowel, referred to as the voice onset time (VOT); or else it may be determined by the distinctive acoustic signal (the formant transition) produced as the tongue moves into the position for the "steady state" portion of a particular vowel.

Another feature of the phonetic mode of perception is that it makes "either–or" interpretations in discriminating between consonants that vary along a particular acoustic dimension. To take the example of the constrast between the "voiced" consonant *d* and its unvoiced neighbor *t,* the chief acoustic marker for this distinction is the duration of the VOT. But the hearer is insensitive to differences in VOT among different pronunciations of either of these consonants, until they cross the critical boundary that makes an absolute difference between a *t* and a *d.* Because of this coding process which, in effect, compresses the acoustic signal, we are able to absorb an astounding amount of changing acoustic information. An average rate of phoneme flow in continuous speech is about 10 phonemes a second. This would be impossible to manage were it not for the phonetic coding of the acoustic signal. The speech sounds that we hear are virtual images constructed by our speech perception apparatus, often after their acoustic basis has gone by in real time. When the acoustic segment that represents a stop consonant is extracted and played on a tape in isolation, it may sound like an unintelligible click or chirp.

One might expect that such a complex system would be highly subject to disruption by a lesion in the auditory association area. This does not appear to be the case; the evidence that impairments in language comprehension are due to impaired speech sound discrimination is scanty. For example, Blumstein *et al.* (1977b) found that four out of four Wernicke's aphasics and four out of five Broca's aphasics showed normal VOT boundary effects for discriminating between *t* and *d*. Baker, Blumstein, and Goodglass (1981) found that in a multiple-choice picture-selection task after having heard a picture name, Wernicke's aphasics were more likely than Broca's aphasics to make errors of picture selection based on close similarity between the first consonant of the erroneous choice and the correct target. However, they made even more errors based on meaning similarity than on sound similarity. Wernicke's aphasics' semantic comprehension disorder placed them at a disadvantage in interpreting the spoken stimulus. It is not clear that their sound-related errors were, in fact, due to actual misperception of the initial consonant, rather than to choosing a response on the basis of incomplete appreciation of the full stimulus, which left them open to being drawn either to the target or to the sound-related foil.

The syndrome of pure word-deafness presents features that may represent a disruption of early phonetic (and possibly presemantic) auditory processing. Auerbach *et al.* (1982) and Miceli (1982) reported on two different patients who had pure word-deafness with a severely impaired ability to discriminate between stop consonants that differed only in place of articulation. Their patients also failed to show the expected enhancement of discrimination between neighboring phonemes (e.g., /p/ versus /b/) at the boundary value of the acoustic variable that distinguishes one from the other. Although their difficulties appear to be confined to aspects of auditory analysis, the precise nature of this impairment is not defined by their failures in acoustic perception tasks. Both of them performed well at discriminating among vowels and among continuant consonant sounds. Although they were poor at discriminating between closely similar stop consonant pairs, they did well at identifying these consonants when they were presented singly. Like most reported word-deaf patients, they could identify some auditorily presented words, but failed many others. It is not known whether there are systematic differences in the acoustic properties of words that are successfully identified and those that are not. From the clinical-experimental evidence available, word deafness is not purely a disorder of speech sound perception. Rather, these patients seem to have a sharply reduced ability to appreciate a string of sounds as being a wordlike auditory stimulus capable of being imitated. The occasional word that is successfully perceived can be promptly repeated and understood. That is, the patients have some access to their prior auditory verbal experience, or "auditory input lexicon."

The traditional approach to such a performance failure would be to postulate a new, intervening process that might be named "speech sound assembly." On the other hand, there may be no such thing as a separate stage of speech sound assembly to be distinguished from a preceding stage of speech sound perception. The reactivation of prior auditory verbal experience through ongoing speech sound perception may be sufficient to account for word recognition in the normal system. Word deafness may simply reflect an impairment of the interaction between these as parallel interacting processes. The point of this suggestion is that there are alternatives to construing language activity as being made up of discrete serial stages. Close analysis of symptoms could result in an ever expanding chain of such postulated stages.

WORD RECOGNITION

A naive serial stage analysis of speech perception would lead us to assume that once the sounds of a word have been perceived, they are recognized as matching the sound pattern of a word in memory which, in turn, activates one or several possible meanings. The proof that the stage of word recognition is intact would be that the individual can make "lexical decisions" that is, correctly report whether a string of sounds is an English word or a nonword. But observations from studies of word recognition in normals raise a serious question as to whether there is a particular point in time when word recognition has been completed and semantic activation begun. A number of investigators (Grosjean, 1980; Marslen-Wilson, 1984) have used the gating procedure in which listeners hear longer and longer segments of a word from its onset. They found that subjects can, on average, identify target words in context when they have heard only 200 msec (less than 50%) of its phonology. The duration of the gated segment that is required before a correct word decision is made depends on the number of other competing words (the "cohort") that share the onset phonology of the target word. Marslen-Wilson's cohort theory holds that as the first sounds of a word are perceived, all the words that share those sounds are activated. As more and more of the phonology is available, the cohort of possible responses shrinks as the activation of nonmatching words is suppressed, until only a single candidate survives. Does the target word as a lexical item emerge at a particular moment from all competitors, and does the activation of its semantic properties begin only at that point? This seems unlikely. Zwitserlood (1985) showed that when experimental subjects heard the opening gated segment of a word, it served to prime lexical decisions on words that were semantically related to nontarget words that were in the cohort for that segment. It appears likely that semantic activity related to the target word is already under way before all competitors have been eliminated, during the unfolding of the word's phonology.

The gating procedure is very similar to a technique that speech pathologists call "phonemic priming," that is, assisting aphasic patients to name a pictured object by providing the opening sound of the object name. Wingfield, Goodglass, and Smith (1990) asked whether successful response to phonemic priming by aphasic patients might occur even if the primes were not preceded by a picture of the object to be named. They applied the gating technique to a population of aphasic patients and to normal controls. Although aphasics required significantly longer gated segments than normals in order to supply the correct target words, this difference was, in absolute terms, surprisingly small (368 msec versus 297 msec for normals). Patients with profound word retrieval difficulty in picture naming tasks were able to supply the correct answer to a gated stimulus at near normal gate durations, even when they had no prior knowledge about the object. Although this study necessarily excluded patients who could not articulate speech sounds, it did indicate that the activation of previously well-known phonological patterns by an initial priming cue is surprisingly robust in the face of word finding problems.

WORD MEANING IN NORMALITY AND PATHOLOGY

In analyzing human language, there seems to be a sharp distinction between the capacity to perceive, encode in memory, and reproduce sequences of speech sounds and the capacity to endow these sound sequences with meaning. (We will shortly see that the concept represented by the word "meaning" is far from clear, but we use it here in its everyday, unanalyzed sense.) Whereas the attachment of significance to words is the essence of communication, the mechanism by which this is implemented has been treated only at the most shallow level of speculation.

In one model, a child is thought to learn the meaning of objects by hearing their names spoken by an adult while their attention is focused on the object being named—the paradigm for learning word meaning is the labeling of animals in a picture book. The mechanism is simply one of association between a spoken and a visual stimulus. The principle of learning by contiguity of stimuli in a child differs from its application to the teaching of an animal pet to respond to a spoken command. The animal must receive reinforcement for the performance of an action (e.g., fetching a slipper), which is specifically triggered by the spoken stimulus. That is, for the dog, the spoken word is an elicitor of immediate behavior; there is no indication that the animal "knows" what "slipper" means in a context where fetching is not possible. The word, then, has the status of a signal for the animal rather than of a symbol, as it has for the human.

Geschwind (1965) proposed that it is the development of cross-modal convergence of multiple sensory inputs in the parietal lobe that makes possible this advance in humans over lower animals. In the animal, the response must be maintained through reinforcement by a limbically driven need satisfaction—that is, food. In the human, Geschwind proposed, the stimulus that is perceived through one modality (e.g., vision) has direct access to auditory, somesthetic, and tactile sensory systems and can activate a polysensory representation of the object in the angular gyrus of the parietal lobe on arrival of the visual stimulus from the visual association area of the occipital lobe.

As Geschwind himself acknowledges (1967), such a model of visual-to-verbal association for learning object names can hardly deal with the acquisition of the vast majority of vocabulary items that refer, not to visually experienced objects, but to abstract nouns, actions, mental states, qualities, and so on. Many of the concrete nouns that we refer to are things that we have not seen ourselves and might not recognize if we did see them (e.g., white corpuscles, viruses, spleens, or tonsils). Because we obviously do not need to experience the contiguity of a visual and verbal stimulus to acquire these words, it is difficult to take visual-to-verbal stimulus contiguity very seriously as a general model for the acquisition of object names. At best, it may have some validity in the object name learning of the very young child, whose evidence of word knowledge is limited to pointing correctly when asked to indicate the object or picture referred to by a particular word, as in "Show me the kitty."

If not association by stimulus contiguity, what model for normal vocabulary acquisition should we turn to? It is clear that visual experience is only one of many ways of building up a representation of a concept; many of the concepts that we refer to derive their primary semantic features from the behavior of the objects, from the way they can be used, by definition, or by inference from the situation in which we have heard them referred to. The label that we attach to the concept must be abstracted from the spoken context. Even when the name of an object is taught in conjunction with a visual presentation or in conjunction with a definition, the name must be extracted from the carrier phrase (e.g., "This is a . . . ."). The association of a new term to its concept is therefore a uniquely linguistic process that cannot be reduced to other forms of nonlinguistic learning.

This brief speculative review has focused as much on what word learning is not as on what it is. It forces us, however, to confront the problem of concepts and their relation to the words that refer to them. In schematic models of language processing, concepts reside in an enclosed area usually labeled as a "semantic system," which denotes the total pool of real-world knowledge of the properties of objects, actions, and abstract entities that our words may represent. Traditional cognitive psychology regards this system as a static store of representations from past experience which exist in a state of low-resting activation until some mental event, externally or internally triggered, causes one or more of them to "light up" or become highly activated. Current views of distributed representation would regard concepts as *potential* patterns of activation that can be partially or totally reinstituted as a result of traces that have been left in various brain structures by prior experience.

One version of distributed representation is that suggested by Damasio (1990). In Damasio's view, the record of prior experiences is encoded at the most peripheral level (e.g., primary sensory or motor cortices), that was engaged in the original experience. Each such record, however, represents but a fragment of the complexity of the total experience, which may involve independent neuronal units for different aspects of form, color, spatial features, and texture in the visual domain alone, to say nothing of the multiplicity of residual traces related to auditory, somesthetic, and other features of the original experience. Neither any individual component nor group of components is a representation of the memory trace without the activating and synchronizing influence of a hierarchical series of "convergence zones." The most peripheral of the convergence zones have both feed forward and feedback connections with the units of a particular modality (e.g., visual, somatosensory, etc.). This arrangement allows for activation of that portion of the network as a result of stimulation arising in either the convergence zone or in one of the peripheral units. The convergence zones that form the most peripheral layer are, in turn, linked in reciprocal relationships with second-order and possibly still higher order convergence zones. The spread of activation through such a network, provided it takes place within a reasonably restricted time window, creates the experience of the unity of the reinstituted memory. For a more detailed explanation and some supporting evidence from neurophysiological research, refer to Damasio (1990).

Although Damasio's model does not provide a full account of the content of past knowledge, it does supply a plausible framework for considering the link between words and their conceptual counterparts. Let us first consider some of the characteristics of the conceptual system as described.

1. The "representation" of a concept is a transient state of neural activity. Whereas the potential for the reactivation of a concept depends on a large number of lasting changes in brain state distributed in many parts of the brain, the ensemble of these states is without effect until the integrating activity of one or more convergence zones reinstitutes the concept.

2. The completeness or depth of activation of a concept on any occasion is a function of the demands of the situation. For example, if the word "dog" occurs in a sentence in running text, only so much of the network for the concept of "dog" is activated as is needed in that sentence context. The spread of activation to all of the components of a concept takes time and focused attention, which are not needed for the level of appreciation that is adequate in running speech or in reading.

3. Although a concept may involve the linking, through activation, of multiple sensory systems, these components are not necessarily equally dominant in its reevocation. Injury to one of the systems that contribute to a concept may degrade or remove that component in the experience of the concept, without the individual's awareness that something is missing from it.

4. Concepts may aggregate additional components in the course of experience. Among such components is the verbal label, which serves as the most effective means of causing the (partial) reactivation of the concept for purposes of communication.

5. Like all other elements in the concept, the word is represented by a transient pattern of neural activity.

LEXICAL SEMANTICS AND CONCEPTUAL ORGANIZATION

The notion of a conceptual "system" as a mechanism for reactivating any one of myriads of potential concepts of concrete or abstract entities is still only a bare skeleton of the mind. It does not deal with higher-order links between concepts to form families related by such features as size, animacy, function, taxonomic category, and so on.

The relationship of object names to the total structure of the concept has been framed as though name representation is simply one more component in the activated network that is the representation of the object. But word-activations, unlike other components, have the property of being rapidly accessible and manipulable. The nature of verbal concepts makes them exceptionally susceptible to linking with each other along a large number of dimensions—some related to semantic features of the concepts that they refer to, others based on purely structural characteristics (prosody, rhyme, spelling similarity, and homophony), and still other on associative relationships that emerge from repeated contiguity of words in daily use. Concepts based on relationships between abstract entities would appear to be entirely dependent on verbal mediation. If their significance is represented entirely in the linguistic domain, is it not possible that even the names of concrete objects have a meaning representation in the language system that is associated with, but autonomous from the nonverbal concept of the object itself? That is, are there two autonomous conceptual domains, each capable of becoming activated without the other, of which one would be the domain of nonverbal sensori-motor based experience that includes object concepts and the other the domain of lexical semantics?

Although there is little basis for one view versus the other in experimental data from normal speakers, there is a whole series of provocative observations from patients with selective dissociations in language involving semantic categories, modality of sensory input and motor output, or a combination of semantic category-specific and modality-specific features. These data save the issue from being one of empty speculation in which anything is possible.

The example of optic aphasia (Chapter 5) is a case in point. In this condition, patients can demonstrate their identification of object concepts visually presented by pantomiming their use, yet are usually unable to name the objects until they experience them through a nonvisual modality, for example, by touch or audition. This phenomenon would seem to be sufficient to rule out a model in which there is a single conceptual representation integrating information from all modalities and (assuming that the patient is not anomic) activating the phonology of the concept name. The phenomenon is compatible with a model in which activation of lexical semantic networks is not totally equivalent to or dependent on nonverbal concept activation. Lexical semantic networks may be sensitive to modality-specific impairments that do not affect the nonverbal concept.

A particularly challenging case is that of Warrington and Shallice (1979) in which optic aphasia was accompanied by an atypical form of alexia without agraphia. The patient could not name objects presented to him visually, but succeeded well in naming them in response to a verbal description. In addition, he retained considerable connotative appreciation of written words that he could neither say out loud nor match correctly to the objects they denoted. A striking feature of this case is that oral word reading could often be correctly elicited by supplying an auditory associate (e.g., "Egypt" for the written stimulus "pyramid"). Such prompting was rarely effective for pictures; that is, the patient's optic anomia was much more resistant to priming than his dyslexia. Not surprisingly, presenting a picture of the object represented by the written stimulus word was ineffective as a prime; it merely reconfirmed the patients severe optic aphasia.

This pattern of behavior is compatible with a model in which processing among various verbal modalities is closely associated with a lexical semantic representation, but has a more tenuous link to the nonverbal (in this case, pictorially activated) concept.

In the majority of cases of optic aphasia, there is anatomically supported evidence of partial disconnection of visual input to the language system. Often, optic aphasia is a residual form of what was initially a visual agnosia, that is, failure of activation of the nonverbal concept through the visual modality. (Rubens, 1979). One way of interpreting this common evolution of the disorder is that the nonverbal concept may be activated by a relatively low level of visual information, but this activation is not sufficient to drive the retrieval of object name phonology. This interpretation obviously is based on the premise that a single conceptual activation is at the core of both the verbal and nonverbal experience of the object. However, this account will not do for the Warrington and Shallice case, because their patient at no time showed evidence of impaired visual recognition. In order to deal with cases of this type, it is necessary to turn to the model, previously suggested, in which the lexical semantic system has a direct link with sensory input systems. The activation of a lexical semantic representation of an object by visual or other sensory input may be autonomous from nonverbal concept activation. It is injury to this source of sensory input that may result in a modality-specific anomia, without agnosia in the corresponding sensory channel.

Warrington and Shallice object to a disconnection account for their patient's disorder, on the grounds that the right hemisphere has not been shown to be capable of the semantic processing of written words of dealing with the recognition of word forms. (Their patient had a complete right hemianopia.) Further, they do not consider it possible for a disconnection from right hemispheric visual input to be compatible with partial access to semantic information. Their account postulates a "word form" system as well as a semantic system specific to written words, both in the left hemisphere. Their patient's reading disorder is attributed to a partial failure of access from the word-form system to the semantic system for written words.

The author believes that Warrington and Shallice's rejection of the disconnection mechanism is faulty for several reasons. The ability of an isolated right hemisphere to recognize written words and extract considerable meaning from them is well established from work with split brain patients and from the fact that patients with pure word-blindness are capable of reading occasional words. An earlier cited case (Coslett and Saffran, 1989; see Chapter 9) illustrates the fact that some patients with pure word-blindness are responsive to the connotative features of words presented briefly to their nonhemianopic left visual field. Furthermore, the poor performance of Warrington and Shallice's patient in making lexical decisions on written words raises a serious question about the integrity of his "word form system," if such a system can be said to exist. The evidence from their patient's pathology would argue for a partial disconnection or degradation of visual input to the language system as a result of intrahemispheric disconnection, rather than a result of a splenial lesion (Greenblatt, 1973). Warrington and Shallice's account cleaves closely to the traditional approach of postulating rigorously demarcated subsystems that are connected to each other serially.

The reader who has followed this somewhat convoluted chain of reasoning may object to beginning by proposing that the concept activated by the verbal label of an object is no more than a "shallow" activation of the original sensorily based experience. That observation is correct within the context of the model of distributed representation that began this section. As the subsequent discussion has attempted to convey, the author does not believe that the single central concept model can account for language behavior. But what about the moment when we first learn the name of an object that has previously been known only through nonverbal, sensory-motor channels? The author suggests that it is inescapable that the representation of the verbal label is incorporated into the original concept and becomes part of its activation. It can be argued that this representation does not function as a linguistic element, but rather as a bit of factual knowledge about the object. The object name as a vocabulary item, capable of being manipulated linguistically and associated with other words (e.g., by category, by sound, etc.) would, in a sense, then be a copy. The meaning activation associated with this word is a partial copy of the original preverbal concept. Although the principle of dual representation may be distasteful from the point of view of parsimony, it appears to be inescapable on the basis of the evidence from modality-specific aphasias without agnosia.

By being liberated, in a sense, from the baggage of the original object concept to which it refers, the word as a linguistic element gains the unlimited flexibility of other words. It can be deliberately used in a nonsensical sense, retrieved for listing as a member of all sorts of categories defined by any of its semantic features, its phonological features, or the features of its orthographic form. It may be redefined to give it a technical meaning or spun-off for metaphorical meanings, in addition to its conventional meaning, and may become a subject for metalinguistic word games, such as puns. For a probing and eye-opening consideration of the notion of "meaning" the reader is referred to Putnam's *Representation and Reality* (1988). In comparison with the uses of the object name as a word, the original nonverbal concept of its referent is an awkward and lumbering mental entity.

Alluded to earlier in this section was the fact that many (in fact, most) of the concepts for which we have one-word labels were never experienced through any nonlanguage sensory input or were learned only through verbal sources. This is true not only for abstract words, but for words that refer to actual objects that we may never have seen (e.g., viruses), or whose physical properties we know only through verbal experience (e.g., Cinderella's glass slipper). Thus, there is *a priori* reason to expect that injury to the language system may dissociate the language-based from the sensory experience-based aspects of concept representation. As we have seen in the review of category-specific lexical comprehension disorders reported by Warrington and her associates (Chapter 7), the dissociation between objects that can be identified from their spoken names and those that cannot, appears to relate to whether they are known primarily by their visual features or by their functional properties. A single case report by Hart and Gordon (1992) illustrates even more concretely the dissociation between the visually based and the language-based aspects of a concept. Their patient could neither report verbally on nor answer questions about the physical attributes (size, number of legs, color) of any animals, although her knowledge of their nonvisual characteristics (habitat, suitability as pets, etc.) was unimpaired. At the same time, she had a fairly severe optic anomia for animals. A complicating factor in the understanding of this case, however, is that her deficiencies were confined to the category of animals.

It is relatively easy to develop a plausible framework for understanding modality-specific impairments of processing at the lexical level, as exemplified by optic aphasia, pure word-blindness, pure word-deafness, or tactile anomia. The starting point for those disorders is the degradation of input from the affected sensory modality. This degradation may be due to disconnection from the association areas, which are the normal source of input to the language zone for the modality involved. Alternatively, it may be due to destruction in the association area itself. Given this starting point, explanatory models to account for the details of symptomatology diverge along two lines. The traditional approach is to postulate discrete stages of processing that are damaged or partially disconnected from each other. In the classical anatomic-associationist models, the stages were relatively coarsely defined; they had a one-to-one correspondence with the injured structure. One example is the model for repetition failure in conduction aphasia or for the reading disorder of pure word-blindness (Geschwind, 1965). In the models of contemporary cognitive psychologists, the stages are finely distinguished in order to accommodate subtle variations in symptomatology, but the stages need have no focal representation in the brain. An example is the case of "semantic access dyslexia" of Warrington and Shallice (1979), just cited. Here, separate, successive stages of word-form recognition and written word semantics are postulated. Because of the variability in the patient's performance on the same words from time to time, a disorder of access from the earlier to the later stage is postulated, as opposed to an impairment of information storage in the later stage. An access disorder is the figurative equivalent of a partial anatomic disconnection, but no anatomic implication is attached to the model.

The approach that most contrasts with that of discrete processing stages is that of parallel processing. In parallel processing, accounts of language acts—units that represent each source of information input and the previously acquired activations to those inputs—send reinforcement or inhibition that spreads to all the units in the network, according to association strengths determined by prior learning. The output that emerges (e.g., the spoken name in response to a written word) is achieved without requiring discrete stages that represent discrete stores of knowledge or rules. A particular spreading activation account for a process (e.g., oral word reading) must be designed with each of the participating units specified so that they can be simulated by computer on the basis of assigned activation strengths. Unlike the stage models, in which the intervening stages have *prima facie* plausibility, spreading activation models must be demonstrated as workable by computer simulation.

Impairments that affect a particular semantic category present a much more difficult problem than those defined by an input modality. The words that we use can be subdivided into innumerable categories, applying the vast number of semantic criteria that are possible. Starting with basic object concepts of animal, vegetable, and mineral types, we can move in the direction of first and second order superordinates and consider categories based on part of speech or animacy, to make only a beginning. There are few clues in the experience of normal language analysis that would predict that any semantic category could be selectively affected by brain injury, or if affected, which one it would be. As a result, the accumulation of cases of category-based dissociations has sent theorists scrambling to find explanations on a *post hoc* basis. Most of these semantic, category-based dissociations have been discussed previously in Chapters 5 and 7. In this section, we consider how these phenomena may relate to normal language and to brain function.

SYMBOL SYSTEM-BASED DISSOCIATIONS

These phenomena are perhaps the ones most understandable in relation to normal language acquisition. The learning of letter names is a byproduct of the invention of alphabetic language systems. The device of transcoding speech phoneme by phoneme into written symbols is a relatively recent innovation, shared by the languages of the western world, but not by Chinese, which uses an idiographic writing system, nor Japanese, which supplements an idiographic system by a syllable-based phonetic system. Thus, letter recognition and letter naming is a skill imposed by a convention of modern civilization—one for which there is no evolutionarily based special mechanism. Whereas written words have an association to the semantics represented in oral language, individual letter identities and their names do not. Letter-name learning places a demand on visual–verbal associative capabilities that is unprecedented and unmatched by any other task in language learning. Not only are letter forms composed of a small set of abstract lines and curves in different, meaningless combinations, but their names are short, phonologically impoverished syllables that have no significance except as labels for the equally meaningless visual forms.

It is remarkable that our language apparatus, as it has evolved, has equipped almost all of us to learn these squiggles as unique visual elements, in association with the short syllables that are their names. It is not surprising that an incapacity for such learning is an early manifestation of one of the most common types of developmental disorder—dyslexia. It takes young children about two years longer to mature in their ability to learn to recognize and name letters than to name objects. Confusion between similarly shaped letters persists well into the age of early reading and may persist some years longer in dyslexic children.

Once acquired by the normal reader, the association of spoken name to letter form is automatized and becomes extremely rapid, possibly because it is the unique verbal association to an otherwise meaningless form. Serial naming of strings of letters is carried out more rapidly than other similar serial naming tasks involving colors or objects by the time a child is six years old (Denckla and Rudel, 1974).

This description makes it plausible that letter recognition and naming may involve different and perhaps more vulnerable associative mechanisms from other visual–verbal learning. However, it does not directly predict the form of abnormalities in letter processing by aphasic patients with different lesions or different aphasic syndromes. Such disorders are among the most common of the category-specific impairments in aphasia. To recapitulate what has been noted in earlier chapters, letter-related dissociations (excluding those associated with more extensive reading disorders) appear in the following forms:

Letter anomia (also termed "literal alexia"). The patient is unable to name individual letters, sometimes producing the name of a common word that begins with the letter (e.g., saying "apple" when asked to name *A*.) It is an uncommon dissociation, more often found in Broca's aphasia than in fluent forms. The correlates of letter anomia have not been investigated systematically. It may appear in people whose reading has always been dominated by whole-word processing and particularly dependent on direct word-to-meaning association. Such a configuration might also be expected to result in features of deep dyslexia after injury to the language zone; however, this correlation has not been reported on or looked for.

Selective preservation of letter naming. This is the converse of letter anomia and was reported by Goodglass *et al.* (1966) to be the most common of the category-based naming dissociations in aphasics, particularly in fluent aphasics. Letter naming is often preserved in patients who are anomic for most other types of visual confrontation naming.

Selectively impaired comprehension of letter names. This symptom was reported by Goodglass *et al.* (1966) as the most common of the category-specific impairments of word comprehension in aphasic patients, also found predominantly in fluent aphasics. Patients with this impairment usually recognize that they have heard the name of a letter, and may repeat it correctly, while selecting the wrong item from multiple choice. It is probably significant that selective *preservation* of letter naming is the most common category-based dissociation in production, whereas selection *impairment* of letters is the most common dissociation in receptive processing. An important question here is why would not the fact that a letter and its name are so intimately and exclusively related cause both directions of associations to be equally resistant to impairment? We cannot presently answer this question.

DISSOCIATIONS AFFECTING BROADLY DEFINED SEMANTIC CLASSES

We reviewed in Chapter 7 the dissociations, first clearly documented by Warrington and her collaborators, between the processing of animate or naturally occurring object concepts and those representing man-made objects. Although these dissociations were seen primarily in the comprehension of the object names, they sometimes included name retrieval and the ability to give a definition or description. The criterion of "naturally occurring" versus "man-made" does not cover all the cases of affected object types, but it is the single best fitting distinction that has been suggested. Warrington and McCarthy (1987) suggest that the underlying reason for this dichotomy lies in the modality of experience through which the different concepts were acquired. Naturally occurring objects are conceptualized primarily by their visual features. These features are constant for all instances of any particular living species. Man-made objects are conceptualized primarily through their functions and are less consistent in their structure, from exemplar to exemplar. In most of the cases in which dissociations have been found following herpes encephalitis, it is the "naturally occurring" items that were most affected, but some cases have shown the reverse dissociation, with manipulable implements more impaired than natural objects. (For a more complete review and discussion of these dissociations, see Caplan, 1992.)

DISSOCIATIONS WITHIN NARROW SEMANTIC CATEGORIES

The most challenging of the cases of semantic dissociation are the very rare cases of anomia for a narrowly defined category: animals (Hart and Gordon, 1992) and fruits and vegetables (Hart, Berndt, and Caramazza, 1985;). Hart and Gordon's case was postencephalitic, with diffuse and patchy temporal lobe pathology. In this respect, it resembled a large number of the previously reported semantic dissociation cases. A few cases, however, have been found in aphasic patients with focal lesions. A third narrow semantic category, that of body parts, is frequently subject to selective impairment of auditory comprehension in aphasic patients (see Chapter 7 for details).

It would be tempting to suggest that language-based representations of object concepts are segregated into a category-specific organization in the brain. There are both logical and empirical objections to this sort of approach. An overarching objection is that the metapsychological capacity of human cognition permits virtually unlimited bases for organizing objects into categories. Categories may be hierarchically stacked (animal→mammal→four-legged→feline→cat→siamese) or grouped by properties (fierceness, size, exotic versus domestic, etc.) to deal with only a small number of possibilities in the realm of living things. It is not plausible that any one of these unlimited varieties of associative networks is organized to be selectively vulnerable to some brain lesion. One empirical objection is that whereas the lesions associated with category dissociations (either broadly or narrowly defined) are generally in the left hemisphere, they are either diffuse or fairly large, and not consistently correlated with a particular affected category. A second empirical objection is that of the many possible narrowly defined object categories that are possible, only three—body parts, animals, and fruits and vegetables—have been found to be selectively impaired. The first of these is usually impaired only for auditory comprehension, the other two for naming, and one of these (animal) only in response to visual presentation. All three of these are biologically based superordinate classes that intuitively seem to have some fundamental semantic coherence.

It is plausible that an inhibitory effect impinging on some aspect of an object's semantic activation spreads, through associative links to salient common features, to involve the entire class to which the object belongs. Except for body parts, such spreading effects are very rare and have to be confined to strongly coherent categories. This account requires acceptance of the notion that "psychological" associations based on common properties are mediated by "real" activation networks that cause a whole group of psychologically interconnected concepts to suffer a similar, organically based effect. An approach of this type spares us from postulating the unlikely model of boxlike categories, any of which may be injured as a whole, or disconnected as a whole from sensory input.

The account just suggested is framed in terms of modality-independent conceptual activation in the language system. To accommodate modality-specific deficits, the suggested model can be elaborated to preserve the modality tagging of the components of the network that arise from each sensory channel—visual, tactile, somatosensory—and to allow preferential spread of inhibitory activation within the network among those components originating from similar sensory inputs.

This line of conjecture is motivated not so much to offer a probable model for modality-sensitive conceptual representation as to illustrate alternatives to boxlike thinking. Modality-tagged components of a concept-activation network would not represent independent modality-specific conceptual stores (Shallice, 1987), but paths by which modality-specific inhibition of concept activation might be mediated.

OTHER BASES FOR DISSOCIATIONS

There remain to be explained category-based dissociations that are related, not to semantic categories, but to the linguistic properties of the words involved. One type that is extremely rare and baffling is anomia for proper nouns as described by Semenza and Zettin (1989) and discussed in Chapter 5. Dissociations related to part of speech take several forms. One is the difficulty of access for verbs that appears in many guises in aphasia (see Chapter 10 for discussion). Although difficulty in verb access is a common feature of agrammatism, we suspect that it is not central to the agrammatic disorder, but a separate category-specific problem that also affects these patients. The difficulty in accessing grammatical functors, which is the prime symptom of agrammatism, is another still unsolved problem.

SENTENCE COMPREHENSION

When a word becomes a sentence constituent, it acquires a new dimension of meaning and may surrender some of the significance that it carried in citation form, that is, as an isolated utterance. For example, in the request "Will you please feed the cat," the word "cat," by serving as the direct object of "feed" also constrains the meaning of "feed" to a set of actions that are appropriate for cats but not for babies or birds, although either of those nouns could fit the sentence frame perfectly well. The significance of "cat" in that sentence is modified by the determiner "the" to refer to a particular cat whose identity is known to the speaker and the listener. If the sentence is spoken in a context in which the cat has been crying for food, the term "cat" is almost redundant. It is only a somewhat more emphatic form of expression than "Will you please feed her." It is little more than a slot-filler that is grammatically obligatory because the verb "feed" is transitive.

Thus, while the word "cat," spoken out of context, may activate a number of the semantic features associated with the quality of "cat-ness," the meaning properties of the same word in a sentence may be quite different. The meaning of the concept "cat" may fade into the background because it is redundant for processing the sentence. At the same time, the word acquires a new aspect of meaning: a grammatical relationship to the verb.

Understanding the sentence, then, becomes a composite of multiple interacting influences. A vital component is the influence of pragmatic factors: the presuppositions dictated by the real life context or by the preceding communicative interchange that limit which of several possible significances of a word applies in a given sentence. Pragmatic influences or verbal contextual influences may make the actual spoken word redundant; that is, so highly predictable that a particular word or words may be muffled by noise without being missed. Equally important is the grammatical role in which the word functions, for example, whether a noun is the agent of the action denoted by a verb or the object of the action. Finally (but not last in importance), is the meaning of the individual words, as they might be defined in a dictionary. In expository messages, the semantics of the individual terms of a sentence, along with their grammatical functions, are likely to override pragmatic influences.

It would be rash, however, to conclude that when a word is redundant in a given context, its meaning has no effect on the language processing system. Swinney (1979) has shown that immediately after a spoken word has been perceived, one can detect its semantic effects, regardless of the preceding context. In particular, if a polysemous word like "bank" is spoken in a sentence context that supports one of its meanings, such as "They sat by the river bank," it facilitates lexical decisions on words related to its other meaning (e.g., "money"), as well as words related to its contextual meaning. Yet, the listener may never become conscious that the other meaning of "bank" has produced an effect on her behavior.

We may state that the problem of sentence comprehension is one of translating the grammatical arrangements of words into a sense of the conceptual relationship between the referents of these words. For example, given the sentence "The truck hit the car," the English speaker will conceive of a truck moving and striking a car.

One approach to this problem is that of theoretical linguistics. Using this approach, the sentence is understood through the assignment of a syntactic role to each of the words according to the rule structure of English syntax. In this simple example, the term "the truck" has to be assigned the role of agent because it begins the sentence and is immediately followed by an active verb. The introduction of generative linguistics by Chomsky (1957) led to efforts to codify all of the possible complexities of English syntax in a system of rules that dictate how words may be ordered in phrases and clauses and how these constituents may in turn be ordered or embedded to convey any kind of meaning relationship. In order to understand how any one word in the sentence relates to the others, the listener must be able to construct a representation of the syntactic structure of the sentence, while it is being perceived, because the relational significance of the words is derived from this representation. For example, if we complicate the original sentence by saying "The truck that ran the light hit the car," the syntactic representation assigns the role of agent of "hit the car" to "the truck" and not to the word "light," even though the sequence "the light hit the car" would make a sentence, if it stood by itself. That is, the listener must, in a sense, parse the sentence as he hears it in order to make sense of it. Because a sentence may consist of a complex arrangement of hierarchically dependent phrases and clauses, such parsing may appear to be a daunting task.

Does this parsing necessarily recreate a mental model of the syntactic structure? From the point of view of the transformational linguist this is the case. That is, knowledge of the rules for constructing syntactic structures underlies both the production and the comprehension of oral language. Ingenious parsing mechanisms have been proposed (e.g., Frazier, 1987) that build up the sentence schema word after word.

Not all theorists are in accord with this view but instead hold that the equivalent of parsing takes place continuously as the listener extracts cues of many different types from semantics, word order, pragmatics, context, and morphological elements (e.g., MacWhinney, 1989). Bates *et al.* (1991) have shown that the importance of cues from word order versus cues from inflectional forms varies as a function of the prominence and constancy of these two factors in the particular language spoken by the subject. Animacy of the referent also plays an important part in the assignment of agency in sentence comprehension. These effects cannot be accounted for by the relatively rigid prescriptions of a syntactic rule-bound sentence parsing.

A further nonsyntactic factor that is generally agreed to play a prominent role in sentence comprehension is the heuristic reliance on word order in interpreting the first noun as the agent of action in simple sentences. Similarly, when one noun is animate and the other is inanimate, the hearer may assume that the animate noun is the agent, without any need to carry out a genuine syntactic parsing. In complex sentences, however, and in sentences in which subject and object have the same animacy property, simple heuristic strategies may yield a misleading or ambiguous interpretation.

As in other instances of competition between a rule-governed account (such as that of transformational grammar) and one based on parallel distributed processing (such as MacWhinney's), the former has the advantage of appealing to logically defined serial steps, whereas the latter must be demonstrated by a computer simulation to explain each construction.

Sentence comprehension impairments in aphasia do not provide decisive evidence for one approach over the other. In Chapter 6 we reviewed some of the factors that make syntactic structures difficult to process for aphasics. One of these is the interpretation of semantically reversible relationships between two terms that are disambiguated by a grammatical morpheme and/or word order. Other factors, such as the separation of a noun from its verb by an embedded construction, can be conceived in terms of cognitive load, including short-term memory demands, with or without reference to a formal analysis of syntactic structure.

FROM CONCEPT TO SPOKEN WORD

Until recently, the process by which a word is accessed for production was not even a topic of research. The assumption was that words with their meanings and phonological forms are stored in a mental lexicon. Once an intended meaning is selected, a lexical search is carried out for the word that fits the meaning. The word is then selected and uttered. The mechanism for this process was an unexamined black box.

In 1966, Brown and McNeil studied the so-called "tip-of-the-tongue" state—the mental condition of being on the verge of retrieving an elusive word that one feels one knows. Brown and McNeil gave definitions of uncommon words to college students with the expectation that students would fail to retrieve a certain proportion of them. They then had the subjects answer questions about their intuitions concerning the sound structure of the words they could not retrieve. They found that the students could often supply correct information about opening sounds, number of syllables, and final sounds. This was evidence that word retrieval was not an all or none event, and that failure to supply a word might conceal considerable partial phonological information that was easily elicited by the proper probes. Goodglass *et al.* (1976) found that some aphasic patients (conduction aphasics) could demonstrate such partial knowledge for about a third of the names of pictures that they could not retrieve, but that other aphasic patients (Broca's, Wernicke's, and anomics) had little success.

In a follow-up of Brown and McNeil's study with normals, Kohn *et al.* (1987) had their subjects talk out loud as they tried to retrieve uncommon words that had been defined for them. Kohn *et al.* analyzed the phonological structure of the guesses that eventually led to a correct response as compared to those that did not. They concluded that whatever partial phonological information the subjects could evoke was already evident in their first erroneous guesses, and that subsequent attempts did not bring them any closer to the target. Successful retrieval after initial wrong responses occurred after either short or prolonged mental effort, but it was predictable only from the degree of phonological match to the target that was already evident in the subject's first wrong guess.

Although the tip-of-the-tongue studies provided some insight into the course of phonological retrieval during prolonged word search in normals, it did not directly illuminate the events during normal rapid word retrieval, which is usually carried out between 500 and 1500 msec after stimulus presentation (Goodglass *et al.*, 1984). Research on word retrieval usually deals with performance on picture naming because it is virtually impossible to harness word retrieval in running discourse for research purposes. Although the time of onset of a picture stimulus for naming can be precisely measured, as can the response latency, there is no signal to tell us when, in the course of running speech, a concept that is to be verbalized begins to activate its phonological form. Thus, in spite of its artificiality, the picture-naming paradigm is virtually without competition as the method of choice for the study of word retrieval.

Any model of picture naming begins with the identification of the picture to be named. There is no agreement as to when in the course of visual picture processing is identification sufficiently advanced to set in motion semantic or phonological activity related to name retrieval. For our purposes at this point, it matters little whether such name-related activity gets under way only after a picture is fully recognized as an exemplar of a familiar object or while its features are still being extracted from the visual display.

The traditional view of normal picture name retrieval is that picture identification leads to the selection of an intended word concept, which in turn activates the phonology of the word. One major body of research on picture naming has come from the Max Planck Institute for Psycholinguistics in Nijmegen, Holland, under the leadership of Levelt (see Levelt, 1989). Levelt's approach is summarized in Chapter 5.

Various models of lexical selection have been proposed that are appropriate for the two-stage naming model. Almost all entail the application of semantic congruency tests to one word candidate (or "lemma" in Levelt's terminology) after another until a match is found with the currently active concept to be named. A widely accepted approach to lexical selection is the "logogen" model, as proposed by Morton (1969). Every word in a person's lexicon is conceived as being represented at all times by a mental device—its "logogen," which exists at some level of resting activation. The resting level of activation depends on the frequency of the word, how recently it was used, and the current context. The logogen is sensitive to both contextual factors and internally generated semantic intentions that meet its selection criteria. When these are met, the logogen "fires." The firing of the logogen makes its phonological form available for production. In cases where there are several competing candidates for naming a particular picture, the logogens for all of the possible candidates would become active, and the first one to reach firing threshold (presumably the one that has the highest valence, derived from its frequency of use, etc.) would become available, in a response buffer, for production.

The parallel activation proposed in the logogen theory is an attractive feature as an alternative to carrying out a series of semantic congruency decisions. However, the all-or-none availability of the phonological form is difficult to reconcile with the "tip-of-the-tongue" phenomenon. It is also difficult to reconcile with the speech errors of aphasics in which partial phonological retrieval figures prominently.

The well regarded theory of Dell (1986), framed in terms of spreading activation, proposes that the attainment of a lemma activates the morpheme or morphemes composing the word, which spreads activation to the onset of the first syllable, which, in turn, spreads its activation to the syllable nucleus as well as back up to the morpheme level. Activation is passed along to each successive syllable component in turn until the phonology has been assembled. It is then read into an articulatory buffer in preparation for motor implementation. For a full and clear account of the theoretical and experimental basis for this version of the two-stage naming model, refer to Levelt (1989).

In Chapter 5, we provided examples of paraphasic errors by aphasic patients that suggest that access to word phonology need not begin with the word onset, but may begin with a noninitial stressed syllable or other phonologically salient element. However, it would be misleading to suggest that priority of noninitial phonology is the usual pattern either in aphasia or in tip-of-the-tongue errors. In both data sets, semantically based errors are the most common, and errors preserving word onset phonology are much more common than those that preserve noninitial phonology. Dominance of the word onset has to be granted, both in word recognition and word retrieval. However, it is not so exclusive as to serve as an obligatory feature in word retrieval models.

The notion of a lemma as a phonologically empty representation is central to the two-stage model, but this notion is weakened by the tip-of-the-tongue evidence that what appears to be an empty sense of a word actually consists of multiple activated components of the phonology, often including its prosody.

A number of spreading activation accounts have been proposed in which competition among two or more semantically close candidate responses interacts with their developing phonology (see, for example,

Humphries *et al.*, 1988). The model offered in Fig. 5.2 and elaborated in Chapter 5 is one that dispenses with the "word node" or lemma as an intervening construct between word semantics and the beginning retrieval of phonology. In this conception, the word is reconstituted on each occasion of use. Observations from aphasia indicate that a schema like this cannot be a totally undifferentiated network, uniformly distributed in the language zone. The "interaction track" of Fig. 5.2 comes closest to being such a uniformly distributed system, but the lexical semantic component is most vulnerable from injury in the posterior speech zone, and the phonological component from injury in the anatomy related to Broca's aphasia and conduction aphasia, as discussed in Chapters 3, 4, 8, and 12.

Empirical evidence has not yet decided between the viability of two-stage as opposed to continuous interaction models of name retrieval. The model suggested in Fig. 5.2 has not been subjected to simulation tests and, for the moment, represents a conjecture as to how word retrieval may come about without postulating a permanent store of words in a low resting activation state.

SENTENCE PRODUCTION

Theorists who have attempted to analyze the process of sentence generation have, with minor variations, postulated the same major steps. At the onset, there is a preverbal message to be conveyed. The speaker must identify key concepts in this message that can be represented by words in his or her language. The speaker must construct, on the basis of the syntactic procedures of the language, a framework that conveys the intended relationship between the lexical terms. Articulatory realization comes last and includes low level rules controlling speech sound production in the speaker's language. All of these components can be found in the schemas proposed by Lordat (1843), Pick (1931), Garrett (1980), and Levelt (1989). There are some differences in the sequence of the stages in Pick's schema compared with the others in that, for Pick, the development of the syntactic frame precedes the selection of lexical terms, whereas this order is reversed in the other schemas. However, it was Garrett who, for the first time, used empirical data that consisted of normal speech errors to deduce a proposed sequence of stages. Garrett's sequence of stages is widely cited and may be summarized as follows:

1. Like all theorists, Garrett starts with the prelinguistic general intent of the message to be uttered: the "message level."
2. As a result of a first pass through the lexicon, the major concepts, that is, verb, subject, object, and goal (if any), are specified along

with their functional relationship to each other. At this stage, the terms are abstractly represented, without phonological form. These are the "lemmas" in Levelt's terminology. This is termed the "functional level."

3. A syntactic structure appropriate to the intended content is selected, according to the grammar of the language. As a result of a second pass through the lexicon, the previously selected lemmas are phonologically specified and inserted into their appropriate slots, along with a representation of all the grammatical morphemes and inflectional specifications of the major lexical items. This is the "positional level."

4. The "phonetic level" is the stage in which the grammatical morphemes as well as the major lexical items are phonetically specified.

5. Articulatory representation.

Levelt (1989) goes beyond the listing of stages to propose a type of processor dedicated to carrying out the functions of each stage. For example, the Grammatical Encoder "retrieves lemmas from the lexicon and generates grammatical relations reflecting the conceptual relations in the message. Its output is called 'surface structure' " (Levelt, 1989, p. 27). A version of a grammatical encoder proposed by Kempen and Hoenkamp (1987) is described by Levelt. In this version the ordering of lexical items is governed by the syntactic demands of each term—properties that are part of its lemma.

How do the observed sentence production difficulties of aphasic patients fit into conceptions of normal sentence generation? Whether one examines the formulation difficulties of a transcortical motor aphasic, the agrammatisms of a Broca's aphasic, the empty speech of an anomic aphasic, or the paragrammatic output of a Wernicke's aphasic, there seems to be a place for every type of breakdown at some point in the comprehensive schemas of such theorists as Garrett and Levelt.

BREAKDOWNS IN SENTENCE INITIATION

Transcortical motor aphasia (Luria's frontal dynamic aphasia) is marked by both a dearth of ideational content and the inability to select the salient concepts in an intended message so as to label them and assign basic functional syntactic roles. Luria, for example, proposes that therapy for these patients begins with assisting them in selecting the terms of a message and focusing on their functional relationships to each other (1970, p. 452). Do these observations permit us to equate the processes of Garrett's "message level," and perhaps some components of the "functional level," with the language functions of the frontal lobe?

Levelt's (1989) analysis of the structure of messages and their generation puts a different perspective on the operations that precede the generation of surface grammatical form—a perspective that blurs the distinction between a preverbal message and the assignment of functional relationships between the terms that will be incorporated in a sentence. Only a skeletal review is possible here, but it will suffice to relate it to the effects of aphasia. The preverbal conception of a message begins with its communicative intent—to inform, direct, inquire, and so on. It takes into account pragmatic considerations, such as what presuppositions are shared by the listener and how cultural conventions may dictate the particular form of expression (e.g., use of a polite question to imply a request or an order). It is founded on the way the human cognitive system parses experience into objects, actions, times, places, sensory features, and states. The terms to be placed in relationship to each other may be assigned priorities that ultimately affect the order in which they are entered into a grammatical frame. The thematic roles among the terms of the message must be conceptualized, but the prelinguistic conceptual elements that are to be encoded are conditioned by the language in which the message is to be uttered. For example, progressive duration versus habitual occurrence in the present tense ("I am working" versus "I work") are necessarily marked in English, but not necessarily in French or Spanish. For a superb and detailed review of the processes leading up to the generation of grammatical form, refer to Levelt (1989).

Although the entire process is analyzable into a great number of factors, no effort has yet been made to assign any of these factors to particular stages of cognition, much less to particular brain mechanisms. It appears that all of the factors that involve selecting, prioritizing, and ordering the lexical terms of the message may be affected by transcortical motor aphasia. It has yet to be determined whether each of these components is selectively vulnerable, or whether they all fall victim together to an impairment of initiation caused by interruption of pathways between limbic and frontal speech zones (Chapter 3).

ANOMIA, PARAPHASIA, AND PARAGRAMMATISM

The fact that anomic patients may embark on well-formed syntactic frames and either balk at the slot to be occupied by a lexical item or insert an indefinite term (e.g., "that there" for a noun or "did that" for a verb) or a more elaborate circumlocution raises a question as to whether the retrieval of a lemma need precede the "positional stage" in Garrett's model. The argument may be made that the lemma has in fact been retrieved because the speaker may have in mind a particular concept with its syntactic functions specified, but is merely blocked in accessing its phonology. For aphasics, this argument founders on the fact that the patient may insert a semantic paraphasia or a weak quasi-synonym (e.g., "animal" for "horse"), that is, a lemma other than that which represents the intended concept. We would therefore propose that the work of the positional stage can proceed without the selection of a lemma, as long as the syntactic properties of the class to which the intended concept belongs is available. The author takes this occasion to argue once more that the construct of a "lemma" that specifies a unique word without any of its phonological content is unnecessary.

In the speech of Wernicke's aphasics we may find well preserved syntactic forms, in spite of the neologistic nature of the terms that occupy the lexical slots. What is most reliably preserved is the inflectional morphology of nouns and verbs and the automatic, correct use of articles and case marking prepositions. Yet in patients with severe paragrammatism verging on jargon, there may be such gross violations of selection restrictions (verbs inserted in noun slots and vice versa) that syntax is inevitably disordered. That is, any two words in sequence taken at a time could be part of a grammatically well-formed construction, but three or more taken at a time become anomalous. Consider the last four words in the example from Caplan, Kellar, and Locke (1972), cited by Schwartz as a violation of auxiliary verb morphology: "Because ya know at one time I didn't have written."

AGRAMMATISM

Among the approaches to the definition of agrammatism that were reviewed in Chapter 6, we referred to

1. The deletion of grammatical functors
2. The loss of the ability to predicate
3. The loss of the knowledge of the rules and procedures of syntax
4. The adaptive simplification of syntactic plans

The last of these is only an effort to account for the surface symptoms of agrammatism, rather than an explanation of the underlying deficit that is being adapted to. This view has been discussed in Chapter 6 and will not be further treated here.

The effect of aphasia on grammatical morphemes accords well with Garrett's deduction, from normal speech errors, that these elements arise as part of the syntactic planning frame in the "positional level" of sentence generation. In normal slips of the tongue that involve word exchanges within a phrase, grammatical morphemes behave as though they are tightly fixed to their position in the syntactic plan, and thus become attached to the wrong lexical item in the case of a word exchange, as in "a hole full of floors" instead of "a floor full of holes" (cited by Levelt, 1989, from Fromkin, 1973). The grammatical morpheme is said to be "stranded" by the movement of the lexical item for which it was intended.

As Schwartz (1987) points out, in addition to the fact that grammatical morphemes are rarely subject to positional reversal, they are not subject to phonological paraphasic errors, as are lexical items. Paraphasias imposed on lexical items arise somewhere in the mapping of a semantic concept to a phonological form. Grammatical morphemes appear to be put into phonological form as part of a syntactic procedure, rather than as an association to a concept. But the same principle that ties the retrieval of grammatical morphemes to the generation of a syntactic planning frame may dictate the vulnerability of these elements when the syntactic planning operation is defective, as is the case in agrammatism.

How are we to relate Luria's (1970) interpretation of agrammatism as an inability to "predicate" with that of a breakdown at the "positional stage" of sentence generation? Garrett refrains from proposing the details of how the syntactic planning frame gains its representation. The Kempen-Hoenkamp (1987) Incremental Production Grammar, as detailed by Levelt, does offer an explicit account of the way the syntactic structure of a sentence is generated in strict left-to-right fashion, beginning with the lead concept in the preverbal formulation. The syntactic demands of each of the lexical terms interact with a set of "categorical procedures" that matches the term with its functional role, while "functional procedures" carry out subroutines that assign the values that will receive morphological marking at each step. Such an algorithm-based model appears to handle normal syntax generation admirably. Within this framework, observed types of slips of the tongue are easily handled. However, because all of the morphological marking procedures are on an equal footing, there is no way of accounting for the selectiveness in aphasia that makes certain kinds of morphological forms much more difficult than others. It may be possible to modify the Kempen-Hoenkamp model to deal with agrammatic phenomena, but these were not considered in its design.

Whether one takes the point of view of Garrett's model or that of Levelt, predication must be accomplished prior to syntax generation, to which it serves as input. Thus, in Luria's view, the basic impairment in agrammatism would be of a conceptual nature, rather than in the later syntax-accessing phase of sentence formulation. His illustrative sample (1970, p. 196) translates a segment of the patient's speech as "I know . . . this guy . . . beer . . . mustache . . . money." Even the patient's efforts to repeat a simple sentence "The weather was nice yesterday," resulted in the fragmented word list: "Was . . . weather . . . sun." In Luria's terms, "The patient's agrammatism [resulted] from retention only of the nominative aspects of words . . . . Behind it there lies a disintegration of the dynamic schemata of speech and a severe disturbance of inner speech which leads to a loss of feeling for language." One may speculate that the source of the agrammatic's incapacity to formulate a message in predicative terms is a pervasive difficulty with verbs that touches not only on the conception of their syntactic roles but on the very ability to retrieve them as lexical items. Zingeser and Berndt (1990) describe the output of a patient who appeared to have just this type of difficulty in producing verbs and verb-dependent syntactic forms, even though in other respects he was fluent rather than agrammatic. This case suggests that the difficulty with verbs that is commonly associated with agrammatism, may be dissociated from that syndrome in occasional instances. (See also Miceli *et al.*, 1984, for further observations on the problem of verb access in agrammatism.) Just as it is possible to find difficulties in verb use outside of the context of agrammatism, there are agrammatic patients who produce a normal proportion of verbs with respect to nouns.

Neither the tendency to omit grammatical morphemes (as discussed earlier) nor the difficulty in expressing verbs and their interactions, nor a combination of these two symptoms, sums up the symptom complex of agrammatism. At this moment we lack a unifying theory that would account for the co-occurrence of these symptoms.

WRITTEN LANGUAGE AND ITS DISORDERS

Reading

In Chapters 9 and 10 on reading and writing, it was argued that a multitude of perceptual and associative processes develop in parallel and interactively as we derive phonology and meaning from written input or activate representations of letter sequences that can be implemented in many media—longhand, print, typing, oral spelling, signed fingerspelling, or even Morse code.

The implications of this position, which derives from the approach of parallel distributed processing (McClelland and Rumelhart, 1986), are different from those that underlie the multiple track model that is most widely accepted in contemporary cognitive psychology. In the multiple track model, word recognition and oral reading may activate a phonological representation, either on a whole-word (lexical) basis or by blend-grapho-phonemic correspondence). The latter procedure is necessarily applied in the reading of nonsense words. Failure of both of these phonological paths leaves available the semantic route—direct activation of meaning through a holistic grasp of the sense of the written word, totally bypassing the phonological value of the graphic form. Evidence of the bypassing of phonology by deep dyslexic patients lies in their production of phonologically unrelated lexical paraphasias (e.g., "happy" for "party") and by their inability to get any sense of the sound structure of non-words. As we have seen in Chapter 9, similar inferences favoring these multiple routes can be made from normal reading performance, which permits us to read regularly spelled words, irregular words, and abbreviations (such as "lbs"), whose letters have no phonological relationship to their pronunciation.

What is lacking in the multiple track models is any role for the interaction between semantic, phonological, and visual perceptual processes. A conspicuous feature of deep dyslexia that is left unexplained by the multiple track model is the large number of visually based, in addition to semantically based, reading errors. McClelland (1992) showed that the principles of parallel processing require us to conceive of the representation of a written word as involving the interaction among visual, phonological, and semantic units. The impairment cannot involve phonological elements without affecting visual elements as well. Consequently, it is reasonable to expect symptoms reflecting the degradation of the visual features.

A more encompassing attack on the multitrack model appears in a summary article by Van Orden, Pennington, and Stone (1990), which argues that the activation of written word phonology always depends on the consistency of the relationship between a particular graphic sequence and its assigned phonology. The notion of holistic perception of irregularly spelled written words is rejected. Van Orden *et al.,* muster experimental evidence that phonological coding always entails the identification of constituent letters. The advantage in recognition speed of most "regularly" spelled words over "exception words" lies primarily in the consistency of the covariance between letter sequences and assigned phonology. When an "exceptional" letter string has an exclusive relationship with a phonological form (e.g., the -tion ending), it is read as quickly as any "regular" English string.

The most extreme example that could be thought of as an illustration of the direct association of meaning to a written form, without phonological mediation, would be Chinese logographs. Yet Seidenberg (1985) has shown that the phonological properties of Chinese characters affect their naming latencies, and Tzeng, Hung, and Wang (1977) found that the phonological properties of Chinese logographs affect both the learning of word lists for graphic reproduction and the detection of grammatical anomalies by Chinese readers. Tzeng and Wang (1983) hold that phonological encoding is not simply a strategic choice, but an automatic and obligatory response to a written symbol, along with the semantic and orthographic information that has co-occurred with that symbol. It is clear, however, that either visual or phonological factors may be dominant, depending on the alphabetic versus logographic character of the symbol. Indeed, impairments in the reading of alphabetic scripts are more likely to be caused by temporal lobe lesions than by occipito-parietal lesions, whereas the reverse is true for the processing of logographs (Hung and Tzeng, 1981).

From the work of Van Orden, Seidenberg, Tzeng and others, we have seen that the best candidates for holistic, nonphonological processing (according to multiple track models) have yielded to experimental data that show them to be subject to a processing of their component letters and to obligatory phonological effects. There remains one instance, however, for which Van Orden has only speculative, indirect evidence of phonological activation: namely, the semantic paralexias of deep dyslexics. Given the other evidence that the constituent letters of a word are always processed, he suggests that phonological activation also figures in the access to a semantic paralexic response, but that the source of errors lies further downstream. In a somewhat similar vein, Van Orden points out that profoundly deaf readers, who have been assumed to read without phonology, nevertheless appear to be sensitive to phonological consistencies between words (e.g., late–fate), which suggests that they have developed something akin to phonological processing.

There appears to be two blind spots in Van Orden's otherwise compelling analyses. One is his occasional failure to distinguish between the obligatory nature of constituent letter analysis and the obligatory nature of phonological activation. The former is convincingly established by his data, but this does not exclude the possibility that activation of phonology may be abolished or nearly abolished in some individuals (particularly deep dyslexics). In the case of profoundly deaf readers, there may be an analogy to phonology in their encoding of certain spelling regularities. However, unless this coding can be mapped to sound, it is not phonology in the sense that has been used in the rest of his discussion.

In the author's opinion, there is no reason to reject the *prima facie* evidence that there are patients who have become unable to achieve the activation of phonology from print, but who still have partially functioning orthographic and semantic representations—that is, they are subject to both visual word-identification errors and semantically based errors. It is curious that while Van Orden is reluctant to acknowledge an acquired deficit in phonological activation in deep dyslexics, he does accept such a deficit in phonological dyslexics but attributes it to a preexisting, developmental condition. In this regard, he comes close to the author's suggestion that the susceptibility of patients to deep dyslexia is also the result of preexisting vulnerability (as discussed in Chapter 12).

The second omission in Van Orden's treatment is his failure to deal with semantic activation, or with variations in the adequacy of such activation, in conjunction with orthography and phonology. This omission may be due to the fact that he is primarily concerned with normal reading processes. Impaired activation of semantics is virtually never an issue in the study of normal reading. It is, however, a major issue in accounting for (1) the semantic errors of deep dyslexics, (2) for the ability to read fluently without comprehension that is sometimes observed in transcortical sensory aphasia and regularly observed in advanced Alzheimer's disease, and (3) in accounting for part-of-speech and concreteness effects in most aphasic alexics, but particularly in deep dyslexics.

An Attempt at Integration

The analysis of aphasia-related reading disorders by multistage and multicomponent models, as reviewed here and in Chapter 9, has been a fruitful enterprise with considerable explanatory power. The most lasting contributions have emerged from the analysis of the cognitive–linguistic impairments and their patterns of co-occurrence. The most flawed aspect of this approach has been the propensity to postulate discrete processing components corresponding to each deficit, with the addition of new components to accommodate variations in symptomatology. The proliferation of syndrome subtypes is the main clue to the fundamental weakness of the multiple component serial-stage approach (see discussion of this point by Ellis, 1987).

The model that is favored by the author is based on the following premises:

1. The acquisition of word reading involves the creation of an associative network linking units from three older, preexisting components of the language system—visual, lexical-semantic, and phonological. (The visual component for alphabetic languages is assumed to be a specialized system of higher visual processing that develops competence in scanning letterlike sequences.) The strength and specificity of the representation

activated by a letter string is a function of the consistency and frequency with which that sequence has been experienced with a particular phonological form and a particular set of semantic specifications.

2. Individual variations in language acquisition skills determine the robustness of connection strengths within components of the network—particularly the relative dominance of the semantic versus the phonological elements. Within the limits set by such individual variation, greater or lesser activation in one component spreads its effects to the others.

3. The skill that, in vulnerable individuals, is most affected by large temporo-parietal lesions is the ability to experience an activated phonological representation on perceiving a pronounceable letter string, whether or not the string is a known word. With this deficiency, there is a concomitant degradation of the semantic and orthographic activations. The most striking result of this impairment is that only some letter strings that have the advantage of prior experience as known words can be correctly reported. The accompanying degradation of semantic activation is manifested in the following:

a. The referential properties of the word's concept assume a disproportionate effect on the activation of the phonological component. Concrete noun stems are most effective, verbs and adjectives less so, and grammatical morphemes the least. Thus, the noun stem may come through intact, but affixes and free grammatical morphemes may be omitted or substituted.

b. The predominance of an imperfectly activated semantic component over a nearly nonfunctional phonological one may result in semantic paralexias, probably by the same mechanism that produces semantic paraphasia in speech.

c. Predominance of underspecified orthographic and phonological activations over still weaker semantic activation may result in structurally based, semantically unrelated paralexias.

d. When the semantic aspect of the activated complex is only minimally affected or recovers, the referential properties of the word concept no longer affect the achievement of phonology. Semantic paralexias are then rare or nonexistent and part-of-speech effects are reduced or disappear, although extreme dependence on the real-word property of the stimulus letter string is still characteristic. This comparatively uncommon variant is called "phonological dyslexia."

Given that the preceding formulation still acknowledges some differentiation between the lexical–semantic, phonological, and visual–orthographic components of an activation network for word reading, what is its advantage over a multiple component, serial-stage model? One advantage is that it recognizes the clinical continuum between the features of mixed aphasic alexia and the relatively rare selective forms, deep dyslexia and phonological dyslexia. It dispenses with separate holistic versus letter-sequence-based mechanisms for the activation of semantics and phonology by letter strings, in accordance with the previously cited evidence summarized by Van Orden *et al.* (1990). This formulation also recognizes that the appearance of one highly selective impairment as opposed to another, or as opposed to a mixed impairment, is unrelated to lesion site within a large peri-sylvian zone. Rather than accounting for such differences by postulating independent, specialized functional organs, it invokes preexisting individual variations in language acquisition skills that result in different patterns of vulnerability. It also avoids the creation of constructs that represent intervening stages of processing (e.g., a word-recognition system), when such constructs may be artifacts of experimental probe procedures, such as the lexical decision task.

This system leaves unexplained two forms of selective reading impairment that result from damage to single components of the reading process without focal injury in the temporo-parietal zone that subserves the preceding associational system. Loss or severe degradation of visual input to the left hemisphere language zone (as in cases of alexia without agraphia) renders the scanning of letter sequences almost useless for activating phonology and semantics, and causes patients to shift to a letter-by-letter strategy. (We now know from recent studies of letter-by-letter readers that partial activation of word semantics, attributable to right hemisphere processing, is sometimes revealed by appropriate probes.)

Severe impairments of lexical semantics, as seen in transcortical sensory aphasia and in Alzheimer's disease, may have little effect on the rest of the reading system, permitting fluent oral reading without comprehension.

Finally, we have not touched on the phenomenon of "surface dyslexia" (see Chapter 9) in the present discussion. In this disorder, as we have seen, patients read aloud as though their prior experience with the words of the language is not consistently available to guide the segmentation of letter strings into morphemes. A possible explanation, in terms of our proposed general model, is that the activation of semantics by the input letter string is inadequate. Consequently, the boundaries of previously experienced real words are underspecified. The result is the generation of phonological output corresponding to haphazard segmentation of the input. The account offered by Marcel (1980), comparing the performance of surface dyslexics to beginning readers comes closest to congruence with our model.

The Writing Process

In our consideration of the normal acquisition of writing (Chapter 10), we proposed that it was built on prior or concurrent acquisition of reading, and that it undoubtedly shared much of the associative substrate of reading and, consequently, was disrupted by the same injuries. But writing, as we recognize it, is constructed around a totally different output system, whose unique properties typically escape our consideration. That is, while we usually associate orthographic output with graphomotor representations and their visual counterpart, normal competence in writing entails a far broader capacity: the rapid and automatic generation of modality-independent, abstract, letter string representations, as in oral spelling. Further, any language-competent individual who acquires skill in another code system, such as signed finger-spelling, Morse code, or typing can "write" in that system, retrieving the spelling of words (or nonwords) at speeds that may be considerably greater than writing on paper. Skilled Morse code operators can allow an incoming message to run a sentence or more ahead of the point at which they are transcribing it on a typewriter. Aside from raising a question about the form of the buffer in which the decoded message is held in temporary storage, this phenomenon illustrates how automatic the retrieval of output orthography is.

We may plausibly contemplate a spreading activation network for word writing that is analogous to the one described for reading. A word representation network would involve a word's phonology, its lexical semantic activation, and its orthographic letter string representation, the latter being mapped onto an output, which is usually graphomotor. There is evidence that the strength of activation of an orthographic output string is a function of the consistency and frequency of its co-occurrence with a particular lexical semantic representation and a particular phonology. The question may then be asked whether orthographic representations for reading and orthographic output activations for any word share a mutual interaction with the word's phonology and lexical semantics.

A consequence of the shared activation of input and output orthographic strings is that disorders of word reading should, as a rule, be paralleled by similar disorders of spelling. In his consideration of this possibility, Caplan (1992) can cite only one reported case (Bub *et al.*, 1986) in which there was considerable overlap between the words subject to errors of reading and errors of spelling. On the other hand, there are many instances in which writing disorders are qualitatively different from reading performance. An example is Bub and Kertesz' (1982a) case of deep dysgraphia. Their patient produced semantically related substitutions to dictated words (e.g., "clock" for "time"). Her writing errors to dictated words showed the semantically based part-of-speech effect on accuracy. Her best performance was on concrete nouns, poorer on verbs, and poorest on grammatical functors. This pattern was not apparent in her reading, as she could correctly read all of the dictated stimulus words as well as immediately detect her writing errors.

An important observation resulted from the author's dictation of polysyllabic pseudowords that included letter sequences of greater or lesser resemblance to English letter sequences, although no real English morphemes were included in these nonword stimuli. The patient's accuracy in transcribing them increased significantly as a function of the increasing approximation of the target to an English letter sequences. This finding is entirely congruent with the principle that the strength of activation of an orthographic sequence depends on the consistency of its past co-occurrence with the corresponding phonological form. The advantage of real words over pronounceable pseudowords was prominent, both in the patient's success rate on the two types of stimuli and in her propensity to assimilate her written output to a real word that was a near neighbor of the dictated pseudoword ("foge" written as "fog"; "wabe" written as "wade").

In spite of the analogies between word reading and word writing, there are obvious differences in the anatomical and functional systems that are tapped by orthographic input and orthographic output. The former is entirely in the visual domain, whereas the latter involves various possible motor realization modes (writing, oral spelling, typing, etc.) Each of these output modes has associated motor and sensory dimensions that may, in turn, acquire a greater or lesser degree of dominance in guiding production. For example, as we have noted in Chapter 10, graphic output involves the dimensions of visual recognition of the written product and motor-kinesthetic encoding of orthographic output sequences. The ability to type brings with it the packaging of certain letter sequences that may result in errors characteristic of this particular mode of output (e.g., typing -ion instead of -ing). It should be no surprise then, that the network of interactions between phonology, semantics, and orthographic output strings may suffer impairments of function that do not overlap with those involving the corresponding orthographic strings on the input side. In particular, partial or full access to word orthography without any evidence of phonological activation is fairly common in patients with severe disorders of word retrieval. They may spontaneously report the first letter of the word, trace the word in the air, or write it on paper, without being able to retrieve it for oral report. However, as we noted in Chapter 10, written word retrieval based on semantics without phonology is usually limited to a small set of words.

Dissociations between the various output modes of orthographic realization have not been systematically studied. Informal observation suggests that this may be a rich source of information because some aphasic patients have considerably more facility in oral spelling than in writing, in the presence of intact elementary graphomotor skills. The performance of patients with premorbid typing skill has not been studied at all. It may be that as a particular output skill (e.g., typing) is acquired, associative networks between phonology, semantics, and that particular mode of orthographic string realization develop to the point where they exercise a significant influence on performance. If this were the case, it might, for example, be possible to detect differences in the adequacy of phonological guidance in typing as compared to writing.

SUMMARY

In this chapter we have returned to the aphasic phenomena that were treated in Chapters 4 through 11; but this time the focus has been on relating them to conceptions of normal language and particularly to models of language processing. Starting with the process of word comprehension, we saw that elementary speech sound discrimination at a prelinguistic level is extremely robust in aphasia but that breakdown in performance becomes manifest in operations that have a semantic component. We went on to consider how the conceptual representation of object names is related to the representation of the object as a physical entity. We concluded from the evidence of such dissociative phenomena as optic aphasia that word-concept activations are part of a system—lexical semantics—that is autonomous from the nonverbal experience of the corresponding objects.

In the subsequent treatment of sentence comprehension, word retrieval, reading, and writing, emphasis was placed on the contrast between two approaches. One is the traditional approach that has characterized classical aphasiology as well as the cognitive neuropsychology of the last 20 years. This approach infers the existence of independently functioning subsystems acting in succession to produce a linguistic act (e.g., oral reading of a word, writing of a word, naming of a picture, etc). Selective impairments in aphasia are taken as evidence of the independence of such subsystems. Characteristic of the traditional approach is the postulation of stored representations of images or memories (e.g., "lexicons") that may be subjected to serial search, and of rules of procedure (e.g., syntactic rules and spelling rules).

The more recent alternatives, represented by parallel distributed processing and neural network models, propose that language behavior is the product of mutual interactions of a reinforcing or inhibitory nature among all the elements that are activated in the course of the acquisition and subsequent performance of the behavior. Consistency and frequency of prior co-occurrence of such elements are the major influences in constraining a behavioral outcome. For example, word reading entails interactive activation of orthographic, phonological, and semantic elements. Impaired activation of the phonological component decreases the activation of orthographic and semantic elements that is normally received from phonological elements. Reduced specification of orthographic and semantic features induces errors along visual and semantic lines.

In adapting a spreading activation model to language, several factors were proposed that might result in highly selective impairments that suggest the independence of subsystems—that is, of multiple independent tracks. One type of effect is due to injury of sensory input to or motor output from the interactive system. Such effects usually correspond directly to lesions that are clearly localized in the respective sensory or motor system. Another effect is the postulation that among the interacting elements, particular associational subclusters may be susceptible to premorbid individual differences in learning facility. That is, some individuals may have a premorbid reading mechanism that relies heavily on semantic activation to enhance the retrieval of phonology, offsetting difficulty in the communication of activation between the orthographic and phonological elements. If such a system suffers injury, that compensatory adaptation may be insufficient; the resulting symptom may be interpreted as the loss of an independent grapho-phonological track. We pointed out that accounts that make use of premorbid individual differences in susceptibility to particular symptoms may explain the absence of anatomic markers distinguishing patients who develop a highly selective psycholinguistic deficit from those who do not.

It was suggested that the complexity of the graphic output channel offered greater possibility for selective impairments in writing than exist in reading. In addition, the existence of individuals with skills in totally different modes of realizing orthographic strings creates unexplored possibilities of further dissociations.

References

Alajouanine, T. (1968). *L'Aphasie et le Langage Pathologique.* Paris: Balliere.

Alajouanine, T., Ombredane, A., and Durand, M. (1939). *Le syndrome de désintégration phonétique dans l'aphasie.* Paris: Masson.

Albert, M. L., and Bear, D. (1974). Time to understand: A case study of word deafness with reference to the role of time in auditory comprehension. *Brain, 97,* 373–384.

Albert, M. L., Sparks, R., and Helm, N. (1973). Melodic intonation therapy for aphasia. *Archives of Neurology, 29,* 130–131.

Alexander, M. P. (1989). Clinical-anatomical correlations of aphasia following predominantly subcortical lesions. In F. Boller and J. Grafman (eds), *Handbook of Neuropsychology,* Vol. 2, pp. 47–66. Amsterdam: Elsevier.

Alexander, M. P., and Lo Verme, S. R. (1980). Aphasia after left hemisphere intracerebral hemorrhage. *Neurology, 30,* 1993–1202.

Alexander, M. P., and Naeser, M. A. (1988). Cortical-subcortical differences in aphasia. In F. Plum (ed.), *Language and Communication.* New York: Raven Press.

Alexander, M. P., Naeser, M. A., and Palumbo, C. (1987). Correlations of subcortical CT lesion sites and aphasia profiles. *Brain, 110,* 961–991.

Alexander, M. P., Fischette, M. R., and Fischer, R. (1989a). Crossed aphasias can be mirror image or anomalous. *Brain, 112,* 953–973.

Alexander, M. P., Hiltbronner, B., and Fischer, R. (1989b). The distributed anatomy of transcortical sensory aphasia. *Archives of Neurology, 46,* 885–892.

Andreewsky, E., and Seron, X. (1975). Implicit processing of grammatical rules. *Cortex, 11,* 379–390.

Annett, M. (1985). *Left, Right, Hand and Brain: The Right Shift Theory.* London: Erlbaum.

Assal, G., Chapuis, G., and Zander, E. (1970). Isolated writing disorders in a patient with stenosis of the left internal carotid artery. *Cortex, 6,* 241–248.

Auerbach, S. H., Allard, T., Naeser, M. A., Alexander, M. P., and Albert, M. L. (1982). Pure word deafness: Analysis of a case with bilateral lesions and a defect at the prephonemic level. *Brain, 105,* 271–300.

Baker, E., Blumstein, S. E., and Goodglass, H. (1981). Interaction between phonological and semantic factors in auditory comprehension. *Neuropsychologia, 19,* 1–15.

Bar Hillel, Y. (1964). *Language and Information.* Reading, Massachusetts: Addison-Wesley.

Basso, A., Luzzatti, C., and Spinnler, H. (1980). Is ideomotor apraxia the outcome of damage in well-defined regions of the left hemisphere? Neuropsychological study of CAT correlations. *Journal of Neurology, Neurosurgery, and Psychiatry, 43,* 118–126.

Bastian, C. (1869). On the various forms of loss of speech in cerebral disease. *British Foreign Medical and Chirurgical Review, 43,* 209, 270.

Bates, E., Wulfeck, B., and MacWhinney, B. (1991a). Cross-linguistic research in aphasia: An overview. *Brain and Language 41,* 123–148.

Bates, E., Chen, S., Tzeng, O., Li, P., and Opie, M. (1991b). The noun–verb problem in Chinese. *Brain and Language, 41,* 203–233.

Bauer, R. M., and Rubens, A. B. (1985). Agnosia. In K. M. Heilman and E. Valenstein (eds), *Clinical Neuropsychology.* New York: Oxford University Press.

Baxter, D. M., and Warrington, E. K. (1987). Category-specific phonological dysgraphia. *Neuropsychologia, 23,* 653–666.

Bay, E., (1964). Principles of classification and their influence on our concepts of aphasia. In A. V. S. De Reuck and M. O'Connor (eds), *Disorders of Language,* pp. 122–138. London: Churchill.

Beauvois, M. F., and Desrouesné, J. (1979). Phonological alexia: Three dissociations. *Journal of Neurology, Neurosurgery, and Psychiatry, 42,* 1115–1124.

Behrman, M., Black, S. E., and Bub, D. (1990). The evolution of pure alexia: A longitudinal study of recovery. *Brain and Language, 39,* 405–427.

Bellugi, U. (1980). The structuring of language: Clues from the similarities between signed and spoken language. In U. Bellugi and M. Studdert-Kennedy (eds), *Signed and Spoken Language: Biological Constraints on Linguistic Form,* pp. 115–140. Dahlem Konferenzen, Weinheim/Deerfield Beach, Florida: Verlag Chemie.

Benedet, M. J., and Goodglass, H. (1989). Body image and comprehension of body-part names. *Journal of Psycholinguistic Research 18,* 485–496.

Benson, D. F. (1979). *Aphasia, Alexia, and Agraphia.* New York: Churhill Livingstone.

Benton, A. L. and Hamsher, K. De S. (1989). *Multilingual Aphasia Examination.* Iowa City: A.J.A. Associates.

Benton, A. L., and Joynt, R. J. (1960). Early descriptions of aphasia. *Archives of Neurology, 3,* 109–126.

Berndt, R. S. (1989). Repetition in aphasia: Implications for models of language processing. In F. Boller and J. Grafman (eds), *Handbook of Neuropsychology,* Vol. 1. Amsterdam: Elsevier.

Berndt, R. S. (1991). Sentence processing in aphasia. In *Acquired Aphasia,* 2nd Edition (M. T. Sarno, ed.). San Diego: Academic Press, pp. 223–270.

Blumstein, S. E. (1988). Approaches to speech production deficits in aphasia. In F. Boller and J. Grafman (eds), *Handbook of Neuropsychology,* Vol. 1. Amsterdam: Elsevier.

Blumstein, S. E., and Cooper, W. (1974). Hemisphere processing of intonation contours. *Cortex, 10,* 146–158.

Blumstein, S. E., Baker, E., and Goodglass, H. (1977a). Phonological factors in auditory comprehension in aphasia. *Neuropsychologia, 15,* 19–30.

Blumstein, S. E., Cooper, W., Zurif, E. B., and Caramazza, A., (1977b). The perception and production of voice onset time in aphasia. *Neuropsychologia, 15,* 371–383.

Blumstein, S. E., Alexander, M. P., Ryalls, J. H., Katz, W., and Dworetsky, B. (1987). The nature of the foreign accent syndrome: A case study. *Brain and Language, 31,* 215–244.

Bouillaud, J.-B. (1825). Recherches cliniques propres à démontrer que la perte de la parole correspond à la lésion des lobules antérieures du cerveau. *Archives Générales Médicales, 8,* 25–43.

Bradley, D. C., Garret, M. F., and Zurif, E. B. (1986). Syntactic deficits in Broca's aphasia. In D. Caplan (ed.), *Biological Studies of Mental Processes,* pp. 269–286. Cambridge, Massachusetts: MIT Press.

Broca, P. (1861). Perte de la parole. Ramollissement chronique et destruction partielle du lobe antérieur gauche du cerveau. *Bulletin de la Société d'Anthropologie, 2,* 235.

Broca, P. (1865). Sur la faculté du langage articulé. *Bulletin de la Société d'Anthropologie, 6,* 337–393.

Brown, R., and McNeil, D. (1966). The "tip-of-the-tongue" phenomenon. *Journal of Verbal Learning and Verbal Behavior, 5,* 325–337.

Bub, D., and Chertkow, H. (1988). Agraphia. In F. Boller and J. Grafman (eds.) *Handbook of Neuropsychology, Vol 1.* Amsterdam: Elsevier.

Bub, D., and Kertesz, A. (1982a). Deep agraphia. *Brain and Language, 17,* 146–165.

Bub, D., and Kertesz, A. (1982b). Evidence for lexicographic processing in a patient with preserved written over oral word naming. *Brain, 105,* 697–717.

Bub, D., Black, S., and Behrmann, M. (1986). Are there two orthographic lexicons? Evidence from a case of surface dyslexia. Paper presented at the Academy of Aphasia, Nashville.

Buckingham, H. W. (1991). Explanations for the concept of apraxia of speech. In M. T. Sarno (ed.), *Acquired Aphasia*. San Diego: Academic Press.

Caplan, D. (1987). *Neurolinguistics and Linguistic Aphasiology*. Cambridge: Cambridge University Press.

Caplan, D. (1992). *Language: Structure, Processing, and Disorders*. Cambridge, Massachusetts: MIT Press.

Caplan, D., Kellar, L., and Locke, S. (1972). Inflection of neologisms in aphasia. *Brain, 95*, 169–172.

Cappa, S. F., and Vignolo, L. (1979). "Transcortical" features of aphasia following left thalamic hemorrhage. *Cortex, 19*, 227–241.

Caramazza, A. (1984). The logic of neuropsychological research and the problem of patient classification in aphasia. *Brain and Language, 21*, 9–20.

Caramazza, A. (1986). On drawing inferences about the structure of normal cognitive processes from patterns of impaired performance: The case for single-patient studies. *Brain and Cognition, 5*, 41–66.

Caramazza, A., and Hillis, A. E. (1991). Lexical organization of nouns and verbs in the brain. *Nature, 349*, 788–790.

Caramazza, A., and Miceli, G. (1990). Structure of the lexicon: Functional architecture and lexical representation. In J. L. Nespoulous and P. Villiard (eds), *Morphology, Phonology, and Aphasia*. New York: Springer.

Caramazza, A., Miceli, G., Villa, G., and Romani, C. (1986). The role of the graphemic buffer in spelling: Evidence from a case of acquired dysgraphia. *Reports of the Cognitive Neuropsychology Laboratory*, No. 17. Baltimore: The Johns Hopkins University.

Chamberlain, H. D. (1928). The inheritance of left-handedness. *Journal of Heredity 19*, 557–559.

Chomsky, N. (1957). *Syntactic Structures*. The Hague: Mouton.

Chomsky, N. (1981). *Lectures on government and binding*. Dordrecht: Foris.

Coltheart, M. (1980). Deep dyslexia: A review of the syndrome. In M. Coltheart, K. Patterson, and J. C. Marshall (eds), *Deep Dyslexia*. London: Routledge and Kegan Paul.

Coltheart, M., Patterson, K., and Marshall, J. C., eds. (1980). *Deep Dyslexia*. London: Routledge and Kegan Paul.

Coslett, H. B., and Saffran, E. M. (1989). Evidence for preserved reading in "pure alexia." *Brain, 112*, 327–359.

Coslett, H. B., Rothi, L. G., Valenstein, E., and Heilman, K. M. (1986). Dissociation of writing and praxis: Two cases in point. *Brain and Language, 28*, 357–369.

Critchley, M. D. (1938). Aphasia in a prelingually deaf woman. *Brain, 61*, 163–166.

Dalin, O. L. (1745). Berättelse om de Dumbe, som Kan siunga. *K. Swenska Wetensk. Acad. Handlingar, 6*, 114–115.

Damasio, A. (1989). Concepts in the brain. *Mind and Language, 4*, 24–27.

Damasio, A. (1990). Synchronous activation in multiple cortical regions: A mechanism for recall. *Seminars in the Neurosciences, 2*, 287–296.

Damasio, A. R., and Damasio, H. (1983). The anatomic basis of pure alexia. *Neurology, 33*, 1573–1583.

Damasio, H., and Damasio, A. R. (1989). *Neuroanatomy and Neuropsychological Disorders: Neuroimaging Procedures and Problems*. New York: Oxford University Press.

Danley, M., de Villiers, J. G., and Cooper, W. E. (1979). The control of speech prosody in Broca's aphasia. In J. J. Wolf and J. J. Klatt (eds.) *Speech Communication Papers Presented at the 97th Meeting of the Acoustical Society of America*. pp. 265–270. New York: Acoustical Society of America.

Danley, M., and Shapiro, B. (1982). Speech prosody in Broca's aphasia. *Brain and Language, 16*, 171–190.

Danley, M., Cooper, W., and Shapiro, B. (1983). Fundamental frequency, language structure, and linguistic processing in Wernicke's aphasia. *Brain and Language, 19*, 1–24.

Dee, H. L., Benton, A. L., and Van Allen, M. (1970). Apraxia in relation to hemisphere locus of lesion and aphasia. *Transactions of the American Neurological Association, 95*, 147–150.

DeBleser, R., and Bayer, J. (1990). Morphological reading errors in a German case of deep dyslexia. In J.-L. Nespoulous and P. Villiard (eds), *Morphology, Phonology, and Aphasia*. New York: Springer.

Dejerine, J. (1891). Sur un cas de cécité verbale avec agraphie, suivi d'autopsie. *Mémoires de la Société de Biologie, 4*, 61–90.

Dejerine, J. (1892). Contribution à l'étude anatomo-pathologique et clinique des différentes variétés de cécité verbale. *Mémoires de la Société de Biologie, 4*, 61–90.

Dejerine, J. (1901). *Anatomie des Centres Nerveux*. Paris: Rueff.

Dell, G. S. (1986). A spreading activation theory of retrieval in sentence production. *Psychological Review, 93*, 283–321.

Denckla, M., and Rudel, R. (1974). Rapid "automatized" naming of pictured objects, colors, letters, and numbers by normal children. *Cortex, 10*, 186–202.

Denes, G., and Semenza, C. (1975). Auditory modality-specific anomia: Evidence from a case of pure word deafness. *Cortex, 11*, 401–411.

Dennis, M. (1976). Dissociated naming and locating of body parts after left anterior temporal lobe resection. An experimental case study. *Brain and Language, 3*, 147–163.

Dennis, M., and Kohn, B. (1975). Comprehension of syntax in infantile hemiplegics after hemidecortication: Left hemisphere superiority. *Brain and Language, 2*, 472–482.

De Renzi, E. (1989). Apraxia. In F. Boller and J. Grafman (eds), *Handbook of Neuropsychology*, Vol. 2, pp. 245–263. Amsterdam: Elsevier.

De Renzi, E., and Lucchelli, F. (1988). Ideational apraxia. *Brain: 111*, 1173–1185.

De Renzi, E., Pieczuro, A., and Vignolo, L. (1966). Oral apraxia and aphasia. *Cortex, 2*, 50–73.

De Renzi, E., Motti, F., and Nichelli, P. (1980). Imitating gestures: A quantitative approach to ideomotor apraxia. *Archives of Neurology, 37*, 6–18.

De Renzi, E., Faglioni, P., Lodesani, M., and Vecchi, A. (1983). Limb apraxia in patients with lesions confined to the left basal ganglia and thalamus. Frontal and parietal injured patients compared. *Cortex, 19*, 333–343.

De Renzi, E., and Vignolo, L. (1962). The Token Test: A sensitive test to detect receptive disturbances in aphasics. *Brain, 85*, 655–678.

Douglass, E., and Richardson, J. C. (1959). Aphasia in a congenital deaf mute. *Brain, 82*, 68–80.

Dubois, J., Hecaen, H., Angelergues, R., Maufras de Chatelier, A., and Marcie, P. (1964). Etude neurolinguistique de l'aphasie de conduction. *Neuropsychologia, 2*, 9–44.

Dubois, J., Hécaen, H., and Marcie, P. (1969). L'agraphie "pure." *Neuropsychologia, 7*, 271–286.

Duffy, R. J., and Duffy, J. R. (1981). Three studies of deficits in pantomimic expression and pantomime recognition in aphasia. *Journal of Speech and Hearing Research, 46*, 70–86.

Ellis, A. (1987). Intimations of modularity, or, the modularity of mind: Doing cognitive neuropsychology without syndromes. In M. Coltheart, G. Sartori, and R. Job (eds), *The Cognitive Neuropsychology of Language*. Hillsdale, New Jersey: L. Erlbaum.

Exner, S. (1881). *Untersuchungen über die Lokalisation der Funktionen in der Grosshirnrinde des Menschen*. Vienna: Wilhelm Braunmuller.

Ferguson, C. A., and Garnica, O. (1973). Theories of phonological development. In E. Lenneberg and E. Lenneberg (eds), *Foundations of Language Development*, Vol. I, pp. 153–180. New York: Academic Press.

Finkelnburg, R. (1870). Vortrag in der niederrheinische Gesellschaft der Aerzte. *Berliner Klinische Wochenschrift, 7*, 449.

Fodor, J. (1983). *The Modularity of Mind*. Cambridge: MIT Press/Bradford Books.

Forster, E. (1919). Agrammatismus (erschwerte Satzfindung) und Mangel an Antrieb nach Stirnhirnverletzung. *Monatsschrift fur Psychiatrie und Neurologie, 46*, 1–43.

Frazier, L. (1987). Theories of sentence processing. In J. Garfield (ed.), *Modularity in Knowledge Representation and Natural Language Processing*, pp. 219–317. Cambridge, Massachusetts: MIT Press.

Freedman, M., Alexander, M. P., and Naeser, M. A. (1984). The anatomical basis of transcortical motor aphasia. *Neurology, 34*, 409–417.

Freund, C. S. (1889). Uber optische Aphasie und Seelenblindheit. *Archiv von Psychiatrie und Nervenkrankheiten. 20*, 276–297.

Friederici, A. D., Schonle, P. W., and Goodglass, H. (1981). Mechanisms underlying writing and speech in aphasia. *Brain and Language, 13*, 212–223.

Friedman, R. B., and Alexander, M. P. (1984). Pictures, images, and pure alexia. *Cognitive Neuropsychology, 1*, 9–23.

Fromkin, V. (1973). *Speech Errors as Linguistic Evidence*. The Hague: Mouton.

Garrett, M. (1975). The analysis of sentence production. In G. Bowers (ed.), *Psychology of Learning and Motivation, Vol. 9*. New York: Academic Press.

Garrett, M. (1980). Levels of processing in sentence production. In B. Butterworth (ed.), *Language Production. Vol. 1, Speech and Talk*. London: Academic Press. pp. 177–220.

Gazzaniga, M. S., Bogen, J. E., and Sperry, R. W. (1965). Observations on visual perception after disconnexion of the cerebral hemispheres in man. *Brain, 88*, 221–236.

Geschwind, N. (1965). Disconnexion syndromes in animals and man. *Brain, 88*, 237–294 and 585–644.

Geschwind, N. (1967). Neurological foundations of language. In H. R. Myklebust (ed.), *Progress in Learning Disabilities*, pp. 182–198. New York: Grune and Stratton.

Geschwind, N. (1969). Problems in the anatomical understanding of the aphasias. In A. L. Benton (ed.), *Contributions to Clinical Neuropsychology*. Chicago: Aldine.

Geschwind, N. (1975). The apraxias: Neural mechanisms of disorders of learned movements. *American Scientist, 63*, 188–195.

Geschwind, N., and Fusillo, M. (1966). Color naming deficits in association with alexia. *Archives of Neurology, 15*, 137–146.

Geschwind, N., and Kaplan, E. F. (1962). A human cerebral disconnection syndrome. *Neurology, 12*, 675–685.

Geschwind, N., and Levitsky, W. (1968). Human Brain: Left–right asymmetries in temporal speech region. *Science, 161*, 186–187.

Geschwind, N., Quadfasel, F. A., and Segarra, J. (1968). Isolation of the speech area. *Neuropsychologia, 6*, 327–340.

Gesner, J. A. P. (1770). Die Sprachamnesie. *Sammlung von Beobachtungen aus der Arzneigelehrkeit und Naturkunde*. Nordlingen.

Gibson, E. J., and Levin, H. (1975). *The Psychology of Reading*. Cambridge, Massachusetts: MIT Press.

Gleason, J. B., Goodglass, H., Ackerman, N., Green, E., and Hyde, M. R. (1975). Retrieval of syntax in Broca's aphasia. *Brain and Language, 2*, 451–471.

Glosser, G., and Friedman, R. B. (1990). The continuum of deep/phonological alexia. *Cortex, 26*, 343–360.

Glushko, R. (1979). The organization and activation of orthographic knowledge in reading aloud. *Journal of Experimental Psychology: Human Perception and Performance, 5*, 675–691.

Goldstein, K. (1948). *Language and Language Disturbances*. New York: Grune and Stratton.

Goodglass, H., Barton, M. I., and Kaplan, E. (1968). Sensory modality and object-naming in aphasia. *Journal of Speech and Hearing Research, 111,* 488–496.

Goodglass, H., and Budin, C. (1988). Category and modality-specific dissociations in word comprehension and concurrent phonological dyslexia: A case study. *Neuropsychologia, 26,* 67–88.

Goodglass, H., and Butters, N. M. (1989). Psychobiology of cognitive processes. In R. C. Atkinson, R. J. Herrnstein, G. Lindzey, and E. D. Luce (eds), *Stevens' Handbook of Experimental Psychology, Second Edition.* New York: Wiley Interscience.

Goodglass, H., and Gleason, J. B. (1960). Agrammatism and inflectional morphology in English. *Journal of Speeceh and Hearing Research, 3,* 257–267.

Goodglass, H., and Hunt, J. (1958). Grammatical complexity and aphasic speech. *Word, 14,* 197–207.

Goodglass, H., and Hunter, M. (1970). Linguistic comparison of speech and writing in two types of aphasia. *Journal of Communication Disorders, 3,* 28–35.

Goodglass, H., and Kaplan, E. (1963). Disturbance of gesture and pantomime in aphasia. *Brain, 86,* 703–720.

Goodglass, H., and Mayer, J. (1958). Agrammatism in aphasia. *Journal of Speech and Hearing Disorders, 23,* 99–111.

Goodglass, H., and Menn, L. (1985). Is agrammatism a unitary phenomenon? In M.-L. Kean (ed.), *Agrammatism.* New York: Academic Press.

Goodglass, H., and Quadfasel, F. (1954). Language laterality in left-handed aphasics. *Brain, 77,* 523–548.

Goodglass, H., and Stuss, D. T. (1979). Naming to confrontation versus oral description in three subgroups of aphasics. *Cortex, 15,* 119–211.

Goodglass, H., Quadfasel, F., and Timberlake, W. (1964). Phrase length and the type and severity of aphasia. *Cortex, 1,* 133–153.

Goodglass, H., Klein, B., Carey, P., and Jones, K. J. (1966). Specific semantic word categories in aphasia. *Cortex, 2,* 74–89.

Goodglass, H., Fodor, I., and Schulhoff, C. (1967). Prosodic factors in grammar: Evidence from aphasia. *Journal of Speech and Hearing Research, 10,* 5–20.

Goodglass, H., Kaplan, E., Weintraub, S., and Ackerman, N. (1976). The "tip-of-the-tongue" phenomenon in aphasia. *Cortex, 12,* 145–153.

Goodglass, H., Blumstein, S. E., Statlender, S., Gleason, J. B., and Hyde, M. R. (1979). The effect of syntactic encoding on sentence comprehension in aphasia. *Brain and Language, 7,* 201–209.

Goodglass, H., Theurkauf, J. C., and Wingfield, A. (1984). Naming latencies as evidence for two modes of lexical retrieval. *Applied Psycholinguistics, 5,* 135–146.

Goodglass, H., Wingfield, A., Hyde, M. R., and Theurkauf, J. (1986). Category-specific dissociation in naming and recognition by aphasic patients. *Cortex, 22,* 87–102.

Goodglass, H., Wingfield, A., and Wayland, S. (1989). The nature of prolonged word finding. *Brain and Language, 36,* 411–419.

Goodglass, H., Christiansen, J. A., and Gallagher, R. S. (in press). Comparison of morphology and syntax in free narrative and structured tests. Fluent versus nonfluent aphasics. *Cortex.*

Green, E. (1969). Phonological and grammatical aspects of jargon in an aphasic patient: A case study. *Language and Speech, 12,* 103–118.

Greenblatt, S. (1973). Alexia without agraphia or hemianopia: Anatomical analysis of an autopsied case. *Brain, 96,* 307–316.

Grodzinsky, Y. (1990). *Theoretical Perspectives on Language Deficits.* Cambridge, Massachusetts: MIT Press.

Grosjean, F. (1980). Spoken word recognition processes and the gating paradigm. *Perception and Psychophysics, 28*, 267–283.

Haaland, K. Y., and Flaherty, D. (1984). The different types of limb apraxia errors made by patients with left versus right hemisphere damage. *Brain and Cognition, 3*, 370–384.

Hart, J., and Gordon, B. (1988). Implications for semantic organization from a case of category-specific anomia. Paper presented at Academy of Aphasia, Montreal.

Hart, J., and Gordon, B. (1992). Neural subsystems for object knowledge. *Nature, 359*, 60–64.

Hart, J., Berndt, R. S., and Caramazza, A. (1985). Category-specific naming deficit following cerebral infarction. *Nature, 316*, 439–440.

Head, H. (1926). *Aphasia and Kindred Disorders of Speech*. New York: Macmillan.

Hécaen, H. (1969). Essai de dissociation du syndrome de l'aphasie sensorielle. *Revue Neurologique, 120*, 229–231.

Hécaen, H., and Ajuriaguerra, J. (1963). *Les gauchers: Prévalence manuelle et dominance cérébrale*. Paris: Presses Universitaires.

Heeschen, C. (1985). Agrammatism versus paragrammatism: A fictitious opposition. In M.-L. Kean (ed.), *Agrammatism*, pp. 207–248. New York: Academic Press.

Heilman, K. M. (1979). Apraxia. In K. M. Heilman and E. Valenstein (eds.) *Clinical Neuropsychology*. New York: Oxford University Press.

Heilman, K. M., Coyle, I. M., Gonyea, E. F., and Geschwind, N. (1973). Apraxia and agraphia in a left-hander. *Brain, 96*, 21–28.

Heilman, K. M., Scholes, R., and Watson, R. T. (1975). Auditory affective agnosia: Disturbed comprehension of affective speech. *Journal of Neurology, Neurosurgery, and Psychiatry, 38*, 69–72.

Heilman, K. M., Rothi, L. G., and Valenstein, E. (1982). Two forms of ideomotor apraxia. *Neurology, 32*, 342–346.

Henderson, L. (1982). *Orthography and Word Recognition in Reading*. New York: Academic Press.

Hofstede, B., and Kolk, H. (1989). Agrammatism and normal ellipsis. Paper presented at Academy of Aphasia, Santa Fe, New Mexico.

Hoit-Dalgaard, J., Murry, T., and Kopp, H. (1983). Voice onset time production and perception in apraxic subjects. *Brain and Language, 20*, 329–339.

Howard, D., and Franklin, S. (1988). *Missing the Meaning?* Cambridge, Massachusetts: MIT Press.

Humphries, G. W., Riddoch, M. J., and Quinlan, P. T. (1988). Cascade processes in picture identification. *Cognitive Neuropsychology, 5*, 67–104.

Hung, D. L., and Tzeng, O. J. L. (1981). Orthographic variation and visual information processing. *Psychological Bulletin, 90*, 377–414.

Isserlin, M. (1922). Uber Agrammatismus. *Zeitschrift fur die gesamte Neurologie und Psychiatrie*, pp. 626–807. Berlin: Springer.

Itoh, M., Sasanuma, S., and Ushijima, T. (1979). Velar movements during speech in a patient with apraxia of speech. *Brain and Language, 7*, 227–239.

Itoh, M., Sasanuma, S., Hirose, H., Yoshioka, H., and Sawashima, M. (1983). Velar movements during speech in two Wernicke's aphasic patients. *Brain and Language, 19*, 283–292.

Jackson, J. H. (1866). Notes on the physiology and pathology of language. *Medical Times and Gazette, 1*, 659.

Jackson, J. H. (1874). On the nature of the duality of the brain. *Medical Press and Circular, 1*, 19, 41, 63.

Jackson, J. H. (1878). On affections of speech from disease of the brain. *Brain, 1*, 304–330.

Jackson, J. H. (1915). Reprints of some of Hughlings Jackson's papers on affections of speech. *Brain, 38*, 28–190.

Jakobson, R. (1941). *Kindersprache, Aphasie und allgemeine Lautgesetze.* Uppsala: Universitet Arsskrift.

Jakobson, R. (1956). Two aspects of language and two types of aphasic disturbances. In R. Jakobson and M. Halle, *Fundamentals of Language.* The Hague: Mouton.

Joanette, Y. (1990). Aphasia in left-handers and crossed aphasia. In F. Boller and J. Grafman (eds), *Handbook of Neuropsychology,* Vol. 2, pp. 173–184. Amsterdam: Elsevier.

Joanette, Y., Keller, E., and Lecours, A. R. (1980). Sequences of phonemic approximation in aphasia. *Brain and Language, 11,* 30–44.

Johns, D. F., and Darley, F. L. (1970). Phonemic variability in apraxia of speech. *Journal of Speech and Hearing Research, 13,* 556–583.

Johnson, D. F., and LaPointe, L. L. (1976). Neurogenic disorders of output processing: Apraxia of speech. In H. Whitaker and H. A. Whitaker (eds), *Studies in Neurolinguistics,* Vol. 1. New York: Academic Press.

Jones, L. V., and Wepman, J. M. (1965). Grammatical indicants of speaking style in normal and aphasic speakers. *Reports of the Psychometric Laboratory of the University of North Carolina,* no. 46, December, 1965.

Kaplan, E., Goodglass, H., and Weintraub, S. (1983). *The Boston Naming Test.* Philadelphia: Lea and Febiger.

Katz, R. B., and Goodglass, H. (1990). Deep dysphasia: Analysis of a rare form of repetition disorder. *Brain and Language, 39,* 153–185.

Kean, M.-L. (1977). The linguistic interpretation of aphasic syndromes: Agrammatism in Broca's aphasia, an example. *Cognition, 5,* 9–46.

Kempen, G., and Hoenkamp, E. (1987). An incremental procedural grammar for sentence formulation. *Cognitive Science, 11,* 201–258.

Kertesz, A., Ferro, J. M., and Shewan, C. M. (1984). Apraxia and aphasia. The functional anatomical basis for their dissociation. *Neurology, 30,* 40–47.

Kimura, D. (1976). The neural basis of language *qua* gesture. In H. Whitaker and H. Whitaker (eds), *Studies in Neurolinguistics,* Vol. 2. New York: Academic Press.

Kimura, D. (1979). Neuromotor mechanisms in the evolution of human communication. In H. D. Stecklis and M. J. Raleigh (eds), *Neurobiology of Social Communication in Primates: An Evolutionary Perspective.* New York: Academic Press.

Kimura, D. (1982). Left hemisphere control of oral and brachial movements and their relationship to communication. In D. E. Broadbent and L. Weiskrantz (eds), *The Neuropsychology of Cognitive Function,* pp. 135–149. London: The Royal Society.

Kimura, D., and Archibald, Y. (1974). Motor functions of the left hemisphere. *Brain, 97,* 337–350.

Kinsbourne, M., and Rosenfield, D. B. (1974). Agraphia selective for written spelling: An experimental case study. *Brain and Language, 1,* 215–226.

Kleist, K. (1916). Uber Leitungsaphasie und grammatische Storungen. *Zeitschrift fur Psychiatrie und Neurologie, 40,* 118–199.

Kohn, S. E. (1984). The nature of the phonological deficit in conduction aphasia. *Brain and Language, 23,* 97–115.

Kohn, S. E. (1989). Verb finding in aphasia. *Cortex, 25,* 57–69.

Kohn, S., and Goodglass, H. (1985). Picture naming in aphasia. *Brain and Language, 24,* 266–283.

Kohn, S., Menn, L., Wingfield, A., Goodglass, H., Gleason, J. B., and Hyde, M. R. (1987). Lexical retrieval: The tip-of-the-tongue phenomenon. *Applied Psycholinguistics, 8,* 245–266.

Kolb, B., and Milner, B. (1981). Performance of complex arm and facial movements after focal brain lesions. *Neuropsychologia, 19,* 491–503.

Kolk, H., Van Grunsven, M., and Keyser, A. (1985). On parallelism between production and comprehension in agrammatism. In M-L. Kean (ed.), *Agrammatism*. New York: Academic Press.

Kussmaul, A. (1881). *Die Storungen der Sprache*. Leipzig: Vogel.

Landis, T., Graves, R. and Goodglass, H. (1982). Aphasic reading and writing: Possible evidence of right hemisphere participation. *Cortex, 8*, 105–112.

Landis, T., Regard, M., Graves, R., and Goodglass, H. (1983). *Neuropsychologia, 21*, 359–364.

Lecours, A-R., Lhermitte, F., and Bryans, B. (1983). *Aphasiology*. London: Balliere Tindall.

Lehmkuhl, G., Poeck, K., and Willmes, K. (1983). Ideomotor apraxia and aphasia: an examination of types and manifestations of apraxic symptoms. *Neuropsychologia, 21*, 199–212.

Leischner, A. (1943). Die "Aphasia" der Taubstummen. *Archiv von Psychiatrie und Nervenkrankheiten, 115*, 469–548.

Lenneberg, E. (1967). *Biological Foundations of Language*. New York: Wiley.

Lesser, R. (1978). *Linguistic Investigations of Aphasia*. New York: Elsevier/North Holland.

Levelt, W. J. M. (1989). *Speaking*. Cambridge, Massachusetts: MIT Press.

Levelt, W. J. M., Schriefers, H., Vorberg, D., Meyer, A. S., Pechman, T., and Haringa, J. (1991). The time course of lexical access in speech production. *Psychological Review, 98*, 122–142.

Liberman, A., Cooper, F. S., Shankweiler, D. S., and Studdert-Kennedy, M. (1967). Perception of the speech code. *Psychological Review, 74*, 431–461.

Lichtheim, O. (1884). On aphasia. *Brain, 7*, 443–484.

Liepmann, H. (1900). Das Krankheitsbild der Apraxie (motorischen Asymbolie). *Monatsschrift fur Psychiatire, 8*, 15–44, 102–132, 192–197.

Liepmann, H. (1905). Die Linke Hemisphäre und das Handeln. *Munchener medezinischer Wochenschrift, 49*, 2375–2378.

Liepmann, H. (1908). *Drei Aufsätze aus dem Apraxiegebiet*. Berlin: Karger.

Liepmann, H., and Maas, O. (1907). Ein Fall von linksseitiger Agraphie und Apraxie bei rechtseitiger Lähmung. *Monatsschrift für Psychiatrie und Neurologie, 10*, 214–227.

Linebarger, M. C., Schwartz, M. F., and Saffran, E. M. (1983). Sensitivity to grammatical functors in so-called agrammatic aphasics. *Cognition, 13*, 361–392.

Linné, C. (1745). Glomska of alla substantica och isynnerheit namm. *Swensk. Wetensk. Akad Handl., 6*, 114–115.

Lordat, J. (1843). Analyse de la parole pour servir à la theorie de divers cas d'alalie et de paralalie. *Journal de la Société Pratique de Montpellier, 7*, 333, 417.

Luria, A. R. (1966). *Higher Cortical Functions in Man*. New York: Basic Books.

Luria, A. R. (1970). *Traumatic Aphasia*. The Hague: Mouton.

MacWhinney, B. (1989). Competition and connectionism. In B. Macwhinney and E. Bates (eds), *A Cross Linguistic Study of Sentence Processing*, pp. 422–457. Cambridge: Cambridge University Press.

Marcel, T. (1980). Surface dyslexia and beginning reading: A revised hypothesis of the pronunciation of print and its impairments. In M. Coltheart, K. Patterson, and J. C. Marshall (eds), *Deep Dyslexia*. London: Routledge and Kegan Paul.

Marcie, P., and Hécaen, H. (1979). Agraphia: Writing disorders associated with unilateral cortical lesions. In K. M. Heilman and E. Valenstein (eds), *Clinical Neuropsychology*. New York: Oxford University Press.

Marie, P. (1906). Révision de la question de l'aphasie: La troisime circonvolution frontale gauche ne joue aucun role spécial dans la fonction du langage. *Semaine Médicale, 26*, 241.

Marshall, J. C., and Newcombe, F. (1973). Patterns of paralexia. *Journal of Psycholinguistic Research, 2*, 175–199.

Marslen-Wilson, W. (1984). Function and process in spoken word recognition. In H. Bouma and D. G. Bouwhuis (eds), *Attention and Performance X*. Hillsdale, New Jersey: L. Erlbaum.

Martin, R. C., and Blossom-Stach, C. (1986). Evidence of syntactic deficits in a fluent aphasic. *Brain and Language, 28*, 196–234.

Martin, R. C., Wetzel, W. F., Blossom-Stach, C., and Feher, E. (1989). Syntactic loss versus processing deficits: An assessment of two theories of agrammatism and syntactic comprehension deficits. *Cognition, 32*, 157–191.

Mateer, C. (1976). "Impairments of nonverbal oral movements after left hemisphere damage: A followup analysis of errors." Research Bulletin #395, Department of Psychology, University of Western Ontario, London, Ontario.

Mateer, C., and Kimura, D. (1977). Impairment of nonverbal oral movement in aphasia. *Brain and Language*, 262–276.

McCarthy, R., and Warrington, E. K. (1985). Category specificity in an agrammatic patient: The relative impairment of verb retrieval and comprehension. *Neuropsychologia, 23*, 709–727.

McClelland, J. L. (1992). Parallel distributed processing and cognitive neuropsychology. Paper presented at International Neuropsychological Society, San Diego.

McClelland, J., and Rumelhart, D. (1986). *Parallel Distributed Processing*. Cambridge, Massachusetts: MIT Press/Bradford Books.

Menn, L. (1979). Toward a psychology of phonology: Child phonology as a first step. In *Applications of Linguistic Theory in the Human Sciences*, pp. 138–179. Linguistics Department, Michigan State University, Lansing, Michigan.

Menn, L. (1981). Theories of phonological development. In H. Winitz (ed.), *Native Language and Foreign Language Acquisition. Proceedings of the New York Academy of Science, 379*, 130–137.

Menn, L., and Obler, L. K. (1990). *Agrammatic Aphasia*. Amsterdam: Benjamins.

Miceli, G. (1982). The processing of speech sounds in a patient with cortical auditory disorder. *Neuropsychologia, 20*, 5–20.

Miceli, G., Mazzucchi, A., Menn, L., and Goodglass, H. (1983). Contrasting cases of Italian agrammatic aphasia without comprehension disorder. *Brain and Language, 19*, 65–97.

Miceli, G., Silveri, M. C., Villa, G., and Caramazza, A. (1984). On the basis of agrammatics' difficulty in producing main verbs. *Cortex, 20*, 207–220.

Miceli, G., Silveri, M. C., Romani, C., and Caramazza, A. (1989). Variations in the omissions and substitutions of grammatical morphemes in the spontaneous speech of so-called agrammatic patients. *Brain and Language, 36*, 447–492.

Michel, F., and Andreewsky, E. (1983). Deep dysphasia: An analog of deep dyslexia in the auditory modality. *Brain and Language, 18*, 212–223.

Milberg, W., and Blumstein, S. E. (1981). Lexical decision and aphasia: Evidence for semantic processing. *Brain and Language, 14*, 371–385.

Miller, D., and Ellis, A. W. (1987). Speech and writing errors in "neologistic jargonaphasia"; A lexical activation hypothesis. In M. Coltheart, G. Sartori, and R. Job (eds), *The Cognitive Neuropsychology of Language*. Hillsdale, New Jersey: L. Erlbaum.

Mills, C. (1904). Treatment of aphasia by training. *Journal of the American Medical Association, 43*, 1940–1949.

Mohr, J. P., Pessin, M. S., Finkelstein, S., Funkenstein, H. H., Duncan, G. W., and Davis, K. R. (1978). Broca aphasia: Pathologic and clinical. *Neurology, 28*, 311–324.

Monrad-Krohn, G. H. (1947). Dysprosody or altered "melody of language." *Brain, 70*, 405–415.

Morgagni, G. B. (1769). *The Seats and Causes of Disease, Investigated by Anatomy*. Translated by B. Alexander. London.

Morris, C. (1938). Foundations of the theory of signs. In M. Neurath (ed.), *International Encyclopedia of Unified Science*. Chicago: University of Chicago Press.

Morton, J. (1969). The interaction of information in word recognition. *Psychological Review,* 76, 165–178.

Morton, J. (1979a). Word recognition. In J. Morton and J. C. Marshall (eds), *Psycholinguistics Series,* Vol. 2. London: Paul Elek.

Morton, J. (1979b). Some experiments on facilitation in word and picture recognition and their relevance for the evolution of a theoretical position. In P. Kolers, W. Wrolstad, and H. Bouma (eds), *Processing of Visible Language.* New York: Plenum.

Morton, J., and Patterson, K. (1980a). Little words—No! In M. Coltheart, K. Patterson, and J. C. Marshall (eds), *Deep Dyslexia,* pp. 270–285. London: Routledge and Kegan Paul.

Morton, J., and Patterson, K. (1980b). A new attempt at an interpretation or an attempt at a new interpretation. In M. Coltheart, K. Patterson, and J. C. Marshall (eds), *Deep Dyslexia,* pp. 91–118. London: Routledge and Kegan Paul.

Myerson, R., and Goodglass, H. (1972). Transformational grammars of three aphasic patients. *Language and Speech, 15,* 40–50.

Naeser, M. A., and Borod, J. C. (1986). Aphasia in left-handers. *Neurology, 36,* 471–488.

Naeser, M. A., Alexander, M. P., Helm-Estabrooks, N., Levine, H. L., Laughlin, S. A., and Geschwind, N. (1982). Aphasia with predominantly subcortical lesion sites: Description of three capsular/putaminal aphasia syndromes. *Archives of Neurology, 39,* 2–14.

Naeser, M. A., Estabrooks, N. H., Haas, G., Auerbach, S., and Srinivasan, M. (1987a). Relationship between lesion extent in "Wernicke's area" on computed tomographic scan and predicting recovery of comprehension in Wernicke's aphasia. *Archives of Neurology, 44,* 73–82.

Naeser, M. A., Mazurski, P., Goodglass, H., Peraino, M., Laughlin, S., and Leaper, W. C. (1987b). Auditory syntactic comprehension in nine aphasic groups (with CT scans) and children: Differences in degree, but not order of difficulty observed. *Cortex, 23,* 359–380.

Naeser, M. A., Palumbo, C. L., Helm-Estabrooks, N., Stiassny-Eder, D., and Albert, M. L. (1989). Severe nonfluency in aphasia: Role of the medial subcallosal fasciculus and other white matter pathways in recovery of spontaneous speech. *Brain, 112,* 1–38.

Nielsen, J. M. (1946). *Agnosia, Apraxia, and Aphasia.* New York: Hoeber.

Ojemann, G., and Whitaker, H. A. (1978). The bilingual brain. *Archives of Neurology, 35,* 409–412.

Ombredane, A. (1951). *L'aphasie et l'élaboration de la pensée explicite.* Paris: Presses Universitaires de France.

Padden, C. A., and Perlmutter, D. M. (1987). American Sign Language and the architecture of phonological theory. *Natural Language and Linguistic Theory, 5,* 335–375.

Paradis, M. (1989). Bilingual and polyglot aphasia. In F. Boller and J. Grafman (eds), *Handbook of Neuropsychology,* pp. 117–140. Amsterdam: Elsevier.

Pate, D. S., Saffran, E. M., and Martin, N. (1987). Specifying the locus of impairment in conduction aphasia. *Language and Cognitive Processes, 2,* 43–81.

Penfield, W., and Roberts, L. (1959). *Speech and Brain Mechanisms.* Princeton: Princeteon University Press.

Peters, A. (1979). Thalamic input to the cerebral cortex. *Trends in Neuroscience, 2,* 183–185.

Pick, A. (1913). *Die agrammatishen Sprachstorungen. Studien zur psychologischen Grundlegung der Aphasielehre.* Berlin: Springer.

Pick, A. (1923). Sprachpsychologie und andere Studien zur Aphasielehre. 1. Zur Psychologie der "Not"-Sprachen. *Schweizeres Archiv fur Neurologie und Psychiatrie, 12,* 105–135.

Pick, A. (1931). Aphasie. In O. Bumke and O. Foerster (eds), *Handbuch der normalen un pathologischen Physiologie.* Vol. 15, pp. 1416–1524. Berlin: Springer.

Pickett, L. W. (1972). An assessment of gesture and pantomime deficits in aphasic patients. *Acta Symbolica, 5,* 69–86.

Pitres, A. (1898). L'aphasie amnésique et ses variétés cliniques. *Progrès Médical, 28,* 17–23.

Poeck, K., DeBleser, R., and Keyserlingk, D. Graf von (1984). Neurolinguistic status and localization of lesion in aphasic patients with exclusively consonant–vowel recurring utterances. *Brain, 107*, 197–217.

Poizner, H., Klima, E. S., and Bellugi, U. (1987). *What the Hands Reveal about the Brain.* Cambridge, Massachusetts: MIT Press/Bradford Books.

Poizner, H., Bellugi, U., and Klima, E. S. (1989). Sign language aphasia. In F. Boller and J. Grafman (eds), *Handbook of Neuropsychology*, Vol. 2, pp. 157–172. Amsterdam: Elsevier.

Porch, S. (1971). *The Porch Index of Communicative Ability.* Palo Alto, California: Consulting Psychologists.

Putnam, H. (1988). *Representation and Reality.* Cambridge: Bradford.

Rife, D. C. (1940). Handedness, with special reference to twins. *Genetics, 25*, 178–186.

Roeltgen, D. P. (1985). Agraphia. In K. M. Heilman and E. Valenstein (eds), *Clinical Neuropsychology*. 2nd ed. New York: Oxford University Press.

Roeltgen, D. P. and Heilman, K. M. (1984). Lexical agraphia. *Brain, 107*, 811–827.

Roeltgen, D. P., Sevush, S., and Heilman, K. M. (1983). Phonological agraphia: Writing by the lexical semantic route. *Neurology, 33*, 755–765.

Rommel, P. (1683). De aphonia rara. *Miscellanea Curiosa Medico-physica Academiae Naturae Curiosorum*, 2 (Ser. 2) 222–227.

Ross, E. D. (1981). The aprosodias: Functional-anatomic organization of the affective components of language in the right hemisphere. *Annals of Neurology, 38*, 561–589.

Rubens, A. B. (1979). Agnosia. In K. M. Heilman and E. Valenstein (eds), *Clinical Neuropsychology*, pp. 233–267. New York: Oxford University Press.

Russell, R., and Espir, M. L. E. (1961). *Traumatic Aphasia.* Oxford: Oxford University Press.

Saffran, E. M., Bogyo, L., Schwartz, M. F., and Marin, O. S. M. (1980). Does deep dyslexia reflect right hemisphere reading? In M. Coltheart, K. Patterson, and J. C. Marshall (eds), *Deep Dyslexia*, pp. 381–406. London: Routledge and Kegan Paul.

Saffran, E. M., Schwartz, M. F., and Marin, O. S. M. (1980). The word order problem in agrammatism: production. *Brain and Language, 10*, 263–280.

Salomon, E. (1914). Motorische Aphasie mit Agrammatismus und sensorisch-agrammatischen Storungen. *Monattsschrift fur Psychiatrie und Neurologie, 35*, 181–275.

Sasanuma, S., and Fujimura, O. (1971). Selective impairment of phonetic and nonphonetic transcription of words in Japanese aphasic patients: Kana versus kanji in visual recognition and writing. *Cortex, 7*, 1–18.

Sasanuma, S., Akio, K., and Kubota, M. (1990). Agrammatism in Japanese: Two case studies. In L. Menn and L. K. Obler (eds), *Agrammatic Aphasia*, Vol. 2, pp. 1225–1283. Amsterdam: Benjamins.

Schenck von Grafenberg, J. (1585). Observationes medicae de capito humano. Lugduni.

Schmidt, J. (1676). De oblivione lectionis ex apoplexia salva scriptione. *Miscellanea Curiosa Medico-physica Academiae Naturae Curiosorum*, 4, 195–197.

Schuell, H. (1953). *Minnesota Test for the Differential Diagnosis of Aphasia.* Minneapolis: University of Minnesota Press.

Schuell, H., and Jenkins, J. J. (1959). The nature of language deficit in aphasia. *Psychological Review, 66*, 45–67.

Schwartz, M. F. (1984). What the classical aphasia categories can't do for us and why. *Brain and Language, 21*, 3–8.

Schwartz, M. (1987). Patterns of speech production deficit within and across aphasia syndromes: Applications of a psycholinguistic model. In M. Coltheart, G. Sartori, and R. Job (eds), *The Cognitive Neuropsychology of Language.* Hillsdale, New Jersey: L. Erlbaum.

Schwartz, M. F., Linebarger, M. C., and Saffran, E. M. (1985). The status of the syntactic deficit theory of agrammatism. In M. L. Kean, (ed.) *Agrammatism.* Orlando, Florida: Academic Press.

Seidenberg, M. S. (1985). The time course of phonological code activation in two writing systems. *Cognition, 19*, 1–30.

Seidenberg, M. S., and McClelland, J. L. (1989). A distributed, developmental model of word recognition and naming. *Psychological Review, 96*, 523–568.

Semenza, C., and Goodglass, H. (1985). Identification of body parts in brain-injured subjects. *Neuropsychologia, 23*, 161–176.

Semenza, C., and Zettin, M. (1989). Evidence from aphasia for the role of proper names as pure referring expressions. *Nature (London), 342*, 678–679.

Seron, X., van der Kaa, M. A., Remits, A., and van der Linden, M. (1979). Pantomime interpretation and aphasia. *Neuropsychologia, 17*, 661–688.

Shallice, T. (1981). Phonological agraphia and the lexical route in writing. *Brain, 104*, 413–421.

Shallice, T. (1987). Impairments of semantic processing: Multiple dissociations. In M. Coltheart, G. Sartori, and R. Job (eds), *The Cognitive Neuropsychology of Language*, pp. 111–127. London: L. Erlbaum.

Shallice, T., Warrington, E. K., and McCarthy, R. (1983). Reading without semantics. *Quarterly Journal of Experimental Psychology, 35*, 111–138.

Shankweiler, D., and Studdert-Kennedy, M. (1967). Identification of vowels and consonants presented to left and right ears. *Quarterly Journal of Experimental Psychology, 19*, 59–63.

Shattuck-Hufnagel, S. R. (1983). Sublexical units and suprasegmental structure in speech production planning. In P. F. MacNeilage (ed.), *The Production of Speech*. New York: Springer.

Shewan, C., Leeper, R., and Booth, J. (1984). An analysis of voice onset time (VOT) in aphasic and normal subjects. In J. Rosenbek, M. McNeil, and A. Aronson (eds), *Apraxia of Speech*. San Diego: College Hill Press.

Spreen, O., and Benton, A. L. (1977). *The Neurosensory Center Comprehensive Examination for Aphasia*. Revised edition. Victoria: University of Victoria, Neuropsychology Laboratory.

Spreen, O., Benton, A. L., and Van Allen, M. (1966). Dissociation of visual and tactile naming in amnesic aphasia. *Neurology, 16*, 807–814.

Sternberg, S., Monsell, S., Knoll, R. L., and Wright, C. E. (1978). The latency and duration of rapid movement sequences. Comparisons of speech and typewriting. In G. E. Stelmach (ed.), *Information Processing in Motor Control and Learning*. New York: Academic Press.

Strub, R., and Gardner, H. (1974). The repetition defect in conduction aphasia: Mnestic or linguistic? *Brain and Language, 1*, 241–255.

Studdert-Kennedy, M. (1978). The beginnings of speech. In G. B. Barlow, K. Immelmann, M. Main, and L. Petrinovich (eds), *The Bielefeld Interdisciplinary Project*. New York: Cambridge University Press.

Swinney, D. (1979). Lexical access during sentence comprehension. (Re)consideration of context effects. *Journal of Verbal Learning and Verbal Behavior, 18*, 645–659.

Tissot, R., Mounin, G., and Lhermitte, F. (1973). *L'Agrammatisme*. Brussels: Dessart.

Trousseau, A. (1864). De l'Aphasie, maladie décrite récemment sous le nom impropre d'aphémie. *Gazette des Hôpitaux, 37*.

Tzortzis, C., and Albert, M. L. (1974). Impairment in memory for sequences in conduction aphasia. *Neuropsychologia, 12*, 355–366.

Tzeng, O., and Wang, D. (1983). The first two R's. *American Scientist, 71*, 238–243.

Tzeng, O., Hung, D. L., and Wang, D. (1977). Speech recoding in reading Chinese characters. *Journal of Experimental Psychology. Human Learning and Memory, 3*, 621–630.

Tzeng, O., Chen, S., and Hung, D. L. (1991). The classifier problem in Chinese aphasia. *Brain and Language, 41*, 184–202.

Tucker, D. M., Watson, R. T., and Heilman, K. M. (1977). Affective discrimination and evocation in patients with right parietal disease. *Neurology, 17,* 947–950.

Vaid, J., and Pandit, R. (1991). Sentence interpretation in normal and aphasic Hindi speakers. *Brain and Language, 41,* 250–274.

Van Orden, G. C., Pennington, B. F., and Stone, G. O. (1990). Word identification in reading and the promise of subsymbolic psycholinguistics. *Psychological Review, 97,* 488–522.

Varney, N. (1978). Linguistic correlates of pantomime recognition in aphasic patients. *Journal of Neurology, Neurosurgery, and Psychiatry, 41,* 564–568.

Vigotsky, L. (1934). Thought and speech. Moscow: Gosizdat.

Von Bonin, G. (1962). Anatomical asymmetries of the cerebral hemispheres. In V. B. Mountcastle (ed.), *Interhemispheric Relations and Cerebral Dominance.* Baltimore: Johns Hopkins Press.

Von Monakow, C. (1914). *Die Lokalisation im Grosshirn.* Wiesbaden: Bergmann.

Wang, L., and Goodglass, H. (1992). Pantomime, praxis, and aphasia. *Brain and Language, 42,* 402–418.

Wapner, W., and Gardner, H. (1979). A note on patterns of comprehension and recovery in global aphasia. *Journal of Speech and Hearing Research, 29,* 765–771.

Warrington, E. K., and McCarthy, R. (1983). Category-specific access dysphasia. *Brain, 106,* 859–878.

Warrington, E. K., and McCarthy, R. (1987). Categories of knowledge: Further fractionation and an attempted integration. *Brain, 110,* 1273–1296.

Warrington, E. K., and Shallice, T. (1969). The selective impairment of auditory verbal short-term memory. *Brain, 92,* 885–896.

Warrington, E. K., and Shallice, T. (1979). Semantic access dyslexia. *Brain, 102,* 43–63.

Warrington, E. K., and Shallice, T. (1984). Category-specific semantic impairment. *Brain, 107,* 829–854.

Warrington, E. K., Logue, V., and Pratt, R. T. C. (1972). The anatomical localization of selective impairment of auditory verbal short-term memory. *Neuropsychologia, 9,* 377–387.

Weigl, E., and Bierwisch, M. (1970). Neuropsychology and linguistics: Topics of common research. *Foundations of Language, 6,* 1–18.

Weisenburg, T., and McBride, K. (1935). *Aphasia.* New York: Commonwealth Fund.

Wepman, J. M. and Jones, L. V. (1961). *The Language Modalities Test for Aphasia.* Chicago: University of Chicago Press.

Wernicke, C. (1874). *Der aphasische Symptomenkomplex.* Breslau: Cohn und Weigert.

Wingfield, A., Goodglass, H., and Smith, K. (1990). Effects of word-onset cuing on picture naming in aphasia: A reconsideration. *Brain and Language, 39,* 373–390.

Witelson, S. F., and Kigar, D. L. (1988). Asymmetry in brain function follows asymmetry in anatomical form: Gross, microscopic, postmortem, and imaging studies. In F. Boller and J. Grafman (eds), *Handbook of Neuropsychology,* Vol. I, pp. 111–142. Amsterdam: Elsevier.

Yamadori, A., and Albert, M. L. (1973). Word category aphasia. *Cortex, 9,* 112–125.

Zaidel, E., and Peters, A. (1981). Phonological encoding and idiographic reading by the disconnected right hemisphere: Two case studies. *Brain and Language, 14,* 205–234.

Zingeser, L., and Berndt, R. S. (1988). Grammatical class and context effects in a case of pure anomia. *Cognitive Neuropsychology, 5,* 473–516.

Zingeser, L., and Berndt, R. S. (1990). Retrieval of nouns and verbs in agrammatism and anomia. *Brain and Language, 39,* 14–32.

Zurif, E. B., Caramazzo, A., and Myerson, R. (1972). Grammatical judgments of agrammatic aphasics. *Neuropsychologia, 10,* 405–417.

Zwitzerlood, P. (1985). Activation of word candidates during spoken-word recognition. Paper presented at Psychonomic Society, Boston.

Author Index

Subject Index

ISBN 0-12-290040-5

90065

9 780122 900402